Trauma, Psychoanalysis and History

Located at the crossroads of psychoanalysis and history, this book investigates the ambiguous concept of trauma and the changes to its formulation and use between the years 1866 and 1939.

Luis Sanfelippo introduces the original conceptions of trauma outlined by Sigmund Freud, Pierre Janet and their contemporaries, before investigating how the meaning of this concept was influenced and informed by large-scale historical events like the First World War. *Trauma, Psychoanalysis and History* investigates the multiple problems linked to this fetishised category and how it has developed over time. Sanfelippo also considers the historiographical and conceptual problems raised by the application of trauma to collective memory and contemporary history, reflecting on what this means for historiography.

Trauma, Psychoanalysis and History will be of great interest to students in training for psychotherapy and mental health practice, trained psychoanalysts, as well as academics and scholars of psychoanalytic studies, the history of psychology, trauma studies and modern history.

Luis Sanfelippo, PhD, is a professor and researcher at the University of La Plata and the University of Buenos Aires, Argentina. He coordinates the Centre for the History of Psychoanalysis at the National Library of Argentina, and has been a practising psychoanalyst since 2001.

"We should be grateful to Luis Sanfelippo for his research on trauma, a concept that over the years since Freud used it to start psychoanalysis, experienced transformations, expansions and bastardizations. His meticulous research of Freud's papers should allow clinicians and theoreticians to stand on more solid ground when attempting to understand the human condition. The exploration of trauma in psychoanalysis is scholarly and complemented by the research on the link with other human sciences and culture that significantly enriches our understanding of the other concept."

Alberto Pieczanski, *MD, psychoanalyst; training and supervising analyst, Washington Baltimore Center for Psychoanalysis; member of the British Psychoanalytical Society, UK; co-editor (with Nydia Pieczanski, MD) of* The Pioneers of Psychoanalysis in South America: An Essential Guide

"Trauma is one of the words most often associated with the experience of the contemporary world: two world wars, crimes and mass violence have originated a growing awareness of psychic injuries, both individual and collective. The interest of Luis Sanfelippo's research lies in the fact that it restores, around Sigmund Freud, a key moment in the genealogy of this notion. Psychologists, psychiatrists and psychoanalysts have not ceased to deepen and reformulate it, but their thinking is inseparable from a history that concerns us all."

Jacques Revel, *Ecole des hautes études en sciences sociales, France*

"Thanks to the recent exhumation of documents and reconstructions of context, which this book helps to bring to light, the canonical version of the reasons for Freud's abandonment of his trauma theory has lost consensus. Pursuing Freud's delays, returns, mutations and perplexities, Luis Sanfelippo highlights unknown subtleties of that inner debate. Observing that whirlwind would allow one to discover, as he says, how 'the past does not determine a necessary direction; but it conditions, it generates conditions of possibility and, also, it determines impossibilities."

Jorge Baños Orellana, *École lacanienne de psychanalyse, Argentina and France*

"The passion for psychoanalysis leads Luis to a rigorous study of the concept of trauma in Freud, given the different versions that emerge from various readings at different times. Luis Sanfelippo's research is already a reference in Latin America for the study of the concept of trauma. His historical, serious and profound journey makes it essential."

Griselda Sanchez Zago, *Instituto Freudiano para el Estudio de las Prácticas Psicoanalíticas (México); Asociación Psicoanalítica de Guadalajara; FEPAL; IPA; co-editor,* Calibán

"A lot has been written in recent years about trauma, either from a psychoanalytical perspective or from a historical point of view. Yet, so far, there were no significant studies dedicated to this capital concept in the history of psychoanalysis and even beyond… Not only does this ground-breaking piece by Luis Sanfelippo show the changing places of trauma in Freudian theory, in different contexts, but it also traces its medical origins back to the first railroad accidents and their objective and subjective consequences. For those willing to know how trauma became a key category to understand our time, this research, as precise as it is lively, will become a must-read."

Alejandro Dagfal, *psychologist and historian; University of Buenos Aires; National Research Council and National Library, Argentina*

Trauma, Psychoanalysis and History

Luis Sanfelippo

Translated by Bruno Colantoni

Routledge
Taylor & Francis Group
LONDON AND NEW YORK

Designed cover image: ChiccoDodiFC © Getty Images.

First published in English
2024 by Routledge
4 Park Square, Milton Park, Abingdon, Oxon OX14 4RN

and by Routledge
605 Third Avenue, New York, NY 10158

Routledge is an imprint of the Taylor & Francis Group, an informa business

Translated by Bruno Colantoni

Published in Spanish by Miño y Dávila, 2018

British Library Cataloguing-in-Publication Data
A catalogue record for this book is available from the British Library

Library of Congress Cataloging-in-Publication Data
Names: Sanfelippo, Luis, author.
Title: Trauma, psychoanalysis and history / Luis Sanfelippo ;
translated by Bruno Colantoni.
Description: 1 Edition. | New York, NY : Routledge, 2024. |
"Published in Spanish by Miño y Dávila, 2018." | Includes
bibliographicalreferences and index. |
Identifiers: LCCN 2023018515 (print) | LCCN 2023018516 (ebook) |
ISBN 9781032460864 (hardback) | ISBN 9781032460826 (paperback) |
ISBN 9781003380016 (ebook)
Subjects: LCSH: Psychoanalysis—History. | Psychic trauma—
History. | Collective memory.
Classification: LCC BF173 .S321413 2024 (print) |
LCC BF173 (ebook) | DDC 150.19/5—dc23/eng/20230722
LC record available at https://lccn.loc.gov/2023018515
LC ebook record available at https://lccn.loc.gov/2023018516

ISBN: 9781032460864 (hbk)
ISBN: 9781032460826 (pbk)
ISBN: 9781003380016 (ebk)

DOI: 10.4324/9781003380016

Typeset in Times New Roman
by codeMantra

To Marina, Leia and Camilo.

Contents

Acknowledgements *xi*

Introduction 1

1 Mechanical Trauma and Psychical Trauma: Railway Accidents and Hysteria (1866–1889) 23

2 Trauma and Memory: The Janet-Freud Debate, 1889–1895/1913–1914 66

3 Sexual Cause and Traumatic Testimonies: The Versions of the Neurotica and Its Abandonment (1896–1933) 112

4 The War Neuroses and a New Economic Conception of Trauma (1914–1920) 161

5 On Collective Traumas: The Persistence and Transmission of Past Experiences (1913 and 1939) 215

Conclusions 238
LUIS SANFELIPPO

Index *257*

Acknowledgements

I would not have been able to write this book without the invaluable help of Hugo Vezzetti and Alejandro Dagfal, who accompanied me as directors throughout the entire investigation. Along with them, I would like to thank Mauro Vallejo and the other members of the Chair I of the History of Psychology at the University of Buenos Aires, of which I have been a member since the year 2000.

I also thank the Faculty of Psychology of the University of La Plata for having received me as Professor of Psychotherapy I, the Álvarez Hospital of the City of Buenos Aires for the years of clinical training, and the Ministry of Culture of Argentina for having awarded me the National Award in Psychological Essay for the period 2015–2018.

I would also like to highlight the meticulous translation work carried out by Bruno Colantoni. I want to give particular thanks to Editorial Miño y Dávila for having trusted the book for its first publication in Buenos Aires (2018) and to Ediciones Nandela for publishing it in Mexico (2022).

Finally, and mainly, I thank my partner Marina Carreiro and my children, Leia and Camilo, for accompanying me on this long journey and for sharing life and dreams.

Introduction

0.1 Issues Surrounding Trauma

In recent years, the term "trauma" has become one of the keywords of Western culture. When a person or a group goes through an experience that seems to shatter the foundations of their lives, its use seems to impose itself as if it were a pristine and self-evident idea. Subjectivities constructed around a past event that continues in the present, or peoples that today experience the present consequences (all too present) of past sufferings; in both spheres, the notion of trauma is called upon to explain a particular alteration of memory and mental functioning, becoming one of the categories derived from "psy" discourses most embraced by contemporary thought.[1]

However, this notion is not clear or univocal, nor did it originate in psychological or psychoanalytic territories. Until the mid-nineteenth century, the term was inscribed in the medical-surgical domain, where it was used to designate (local or generalised) *somatic damage* which was not caused by an infectious disease or by hereditary factors (Hacking, 1995; Leys, 2000; Micale & Lerner, 2001; Young, 1995). The trauma, therefore, corresponded to an area of pathology which established an accident as its cause. The accident exerted on the organism a mechanical action such that it produced an injury and created the conditions for the emergence of morbid phenomena. Broken bones, internal or external haemorrhages, perforated organs and functions disturbed by the material deterioration of tissues: these constituted the injuries that were most frequently encompassed – along with the event that caused them and the subsequent consequences – in the semantic field of the notion. Such meaning still exists in certain sectors of medicine; above all, within emergency teams in hospitals and in the speciality named "traumatology".

However, it is clear that this meaning is no longer the most common one. Currently, the notion of trauma generally remits to the idea of *psychical damage*, to a wound that is impossible to locate in the body that, nevertheless, affects the mind in a lasting way (that is, not only during the course of the event considered traumatic but also, and fundamentally, after its conclusion). It is as if the cessation of the situation does not prevent its effects from lasting continuously, or, more precisely, as

DOI: 10.4324/9781003380016-1

if the cause of the damage becomes independent of the past event and becomes a source that is still present, capable of generating malaise.

This *shift* in meaning also entailed an *extension* of the term's use. If its use was not limited to cases in which it was possible to demonstrate the existence of a material injury, then it could be used in reference to other situations. The range of these currently seems to expand from exceptional events (such as the extermination camps) to more everyday or banal experiences that generate suffering (Hacking, 1995; Leys, 2000).

Along with its shift and extension, there has been an *insertion* of this category in new areas. It is not only fully implanted in the medical and psychopathological domains but also in the legal domain – generally associated with the categories of damage and abuse – and, for at least 30 years, in the field of studies on social memory and the history of the recent past. There, it is used to refer to the collective effects of certain historical experiences such as the Shoah, the Vietnam War, some wars and some Latin American dictatorships (Caruth, 1995; Franco & Levín, 2007; Friedlander, 1992; LaCapra, 2008, 2009, 2014). It can also be affirmed that the notion has been installed in common sense and the colloquial language of a good part of Western culture. Here, it is often used to legitimise demands for reparation or exceptions for damages allegedly suffered. This type of petition or complaint (not necessarily understood in legal terms) has grown considerably in recent years (Assoun, 2001; García, 2008).

Finally, we wish to highlight the high degree of *institutionalisation* of the notion in certain sectors of the "psy" disciplinary field. For example, since the third version of the influential *Diagnostic and Statistical Manual of Mental Disorders* (*DSM*) of the American Psychiatric Association (APA), edited in 1980, a specific nosographic category has been included to account for the pathological effects of trauma: post-traumatic stress disorder (PTSD). For its part, in the equally powerful American Psychological Association, there is a section fully dedicated to the investigation and dissemination of this subject: Division 56, called "Trauma Psychology".[2] Furthermore, in the United States, there are periodic academic publications specifically dedicated to the subject, such as *Psychological Trauma: Theory, Research, Practice and Policy*, the *International Journal of Stress Management* or *Traumatology*.

However, the high degree of institutionalisation has not prevented the *multiplication of conceptions* regarding trauma. There is no consensus on its definition or a homogeneous field of problems to which this notion can refer. It is not even possible to find a conceptual agreement between the works that claim to be inscribed within the Freudian legacy. It is possible to indicate some common features that differentiate the psychoanalytic notions of trauma from those of other theoretical or therapeutic orientations. However, in the strict sense, multiple psychoanalytic conceptions of trauma exist.

In the face of so much diversity, it does not seem possible to speak of trauma in the singular. Nevertheless, some continue to refer to it as a single concept, valid for all times and places. According to these approaches to the subject, often linked to practitioners of "psy" disciplines who adhere to some of the contemporary conceptions, history only allows us to see the past *errors* and the *antecedents* that led to current knowledge. For example, in the paragraphs introducing a historical perspective in the widely read *Traumatic Stress: The Effects of Overwhelming Experience on Mind* (Van der Kolk, McFarlane & Weisaeth, 1996), the authors seem to conceive trauma as a transhistorical and universal phenomenon, with a short psychiatric history that advances without a solution of continuity from the end of the nineteenth century to the present day.

> People have always known – the authors say – that exposure to overwhelming terror can lead to troubling memories, arousal and avoidance. This has been a central theme in literature, from the time of Homer to today. In contrast, psychiatry as a profession has had a very troubled relationship with the idea that reality can profoundly and permanently alter people's psychology and biology. Psychiatry itself has periodically suffered from marked amnesias in which well-established knowledge has been abruptly forgotten, and the psychological impact of overwhelming experiences has been ascribed to constitutional or intrapsychic factors alone.
>
> (Van der Kolk, Weisaeth & Van der Hart, 1996, p. 47)

The paragraph is eloquent: trauma would seem to be a universal experience and a real object that, despite being known by common sense, could not be seen or was forgotten many times by psychiatric knowledge. According to these authors, the weight given to constitutional or intrapsychical theories prevented the recognition of a truth (considered unquestionable) that, nevertheless, had already been perceived by "well-established" knowledge (addressed in the historical chapter) which served as an antecedent of current knowledge (which would be the object of the book).

To this type of approach, we can apply the same criticisms that concern the traditional history of the "psy" disciplines. In this case, the authors seem to naturalise their objects of study, justify and celebrate the present as the moment of greatest epistemic development, believe in the linear and necessary progress of knowledge and be unaware of the existence of immeasurable discontinuities. The traditional perspective also sometimes constructs myths of origin, according to which a prestigious figure created a new discipline or branch of knowledge on their own initiative and thanks to their genius, without the intervention of collective factors, be these epistemic, cultural or political.

In an attempt to distance ourselves from these perspectives, we seek to conceive trauma as a strictly historical object of investigation and, therefore, as being contingent, transformable and diverse. Thus, the term's current dispersion is not a mere illusion that hides the true notion of trauma; rather, it illuminates the web of problems, theories, practices and uses that this term covers.

For our part, in our investigation on trauma, we have emphasised the works of Sigmund Freud. Nevertheless, we have not done so intending to consecrate his ideas as the only truth on the matter. We consider, rather, that the path this category took in the writings of the founder of psychoanalysis *and his interlocutors* allows us to illustrate many of the central problems and the most famous debates that accompanied its historical transformations, such as:

- What is the nature of trauma?
  (Is it somatic or psychical? Is it anatomical or physiological? Is it the product of ideas or affects?, etc.)
- What are the determining factors of a traumatic experience? Are they the objective and/or external conditions of the situation or the subjective and/or internal particularities of the person going through it? Are they the current elements or the predisposition?
- What relationship exists between trauma and memory?
- What role does trauma play in aetiology?
- How should trauma narratives be interpreted? (Reality or phantasy?)
- What is the relationship between trauma and sexuality?
- Can a trauma be inscribed into a web of representations? Or, rather, does it circumscribe the limits of these webs?[3]
- Could a community be affected by collective trauma and remain fixed ('petrified') to that past experience?
- Can trauma be transmitted and affect those who have not lived through the traumatic experience?

In other words, the fact that this book on trauma is focused on Freudian ideas does not imply that it follows the guidelines of an *internal* history, which considers conceptual transformations to be the result of the development of ideas in an author, in their works or in a professional community. Just as trauma seems to interrogate the limits between the internal and the external, the history of this notion forces us to question the borders – which are often judged as precise and invariable – between different discourses and between each disciplinary field and its context. Therefore, to address it, we believe it necessary to reconstruct the *web* of interlocutors, knowledges, practices and cultural processes, within which the Freudian conceptualisations of trauma found their conditions of possibility. In this sense, we seek to base our research within the framework of *intellectual history* (Vezzetti, 2007). We consider that the transformations in the field of trauma do not depend only on the conceptual discussions but also on the clinical problems and technical and therapeutic procedures through which the notion of trauma found its place, as well as on the impact that certain social and cultural experiences had on the field of psychopathology.

For example, during the final decades of the nineteenth century, a process of "psychologization" of trauma took place (Gauchet & Swain, 2000; Hacking, 1995;

Leys, 2000; Micale & Lerner, 2001). The different forms of this process were determined by epistemic transformations within medical knowledge but also by the legal and economic problems associated with the expansion of a crucial technological advancement: the railway. The accidents caused by this revolutionary mode of transport and the expansion of health insurance in some European countries generated a great debate around a class of cases in which it was not easy to find the injury that justified the symptoms, but where the existence of simulation or fraud was not evident either.

Following this, around the 1880s, this medical-expert debate intersected with two other fields of problems. On the one hand, with discussions about the status of hysteria. This nosographical category not only posed clinical and epistemic enigmas regarding its ultimate nature and its mechanisms but also entailed a moral dimension (accusations of deceit, lies and simulation) and a gender issue (the rapid association of hysteria with the female sex) (Edelman, 2003; Foucault, 2006; Gauchet & Swain, 2000). On the other hand, railway accidents and cases of hysteria converged, in the same period, with the history of hypnosis and suggestion. This history not only referred to the development of new research and therapeutic techniques but also brought with it ethical and political debates (which reached journalistic coverage and a public dimension) about the dangers of the excessive influence that some men could exercise over others (Carroy, 1991; Edelman, 2003).

By the 1890s, the notion of trauma had not only reached a high degree of psychologisation, but was also beginning to be related, for the first time, to the question of *memory* (Hacking, 1995; Leys, 2000). Both Janet and Freud conceived trauma and its therapy as a novel articulation between different forms of forgetting and remembering (Assoun, 1981; Dagfal, 2013; Ellenberger, 1970; Gauchet & Swain, 2000). In doing so, they not only intervened in the limited scope of the clinic of the neuroses but also inscribed their work in a broader territory, that of the problematisation of memory. At the same time that tradition (understood as the transmission of past teachings still in force) was beginning to lose importance in the face of an increasingly accelerated rate of transformation (Hartog, 2003; Koselleck, 1993), different scientific conceptions of memory were developed in Europe. Among these, we can find clinical approaches to neurotic and traumatic amnesia, neurological studies on the localisation of different types of memory and experimental research on different memory functions (Hacking, 1995). To these three approaches, we must add the hereditarian psychiatric tradition, which assumes the existence of a biological memory whose traces can be passed down from generation to generation.

In the following century, several of the conceptual transformations and the variations in the relative significance given to the issue of trauma were linked to major war events, fundamentally, the World Wars and the Vietnam War (Friedlander, 1992; Hermann, 1992; Leys, 2000; Ramirez Ortiz, 2007; Young, 1995). For example, the First World War newly forced a discussion about the somatic or psychical nature of trauma, led to rethinking the role of sexuality in trauma and in the aetiology of the neuroses and pushed Freud towards developing a fundamentally "economic" conception of trauma (Leys, 2000; Ramirez Ortiz, 2007). The Second World War influenced this theme in two moments. First, shortly after it ended, it generated a debate on the illnesses of the survivors of the concentration camps (Bonomi, 2007). Afterwards, around the 1980s, the insertion of the notion of trauma in the field of collective memory studies coincided with the reinterpretations of the Shoah as a key event in Western culture (Badiou, 2009; Franco & Levin, 2007; Friedlander, 1992; Hartog, 2003). Finally, the demands of the Vietnam veterans for the recognition of the psychological consequences of war prompted the trauma category to be included in the third version of the DSM (Borch-Jacobsen, 1996; Hacking, 1995; Hermann, 1992; Young, 1995).

In other words, the complexity of knowledge, practices and interests tied to the category of trauma led us to approach this topic from the perspective of intellectual history. Hugo Vezzetti understands this perspective as "an approach and inclusive domain which receives something from different historiographic genres" (2007, p. 161). We consider that different historiographic methodological tools become necessary to address an object such as trauma and place it

> in a web that inevitably exceeds the limits of the discipline or the institution. A history conceived in this way is characterised by a plural placement, disposed to shift to the extent that its 'objects' are organised into constructions that can be differentiated into two spheres: sociocultural and conceptual.
>
> (Vezzetti, 2007, p. 162)

Following the suggestion of this author, we attempt to avoid the "reduction to the logic of scientific thought", which ignores the context and only constructs "internal" histories; however, neither do we aspire to develop an "external" history, which limits itself to the "description of the uses and the social forms" and is unaware of conceptual problems (Vezzetti, 2007, p. 162). At the same time, we attempt to submit to a certain standard of precision in the handling and analysis of psychoanalytic concepts and practices (precision that is often lost in certain histories of psychoanalysis elaborated by professional historians without a psychoanalytic background). Simultaneously, we try not to leave aside the critical distance that a historical investigation must have with respect to the object of its inquiry (a distance that is usually missing when insiders interested in legitimising the domain to which they belong, develop narratives on the history of a discipline or discourse).

By basing our research on the framework of intellectual history and making use of its historiographical tools, we attempt to reconstruct *the different models, the diverse conceptual configurations* (theoretical and practical) and *the varied images* that have been used to think about trauma or to guide the interventions conducted on those who have gone through a traumatic experience. We identified these models, configurations and images at different moments of the historical route we set out to cover, extending from the decade of 1860 until the end of the thirties of the following century. Such periodisation reflects our intention to analyse the totality of the Freudian work, although without reducing our research's scope to it. We consider that the conceptions of the Viennese psychoanalyst discovered their field, found their interlocutors and defined their particular features in relation to broader problems (that exceed an author's ideas) and with the contribution of some of his colleagues (Erichsen, Page, Oppenheim, Charcot, Janet, Jung, Jones, Abraham, Ferenczi, among others), whose ideas influenced Freud or with whom he discussed. At the same time, the periodisation we put forward does not develop linearly and continuously from the mid-nineteenth century to 1939. Instead, each chapter circumscribes a series of different problems, the reason for which it is possible to find temporal overlaps, recapitulations and fragmented developments that respond to the problem that was intended to be analysed at each moment.

0.2 Previous Approaches

Developing an intellectual history of the notion of trauma based on the works of Freud and his interlocutors implies delving into heterogeneous bibliographical sources, which constitute different corpora: the history of psychoanalysis, the history of the clinic and psychotherapies, the historiographical reflections on the forms of producing disciplinary, intellectual and cultural history. To this, we must add, obviously, the primary sources of research: the psychoanalytic, medical and psychopathological writings that address the problem of trauma.

Regarding the history of Freudian psychoanalysis, the bibliography is extensive and heterogeneous. For many years, the reference text has been the biography written by Ernest Jones (1953–1957). This work had the merit of considering not only the texts included in the *Standard Edition* but also a large part of the unpublished manuscripts and correspondences. In addition, the Freudian trajectory was included in a web of relationships, collaborations and disputes with those who accompanied him or with whom he rivalled, establishing the idea that in order to understand the Freudian conceptual developments better, it was also necessary to be familiar with the history of the psychoanalytic movement. His text established a tradition of reading that became canonical in the International Psychoanalytic Association, characterised by holding an idealised vision of the father of psychoanalysis and circumscribing research within the interior of the analytic movement, leaving aside the different (epistemic, clinical and cultural) contexts in which it was able to develop.

From the 1960s onwards, the historical works on psychoanalysis multiplied and differed from the previous tradition. Firstly, because many of these works abandoned the aim of addressing the entire Freudian trajectory or the entirety of psychoanalysis in favour of focusing on specific aspects of each one of them. Secondly, because several of these works were written by people external to psychoanalytic practice. This novel situation made it possible to better highlight the continuities and differences between Freud's works with previous or contemporary authors

(Ellenberger, 1970), to address the relationship of his thought with his time (Gay, 1989) or to show in more detail the connection of his ideas with scientific traditions and epistemic discourses alien to strictly psychoanalytic problems, such as neurophysiology, pathological anatomy, energetics or evolutionism (Assoun, 1981; Gauchet, 1994; Sulloway, 1979, 1991).

However, it is necessary to clarify that, up to now, no book on the history of psychoanalysis has focused its research on the various notions of trauma. In the state of the art, it is possible to find work on the history of psychoanalysis that only deals with certain aspects related to the topic, or books on the history of trauma in which the psychoanalytic point of view is just one more among a series of theories used to address the subject.

For example, the now-classic book by Kenneth Levin (1985), *Freud's Early Psychology of the Neuroses*, addresses in depth the early years of Freud's work from a historical perspective without making trauma the centre of its research. For his part, the psychoanalyst Guy Le Gauffey includes, in some of his works, certain historical references that allow the psychoanalytic practice to be situated in relation to other techniques and therapeutic orientations (2001) or that make it possible to understand that certain features of Freudian thought depend on the characteristics of the scientific discourse of its time (1995). The connection of these references with the subject of our research exists but is limited. On the other hand, the work of Ramirez Ortiz, *Psicoanalistas en el frente de batalla. Las neurosis de guerra en la Primera Guerra Mundial* (2007), and Kurt Eissler's work, *Freud sur le front des névroses de guerre* (1992), constitute some of the few books specifically dedicated to addressing the question of the involvement of psychoanalysts in the First World War. Furthermore, the Argentine historian Omar Acha studied the psychoanalytic conceptions of time and history, which are closely related to the problem of trauma, but without being equivalent (Acha, 2007, 2010).

There is abundant literature with a historiographical perspective that deals with the Freudian hypotheses referring to childhood sexual trauma, often classified under the title of "Seduction Theory" (Carter, 1980; Esterson, 1993, 2001; Gelfand, 1989; Good, 1995; Israel & Schatzman, 1993; Triplett, 2004). Among these texts, on the one hand, Masson's book *The Assault on Truth* (1984) stands out, in which Freud is accused of abandoning an alleged complaint about the existence of child sexual abuse for fear of reprisals from his colleagues. On the other hand, some works by Borch-Jacobsen also stand out, which highlight the involvement of suggestion in the Freudian practice of that time and conjecture the possibility that the patients' reports of childhood sexual trauma may have been induced by Freud using suggestion (Borch-Jacobsen, 1996; Borch-Jacobsen & Shamdasani, 2006). More recently, several works by Mauro Vallejo (some written in collaboration with the author of this book) have contributed to making these debates more complex. They did so by placing the Freudian postulates within the context of his search for an aetiological factor that could displace heredity from the central role it had until then, and by relativising the classic opposition between phantasy and reality, with which the problem of seduction was usually approached (Sanfelippo & Vallejo, 2013a,b; Vallejo, 2011, 2012).

The works mentioned in the two previous paragraphs are among those that address, from a historical perspective, some aspects of psychoanalysis related to trauma. Now we wish to mention some historiographical texts whose primary object of inquiry is trauma itself and no longer psychoanalysis.

Ian Hacking explicitly addresses the issue of psychical trauma in one of the chapters of his book *Rewriting the Soul: Multiple Personality and the Sciences of Memory* (1995). In this chapter, this category is inserted into a web of clinical (nosographic discussions), cultural (the effects of the emergence of the railway) and conceptual problems (the debate between Freud, Charcot and Janet regarding therapy, memory and truth). However, his analysis is reduced to early moments of the Freudian works, leaving out both later conceptual modifications and critical historical events in the history of this notion (such as the First World War).

Probably one of the most important books on the notion that we set out to investigate is *Trauma: A Genealogy* (Leys, 2000). In this book, the author intends to examine the history of the term by placing it at the crossroads of knowledges, practices and social events, without neglecting the conceptual and technical debates within the doctrines, the disputes over therapeutic approaches or the impact of events such as wars and the Holocaust. However, given its claim to address the notion from the perspectives of the different psychological schools over a period of more than a hundred years, the chapter dedicated to Freud ends up losing precision and reflects more work on commentators rather than on primary sources (Leys, 2000, pp. 18–40).

In 2001, an important collective work on the issue was published, articulating the psychiatric notion of trauma with the cultural processes that took place towards the end of the nineteenth century and the beginning of the twentieth. Entitled *Traumatic Past: History Psychiatry and Trauma in the Modern Age, 1870–1930*, the book includes several articles that allow for the weighing of the relationship of the category of trauma with the changes in means of transport, with the constitution of a Welfare State, with hysteria and certain gender issues and with the First World War (Micale & Lerner, 2001).

For their part, some of the most important theorists of the neurobiological conceptions of PTSD have written several historical texts on the subject (Van der Hart & Horst, 1989; Var der Kolk & Van der Hart, 1995; Van de Hart, Brown & Van der Kolk, 1989; Van der Kolk, McFarlane & Weisaeth, 1996). The problem with this type of approach usually lies in the assumption of the ahistorical nature of the object being investigated (in this case, trauma). These kinds of works are usually developed as if the only modification that time and humankind could make to the object was introducing a new way of conceiving it.

There are also historical studies that address problems linked to the clinic and psychopathology without specifically focusing on psychoanalysis or on trauma, but which have contributed enormously to this present research. We would first like to mention Gladys Swain and Marcel Gauchet's book on Charcot (Gauchet & Swain, 2000). To the exhaustive, original and rigorous nature of their work based on Charcotian sources, a detailed analysis of the French clinician's trajectory is added, allowing us to understand his impact on the psychologisation of trauma. Also, Swain's article "*Du traitement moral aux psychothérapies*" (1994) constitutes an essential synthesis of the main characteristics of the therapeutic orientations of the beginning of the twentieth century.

Furthermore, Nicole Edelmann's book on the transformations of hysteria in the nineteenth century and Jacqueline Carroy's on hypnosis and suggestion, provide relevant data on the relationship between gender and hysteria, the role given to sexuality, the different images of trauma and the role of research techniques in conceptual transformations (Carroy, 1991; Edelman, 2003). Danziger's works (1984 and 1990) are also relevant to thinking about the role of research practices in the history of trauma. Moreover, an extensive article by Alejandro Dagfal (2013), clearly presents the state of the art of historical research on Pierre Janet and makes a precise analysis of the debates between the French author and the founder of psychoanalysis. All of these works illuminate certain aspects essential to thinking about the origins of psychoanalytic conceptualisations.

The hypotheses of Michel Foucault (1978) on the existence of "devices of sexuality" in the West allow us to better weigh the influence of sexuality in the conceptions of trauma in the work of Freud and his contemporaries. In addition, the French philosopher approached our theme more directly by proposing the connection between the medicalisation of hysteria, the problem of simulation and the medical and expert controversies on the nature of the symptoms of traumatised people (Foucault, 2006).

In this way, by connecting clinical and judicial discussions, another of the great contemporary problems related to trauma opens up: the nature of victims of traumatic experiences and the claims and attempts for reparation, which many authors have approached from different perspectives (Assoun, 2001; García, 2008; Hermann, 1992; Leys, 2000).

We also wish to mention some of the countless works on trauma written by psychoanalysts. At the very moment in which this investigation was coming to an end, Sandra Leticia Berta's doctoral thesis, defended in Brazil, entitled "*Escrbir el trauma, de Freud a Lacan*" (2014), was published in Argentina. This work provides valuable insights into the temporality of trauma and its psychical inscription. It probably constitutes one of the most ambitious and systematic attempts to approach the conceptions of trauma in the works of both psychoanalysts. Unlike our research, it focuses its attention solely on the interior of their respective works, excluding from its objectives the study of the epistemic, cultural or political contexts of psychoanalytic ideas.

In an article published in the *Revue Francaise de Psychanalyse*, Francoise Brette (1988) posits the existence of three theories of trauma in Freud's work. The first is of Charcotian inspiration; the second is constituted by the seduction theory; the third takes the war neuroses as a model. The author seeks to underline a common characteristic between the three: the persistence of an economic perspective. Although her analysis could help to organise these issues, her reading simplifies conceptual transformations of great complexity and does not consider the context of debates and authors in which the Freudian work is immersed.

In a very interesting publication, H. Thoma and N. Cheshire (1991) differentiate the Freudian notion of *nachträglichkeit* from Strachey's supposedly analogous conception called "deferred action". The axis of this article resides in the way of conceiving the temporality of trauma in both authors. Similarly, we also wish to mention a text by Javier Alarcón, entitled *Trauma y apres-coup* (1996), and a brief paper by Gerhard Dahl, called "The Two Time Vectors of Nachträglichkeit in the Development of Ego Organization: Significance of the Concept for the Symbolization of Nameless Traumas and Anxieties" (2010). Other articles, such as those written by Thierry Bokanowski (2005) and Alicia Lowenstein (1996), also distinguish between terms that are usually equated: *traumatism*, the *traumatic* sphere and *trauma*.

For his part, Paul-Laurent Assoun refers to the topic of trauma in several of his books. In addition to having posed the relationship of trauma with the body and with anxiety (Assoun, 1998, 2003), this author set out to study the topic from the feeling of prejudice (Assoun, 2001). For this author, the "prejudiced" is considered "exceptional" because of the damage received and, therefore, is reluctant to abandon a victim position that tends to be idealised, despite the suffering that it could entail. The book presents an original approach to pointing out the links between trauma, the victim position and the demands for reparation. However, unlike our research, it does not carry out a detailed historical analysis of Freud's work.

In the publications mentioned above (and in most of the writings of practitioners of psychoanalysis who deal with the issue of trauma) we can observe that in the corpus of sources and secondary bibliography many texts written by psychoanalysts are included, in which almost no attention is paid to the works of authors with other clinical orientations or to the historical studies on psychoanalysis written by authors outside the psychoanalytic movement. We believe that, in this way, a great risk is run: that of adhering (implicitly or explicitly) to the assumption that ideas can only arise from the internal development of an author's work or a professional community. Furthermore, on many occasions, the works cited are concerned with determining and making explicit what they consider trauma to be. Our purpose is another: to investigate the transformations that the notions of trauma have undergone at different times, transformations that not only depend on motives which are "internal" to Freudian thought but also depend on factors usually considered to be "external", which exceed the restricted framework of an author's work. In other words, we are not trying so much to provide an answer to a problem as to reconstruct a "problematic" (Danziger, 1984) in the frame of which Freud's proposals not only found interlocutors, allies or detractors but also their conditions of enunciability. In order to achieve this, it is necessary to consider the context (intellectual, professional, cultural, etc.) as an essential element in understanding the construction process of a category.

Finally, given that the notion of trauma has not extended its reach from the médical-surgical field to the psychological field but has also been incorporated into the domain of social memory and the history of the recent past, we wish to point out some of the literature that has analysed the problems linked to the consideration of past experiences such as "collective traumas".

Firstly, a vast amount of literature deals with Freud's ventures into group psychology. In particular, we are interested in mentioning those researchers who analysed "Moses and Monotheism" (Freud, 1939), the only text by the founder of psychoanalysis that deals explicitly with the issue of the transgenerational transmission of collective traumas. Without claiming to be exhaustive in our enumeration, this Freudian text was approached from historiography (Acha, 2007; De Certeau, 1999), philosophy (Derrida, 1987, 1997), literary criticism (Assmann, 1999; Blum, 1991), psychoanalysis (Le Gaufey, 1995), the history of psychoanalysis (Gay, 1989; Jones, 1953–1957) and the studies on Judaism (Yerushalmi, 1996).

Secondly, other investigations have dealt with analysing the presence of the notion of trauma (and of the related field of problems) in the specific field of historical studies of the recent past. Some of them intend to account for the historical conditions that made possible the displacement of the notion from psychology and psychoanalysis to historiography (Acha & Vallejo, 2010; Badiou, 2009; Ricoeur, 2008; Sanfelippo, 2011a). Others try to investigate the possibilities and limits of the utilisation of these concepts in the field of history (Franco & Levin, 2007; LaCapra, 2008, 2009, 2014; Mudrovcic, 2005, 2009; Sanfelippo, 2011b; Vezzetti, 2002, 2009).

0.3 Preliminary Hypotheses

In order to better organise and make more explicit some of the ideas expressed in the presentation of the issue at hand, we would like to introduce the general orientations that we have adopted and the main hypotheses we have tested in our research.

First, as we have already anticipated, we do not consider trauma to be a natural object, identical in all times and places, waiting to be discovered. Therefore, the transformations it has undergone should not be understood as changes in the interpretation of the concept or the discourses about the object, but as variations in the object itself (Canguilhem, 2009). The same term refers to different objects at different times and is linked to dissimilar problems, uses and domains.

Second, if the object "trauma" has changed over time, then the history of its variations cannot be thought of as a unique and necessary development (Leys, 2000, p. 8). The fact that trauma has changed meanings, extended its uses and been displaced towards other domains and problems is not due to a natural evolution or to the flourishment of its supposed essence (nor is it due to the intention or genius of certain well-known authors). Instead, these variations are due to multiple heterogeneous and contingent factors: the internal obstacles of each author's theory, the works of their colleagues; epistemic changes that exceed the specific territory of the clinic of the neuroses; historical processes independent of psychopathological knowledge (such as railway accidents or wars), etcetera. Therefore, the study of these transformations should not be reduced to the description of a linear journey but instead should reconstruct the web of knowledges, practices and institutional and cultural processes which generated the historical conditions of possibility for the different notions of trauma to appear. This historical web provided the interlocutors and propitiated the debates that allowed for the transformations of "trauma" to occur.

Third, regarding Freud's ideas, we aim to test the following hypotheses:

- A single Freudian conception of trauma does not exist; there are several, whose differences are usually avoided by using a single term that, nonetheless, carries very different meanings and referents.
- Contrary to the thesis that arises from certain readings that understand psychoanalysis as a theory of desires and internal impulses that disregards the trauma (Van der Kolk & Van der Hart, 1995), we believe this notion has always played an important role in the Freudian conceptual edifice and was linked to many of its central problems and concepts: the unconscious and psychical conflict, sexuality and aetiology, non-linear temporalities, repetition in transference, the drives and the unbound energy.[4]
- Despite the transformations undergone by the notion, there is a common factor among all the conceptual configurations constructed by Freud. The trauma has always been defined in *relative* and never in absolute terms. In other words, it depends on the type of relationship established between an element and an entity that intends to function as an organised totality (and not on the intrinsic characteristics of the element or the entity).
- The characteristics attributed to the trauma stemming from the clinical experience with neurotics can be applied to group psychology. In particular, for Freud, the traces of past traumas persist beyond the situation that caused them and could produce posthumous effects, either in the life of an individual or in the life of a people, thanks to a process of transgenerational transmission.

Fourth, there are other recurrences despite the numerous changes that the notion has undergone. We are referring to the existence of two significant tensions in the debates about what determines that an experience becomes traumatic. On the one hand, the objective/subjective tension. Would an experience be traumatic due to the objective conditions of the situation (supposedly identical for all participants)? Or would it depend on the subjective particularities of the person who goes through it? On the other hand, the tension between the past and the present. Does an experience become traumatic because of its current characteristics? Or because of the background of the protagonists? Both axes can be combined, but they must be distinguished since the four alternatives could be possible. In addition, extreme positions are sometimes derived from these tensions. These positions are presented as exclusive oppositions, since they take into consideration only one of the two possible poles of each axis (for example, when affirming that the trauma solely depends on the objective conditions but not on the subjective ones; that it is entirely determined by the antecedents, but not by the current characteristics of the experience, etc.) Throughout this book, we will attempt to analyse the consequences of such dichotomous positions, and we will also aim to investigate if the Freudian conceptions have been able to avoid this type of exclusive disjunctions.

0.4 Brief Methodological Clarifications

As anticipated, we attempt to inscribe our research on the notion of trauma within the framework of intellectual history. Therefore, it does not seek to address the – supposed – "totality" of facts involved in the history of trauma but, instead, to organise the historical narrative around different "problems" (Vezzetti, 2007, p. 161): the emergence of psychological conceptions of trauma at the crossroads between railway accidents and clinical hysteria (Chapter 1), the – conceptual and therapeutic – relationship between trauma and memory (Chapter 2), the search for the ultimate cause of the neuroses and the intersection between reality and phantasy in the stories of trauma (Chapter 3), the debates surrounding the war neuroses and the limits of representation (Chapter 4), the persistence and transmission of collective traumas (Chapter 5).

At the same time, the fact that our analysis deals with the works of Sigmund Freud does not imply limiting the investigation to his texts, his work or his image; we do not even reduce it to the movement that he founded. Instead, we attempt to reconstruct the web of interlocutors, knowledges, practices, institutional developments and cultural processes that constituted the *field of problems* in which the Freudian ideas and practices (as well as the different notions of trauma) found their conditions of possibility.

This intellectual history of trauma exceeds the reduced framework of enumerating and describing the "ideas" about trauma. It also does not solely address merely epistemic considerations (although it does not neglect this dimension, thus avoiding the risk of becoming a social or cultural history). Clearly, it is not a history "of the intellectuals" or of the "intellectual field" (Bourdieu, 2008). Rather, it is a history that deals with the conceptual and practical transformations of the notion of trauma, understanding that these depend on both epistemic issues and sociocultural factors (Vezzetti, 2007, p. 162).

To better address the complexity of this web, we have resorted to three axes, with the expectation of them allowing us to structure the material better and more clearly illuminate the characteristics of the transformations produced. On the one hand, we study the impact of other problems, discourses, practices, instruments or disciplines that came to function as *models* (in the broadest sense of the term) for conceiving different forms or different aspects of trauma.[5] Then, we outline and explain the different *conceptions or conceptual configurations* of trauma. With the latter term, we intend to refer to the fact that none of the notions of trauma constitutes a simple entity; rather, it is composed of at least three elements. First, an *element* that is determined as being traumatic (such as a mechanical action, an idea or an affect). Second, the *organisation* that is affected by the element (the organism, the nervous system, the ego, the psychical apparatus, etc.). Finally, the *type of relationship* that is established between that element and this organisation. As we will see, the variations in these *configurations* or *conceptions* have depended both on theoretical and doctrinal developments and on the practices put forward to mitigate the effects of trauma (since changes in the practices generally imply conceptual alterations and vice versa). Lastly, we rely on a third axis: the *images* of the traumatised subject (the injured person, the hysteric, the hypnotised individual, the abused child, the neurotic soldier, etc.) We consider that these images (which constitute the objects of the different knowledges and practices on trauma) help to better understand the variations in the conceptions of trauma. But in addition, they illuminate the social place that has been given to those who lived through an experience considered traumatic, as well as the strategies that have been implemented to mitigate the latter's effects. In summary, *models*, *conceptual configurations* and *images* will be some of the tools we will use to address the history of the notion of trauma.

0.5 Internal Organisation

This book is organised into five chapters that refer to different periods and problems. The first chapter addresses the process known as the "psychologization" of trauma (Gauchet & Swain, 2000; Hacking, 1995; Leys, 2000; Micale & Lerner, 2001). In it, we attempt to justify why this process cannot be considered a homogeneous development or a clear jump from a somatic to a psychological conception of trauma. Instead, different authors (especially Erichsen, Page, Oppenheim and Charcot) introduced different elements that are now associated with the idea of psychical trauma (such as suspicions of simulation, latency in the appearance of symptoms, the role of emotions and ideas in its development and the impossibility of eliminating symptoms through consciousness and willpower) but which at that time were still inscribed in an eminently medical (anatomical or physiological) field. We also seek to highlight the successive changes in the boundaries between the organic and the psychological spheres, as well as the role played by forensic and clinical techniques and practices in conceptual transformations.

In the second chapter, we try to explain the historical origin of the relationship between trauma and memory. Although both terms seem, at present, inconceivable without the other, they were first linked together in the early works on neuroses by Janet and Freud. These famous disciples of Charcot were who began to think of trauma as a pathological experience that depends on a particular interplay between remembering and forgetting. At the same time, in this section, we discuss contemporary historiographical approaches that, by recovering Janet's reading, consider him the founder of a traumatic theory of psychopathology; while Freud is seen as someone who impeded the reflection on trauma due to the importance he gave to drives and phantasies. However, the first works of both authors allow us to observe that the French doctor and philosopher relativised the traumatic situations by virtue of the weight given to heredity. At the same time, his Viennese colleague much more clearly defended pathology's accidental and contingent nature. Lastly, the analysis of their respective therapeutic approaches allows us to identify the original responses that each one was able to formulate in the face of a clinical obstacle they encountered: to overcome trauma, remembering was not enough.

Chapter 3 is dedicated to analysing the construction and abandonment of the Freudian theory known as "seduction". We aim to highlight three aspects that have not been considered in depth by other authors who dealt with it. First, the objective behind Freud's *Neurotica*: to establish an aetiological theory that could displace hereditarian theories and that could establish a specific sexual cause for each clinical picture. Second, the *nachträglich* temporality of trauma, which is distinguished both from the conceptions that establish a linear, causal and deterministic relationship between the trauma and the symptoms, and from those that emphasise an a posteriori resignification, thus relativising the weight of the experience. Lastly, the different versions of the abandonment of the theory, where we still find the debate between the real or phantasist nature of the narratives about past traumas. Unlike the usual theses, we attempt to justify that the opposition between reality and phantasy is very much relativised in many passages of the Freudian work.

Chapter 4 focuses on the war neuroses. The First World War once again put the problem of psychical trauma at the centre of the scene for those who dealt with the treatment of the neuroses, after a period of 15 years in which this illness had lost the significance it had gained during the final decades of the nineteenth century. This chapter is divided into two parts. Initially, we aim to analyse three major debates that arose regarding the war neuroses during the armed conflict. The first of these consisted of a new discussion on the nature of trauma: somatic or psychical? Was it a new disease or new forms of the old neurotic illnesses? Sexual or non-sexual? In this context, psychoanalytic hypotheses (and psychoanalysts) were met with the possibility of achieving greater visibility and acceptance in the medical world. The second controversy revolved around the attribution of the determining power in the production of symptoms: either to the objective conditions of the situation or to the subjective particularities of the ill person. The third debate was on the efficacy of the different therapies: faradisation, isolation, active therapies, hypnosis, suggestion, persuasion, catharsis and some versions of psychoanalysis.

The second part of the chapter limits its attention to the ethical and conceptual resonances of the war on Freudian thought after 1920. In particular, we attempt to analyse his position regarding the ethical implications of the treatments used in the wartime context. We also try to develop the main characteristics of a new economic conception of trauma. We hypothesise that this conception not only implied a conceptual rearrangement of some key principles of his theory but also introduced a new problem linked to the limits of the field of representations in processing the quantities of excitation it faced.

The final chapter attempts to circumscribe (within the Freudian excursions into the realm of group psychology) the problem of collective traumas. This problem appears fundamentally in two books: *Totem and Taboo* (1913) and *Moses and Monotheism* (1939). In these texts, we do not find new conceptual configurations of trauma but rather a recapitulation and application (in the collective field) of the different conceptions that the Viennese psychoanalyst had devised from his psychoanalytic practice. This application was possible given his assumption that the same laws govern individual and group psychology. For Freud, certain collective experiences from humanity's past, despite being excluded from the explicit narratives about past times, persist in social memory, insist on compulsively returning and contain elements that resist being bound to the webs of shared representations. In particular, Freud conjectured the existence and permanence of two traumas: on the one hand, the murder of the violent leader of the primal horde at the hands of his sons, which would have led to clan organisation and the transition from nature to culture; on the other hand, the repetition of that crime in the murder of Moses, founder of the Jewish people, who tried to impose a monotheistic religion of Egyptian origin. The preservation of these traumas supposedly experienced by our ancestors introduced another relevant issue: the transgenerational transmission of past experiences, which would end up affecting those who did not directly participate in the experience.

It can be seen that the ordering of the chapters does not respond strictly to a chronological criterion but to the consideration of certain key problems: the tension between the event as an objective fact and its subjective representation; the relationship between trauma and memory; the question of causality; the problematic nature of narratives (or testimonies) of past traumatic experiences; the problem of sexuality; the link between trauma and war; the limits of the webs of representations; and collective trauma and its transmission.

We consider that these problems are not only central in the psychopathological and clinical field but also have relevance in the debates on trauma in the field of collective memory and the history of the present. As some of Europe's most renowned historians point out, we live in an era characterised by a "great wave of memory" (Hartog, 2003, p. 16), by an "obsession" with memory (Traverso, 2007, p. 69), by a "proliferating and multiform commemorative endeavour" (Revel, 2005, p. 271). From a Freudian perspective, not only some individuals but also some peoples seem to have been "absorbed in mental concentration upon the past" and have abandoned "all interest in the present and future" after having gone through "a traumatic event" which shattered the foundations of their lives (Freud, 1916–17a, p. 276). Addressing these problems historically without reducing them to the strict domain of the clinic is our way of being explicitly consistent with the context in which our work is produced,[6] and of building bridges between psychoanalysis, the history of psychoanalysis and the history of the recent past.

Notes

1 In this regard, Dominick LaCapra refers to the question of trauma in the following way: "This problem has become crucial in modern thought in general and is especially prominent in post-World War II thought bearing on the present and the foreseeable future" (2005, p. xxix).
2 See: http://www.apatraumadivision.org.
3 *Translator's note*: We have translated the author's original notion of "*trama de representaciones*" as "web(s) of representations". This decision implies a double compromise. The vital Freudian notion that in Strachey's translations is referred to as "idea", in José Luis Etcheverry's translation into Spanish is called "*representación*". Throughout this book, we have attempted to adhere to the use of "idea" as a replacement for the Spanish "*representación*", despite the semantic implications this may have. Therefore, we wish to advert the readers that when the word "representation" and its derivatives appear, it has connotations to the Freudian "idea"; and vice-versa, "idea" alludes to the semantically richer "*representación*". Furthermore, we believe "web/webs" is the English word that most suitably substitutes the Spanish term "*trama*" and its variety of condensed meanings and connotations. This term stems from the infinitive verb "*entramar*", similar to the English "to weave". "*Trama*" also means "plot", as in the development of a story, which fits well with this book's themes. Lastly, note the formal likeness of this word ("*trama*") with the one that is central throughout this book ("trauma"); this will become especially relevant in the book's final chapters.
4 We agree on this point with the opinion of Sandra Berta, who stated that "without it being a fundamental concept, the trauma continues to be a central issue for psychoanalysis, around which revolves an extensive discussion that involves crucial issues such as causality, sexuality, structure and temporality" (Berta, 2014, p. 19; italics in original).
5 Some of the models that we come across are pathological anatomy, faradisation, the technique of hypnosis, the hypothesis of a cerebral unconscious and Herbart's ideas about the conflict between ideas, among others.
6 This is something which the traditional "historiographical operation" tries to avoid, although, as De Certeau (from whom we took the previously quoted syntagma) puts it, there are no technical devices that are totally "capable of effacing the *specificity* of the place, the origin of my speech, or the area in which I am researching" (De Certeau, 1988, p. 56; italics in original).

References

Acha, O. (2007). *Freud y el problema de la historia*. Buenos Aires: Prometeo.
Acha, O. (2010). No todo es historia. Lacan y los entretiempos freudianos. In O. Acha & M. Vallejo (Eds.), *Inconsciente e historia después de Freud. Cruces entre filosofía, psicoanálisis e historiografía* (pp. 267–282). Buenos Aires: Prometeo.
Acha, O. & Vallejo, M. (2010). *Inconsciente e historia después de Freud. Cruces entre filosofía, psicoanálisis e historiografía*. Buenos Aires: Prometeo.
Alarcón, F. (1996). Trauma y après coup. *Revista de Psicoanálisis de la Asociación Psicoanalítica de Madrid.* Extra 1996, 123–142.
Assmann, J. (1999). Monothéisme et mémoire: Le Moïse de Freud et la tradition biblique. *Annales. Histoire, Sciences Sociales, 54 Année, 5* (September–October), 1011–1026.
Assoun, P.-L. ([1981] 1987). *Introducción a la epistemología freudiana.* México: Siglo XXI.
Assoun, P.-L. (1998) (Ed.) *Lecciones psicoanalíticas sobre Cuerpo y Síntoma.* Buenos Aires: Nueva Visión.

Assoun, P.-L. (2001). *El perjuicio y el Ideal. Hacia una clínica Social del trauma.* Buenos Aires: Nueva Visión.

Assoun, P.-L. (2003). Lo real y la angustia: el trauma. In P.-L. Assoun (Ed.), *Lecciones psicoanalíticas sobre la angustia* (pp. 55–62). Buenos Aires: Nueva Visión.

Badiou, A. (2009). *El Siglo.* Buenos Aires: Manantial.

Berta, S. (2014). *Escribir el trauma, de Freud a Lacan.* Buenos Aires: Letra Viva.

Blum, H. (1991). Freud and the figure of Moses: The Moses of Freud. *Journal of American Psychoanalitic Association, 39*, 513–535.

Bokanowski, T. (2005). Variaciones sobre el concepto de traumatismo: Traumatismo, lo traumático, trauma. *Revista de Psicoanálisis, 62* (1), 11–28.

Bonomi, C. (2007). *Sulla Soglia Della Psicoanalisi.* Torino: Bollati Boringhieri.

Borch-Jacobsen, M. (1996). Neurotica: Freud and the Seduction Theory. *October, 76*, 15–42.

Borch-Jacobsen, M. & Shamdasani, S. (2006). *Le dossier Freud. Enquête sur l'histoire de la psychanalyse.* París: Les Empêcheurs de penser en rond.

Bourdieu, P. (2008) *Los usos sociales de la ciencia.* Buenos Aires: Nueva Visión.

Brette, F. (1988). Le traumatisme et ses théories. *Revue Française de Psychanalyse, 52* (6), 1259–1284.

Canguilhem, G. (2009). El objeto de la historia de las ciencias. In G. Canguilhem (Ed.), *Estudios de historia y de filosofía de las ciencias* (pp. 11–26). Buenos Aires: Amorrortu.

Carroy, J. (1991). *Hypnose, Suggestion et Psychologie. L'invention des sujets.* Paris: PUF.

Carter, C. (1980). Germ theory, hysteria, and Freud's early work in psychopathology. *Medical History, 24*, 259–274.

Caruth, C. (Ed.). (1995). *Trauma: Explorations in Memory.* Baltimore, MD: The Johns Hopkins University Press.

Dagfal, A. (2013). 1913–2013: A un siglo de "El psico-análisis' según Janet. *Estudos e Pesquisas em Psicología, 13* (1), 320–376. Dahl, G. (2010). The two time vectors of Nachträglichkeit in the development of ego organization: Significance of the concept for the symbolization of nameless traumas and anxieties. *The International Journal of Psychoanalysis, 91*(4), 727–744.

Danziger, K. (1984). Towards a conceptual framework for a critical history of psychology. *Revista de Historia de la Psicología, 5* (1/2), 99–107.

Danziger, K. (1990). *Constructing the Subject. Historical Origins of Psychological Research.* Cambridge: Cambridge University Press.

De Certeau, M. (1988). *The Writing of History.* New York: Columbia University Press.

Derrida, J. (1987). Freud y la escena de la escritura. In J. Derrida (Ed.), *La escritura y la diferencia* (pp. 271–317). Barcelona: Anthropos.

Derrida, J. (1996). *Archive Fever. A Freudian Impression.* Chicago, IL and London: The University of Chicago Press.

Edelman, N. (2003). *Les métamorphoses de l'histérique. Du debut du XIX siècle à la Grande Guerre.* Paris: La Découverte.

Eissler, K.R. (1992). *Freud sur le front des névroses de guerre.* Paris: Presses Universitaires de France.

Ellenberger, H. (1970). *The Discovery of the Unconscious: The History and Evolution of Dynamic Psychiatry.* New York: Basic Books.

Esterson, A. (1993). *Seductive mirage. An exploration of the Work of Sigmund Freud.* Chicago, IL: Open Court.

Esterson, A. (2001). The mythologizing of psychoanalytic history: Deception and self-deception in Freud's accounts of the seduction theory episode. *Hystory of Psychiatry, XII*, 329–352.

Foucault, M. (1978). *The History of Sexuality. Volume 1: An Introduction.* New York: Pantheon Books.

Foucault, M. (2006). *Psychiatric Power. Lecture at the Collège de France, 1973–1974.* New York: Palgrave Macmillian.

Franco, M. & Levín, M. (Ed.). (2007). *Historia reciente. Perspectivas y desafíos para un campo en construcción.* Buenos Aires: Paidós.

Freud, S. ([1916-1917] 1963). XVIII. Fixation to traumas – The unconscious. In S. Freud (Ed.), *The Standard Edition of the Complete Psychological Works of Sigmund Freud, Vol XVI. Introductory Lecture on Psychoanalysis (Part. III)* (pp. 273–285). London: The Hogarth Press and the Institute of Psycho-Analysis.

Freud, S. ([1939] 1964). Moses and monotheism: Three essays. In S. Freud (Ed.), *The Standard Edition of the Complete Psychological Works of Sigmund Freud, Vol XXIII: Moses and Monotheism, an Outline of Psycho- Analysis and Other Works* (pp. 1–137). London: The Hogarth Press and the Institute of Psycho-Analysis.

Friedlander, S. (Ed.). (1992). *Probing the Limits of Representation. Nazism and the 'Final Solution'.* Cambridge and London: Harvard University Press.

García, G. (2008). *Actualidad del trauma.* Buenos Aires: Grama.

Gauchet, M. (1994). *El inconsciente cerebral.* Buenos Aires: Nueva Visión.

Gauchet, M & Swain, G. (2000). *El verdadero Charcot.* Buenos Aires: Nueva Visión.

Gay, P. (1989). *Freud. Una vida de nuestro tiempo.* Buenos Aires: Paidós.

Gelfand, T. (1989). Charcot's Response to Freud's Rebellion. *Journal of the History of Ideas, 50* (2), 293–307.

Good, M. (1995). Karl Abraham, Sigmund Freud, and the fate of the seduction theory. *Journal of the American Psychoanalytic Association, 43* (4), 1137–1167.

Hacking, J. (1995). *Rewriting the Soul: Multiple Personality and the Sciences of Memory.* Princeton, NJ: Princeton University Press.

Hartog, F. (2003). *Régimes d'Historicité. Présentisme et expériences du temps.* Paris: Seuil.

Hermann, J. (1992). *Trauma and Recovery.* New York: Basic Books.

Israel, H. & Schatzman, M. (1993). The seduction theory. *History of Psychiatry, 4*, 23–59.

Jones, E. (1953–57). *The Life and Work of Sigmund Freud. Volume I, II & III.* New York: Basic Books.

Koselleck, R. (1993). *Futuro pasado. Para una semántica de los tiempos históricos.* Barcelona: Paidós.

LaCapra, D. (2008). *Representando el Holocausto. Historia, teoría y trauma.* Buenos Aires: Prometeo.

LaCapra, D. (2009). *Historia y memoria después de Auschwitz.* Buenos Aires: Prometeo.

LaCapra, D. (2014). *Writing History, Writing Trauma.* Baltimore, MD: John Hopkins University Press.

Le Gaufey, G. (1995). *La evicción del origen.* Buenos Aires: Edelp.

Le Gaufey, G. (2001). *Anatomía de la tercera persona.* Buenos Aires: Edelp.

Levin, K. (1985). *Freud y su primera psicología de las neurosis.* México, MX: F.C.E.

Leys, R. (2000). *Trauma. A Genealogy.* Chicago, IL: The University of Chicago Press.

Lowenstein, A. (1996). Trauma y pulsión. *Revista del Seminario Lacaniano, 7*, 20–23.

Masson, J.M. (1984). *The Assault on Truth: Freud's Suppression of the Seduction Theory.* Penguin Press.

Micale, M. & Lerner, P. (Eds.). (2001). *Traumatic Past: History, Psychiatry, and Trauma in the Modern Age, 1870–1930.* Cambridge: Cambridge University Press.

Mudrovcic, M.I. (2005). Alcances y límites de perspectivas psicoanalíticas en historia. In M. I. Mudrovcic (Ed.), *Historia, narración y memoria. Los debates actuales en filosofía de la historia* (pp. 139–154). Madrid: Akal.

Mudrovcic, M.I. (2009). Trauma, memoria e historia. In D. Brauer (Ed.), *La historia desde la teoría. Vol. 2. Una guía de campo por el pensamiento filosófico acerca del sentido de la historia y del conocimiento del pasado* (pp. 105–126). Buenos Aires: Prometeo.

Ramirez Ortiz, M.E. (2007). *Psicoanalistas en el frente de batalla. Las neurosis de guerra en la Primera Guerra Mundial.* Antioquía: Editorial Universidad de Antioquía.

Revel, J. (2005). La carga de la memoria: historia frente a memoria en Francia hoy. In J. Revel (Ed.), *Un momento historiográfico. Trece ensayos de historia social* (pp. 271–283). Buenos Aires: Manantial.

Ricoeur, P. (2008). *La memoria, la historia, el olvido.* Buenos Aires: Fondo de Cultura Económica.

Sanfelippo, L. (2011a). El trauma en la historia. Razones y problemas de una importación conceptual. *Usages publics du passé.* See http://ehess.dynamiques.fr/usagespublicsdu-passe/rubriques/reflexions-critiques/luis-sanfelippo-el-trauma-en-la-historia.html. Also published in *Pasajes. Revista de Pensamiento Contemporáneo,* n° 40. Valencia: Universidad de Valencia, 2013 (pp. 24–37).

Sanfelippo, L. (2011b). La utilización de la noción de trauma en la historiografía y la memoria social. In Facultad de Psicología (Ed.), *Memorias de las XVIII Jornadas y III Congreso Internacional de Investigación y Práctica Profesional* (pp. 130–136). Buenos Aires: Fac. de Psicología. U.B.A. Sección Historia de la Psicología.

Sanfelippo, L. & Vallejo, M. (2013a). Los orígenes de la teoría de la seducción. Etiología específica y herencia en los primeros escritos de Sigmund Freud. *Revista de la Sociedad Argentina de Psicoanálisis, 17,* 257–276.

Sanfelippo, L. & Vallejo, M. (2013b). Disparidades entre las distintas miradas que Sigmund Freud dirigió hacia su teoría de la seducción. Realidad o fantasía? *Perspectivas en Psicología, 10,* 33–41.

Sulloway, F. (1979). *Freud Biologist of the Mind. Beyond the Psychoanalytic Legend.* New York: Basic Books.

Sulloway, F. (1991). Reassessing Freud's case histories: The social construction of psychoanalysis. *Isis, 82,* 245–275.

Swain, G. (1994). Du traitment moral aux psychothérapies. Remarques sur la formation de l'idêe contemporaine de psychothérapie. In G. Swain (Ed.), *Dialogue avec l'insensé* (pp. 237–262). Paris: Gallimard.

Thoma, H. & Cheshire, N. (1991). Freud's Nachträglichkeit and Strachey's 'deferred action': Trauma, constructions and the direction of causality. *The International Review of Psycho-Analysis, 18* (3), 407–427.

Traverso, E. (2007) Historia y memoria. Notas sobre un debate. In Franco, M. y Levín, M. (Ed.), *Historia reciente. Perspectivas y desafíos para un campo en construcción* (pp. 67–96). Buenos Aires: Paidós.

Triplett, H. (2004). The misnomer of Freud's "Seduction Theory". *Journal of the History of Ideas, 65* (4), 647–655.

Vallejo, M. (2011). *Teorías hereditarias del siglo XIX y el problema de la transmisión intergeneracional. Psicoanálisis y Biopolítica.* Doctoral Thesis. UNLP.

Vallejo, M. (2012). *La seducción freudiana (1895–1897). Un ensayo de genética textual.* Buenos Aires: Letra Viva.

Van der Hart, O. & Horst, R. (1989). The dissociation theory of Pierre Janet. *The Journal of Traumatic Stress, 2* (4), 397–412.
Van der Hart, O., Brown, P. & Van der Kolk, B. (1989). Pierre Janet's treatment of post-traumatic stress. *The Journal of Traumatic Stress, 2* (4), 379–395.
Van der Kolk, B. & Van der Hart, O. (1995). The intrusive past: The flexibility of memory and the engraving of trauma. In C. Caruth (Ed.), *Trauma: Explorations in Memory* (pp. 158–182). Baltimore, MD: The Johns Hopkins University Press.
Van der Kolk, B., McFarlane, A. & Weisaeth, L. (Eds.). (1996). *Traumatic Stress: The Effects of Overwhelming Experiences on Mind.* New York: Guilford Press.
Van der Kolk, B., Weisaeth, L. & Van der Hart, D. (1996). History of trauma in psychiatry. In B. Van der Kolk, A. McFarlane & L. Weisaeth, L. (Eds.), *Traumatic Stress: The Effects of Overwhelming Experiences on Mind* (pp. 47–76). New York: Guilford Press.
Vezzetti, H. (2002). *Pasado y presente*. Buenos Aires: Siglo XXI.
Vezzetti, H. (2007). Historias de la psicología: Problemas, funciones y objetivos. *Revista de historia de la psicología, 28* (1), 147–165.
Vezzetti, H. (2009). *Sobre la violencia revolucionaria.* Buenos Aires: Siglo XXI.
Yerushalmi, Y. (1996). *El Moisés de Freud. Judaísmo terminable e interminable*. Buenos Aires: Nueva Visión.
Young, A. (1995). *The Harmony of Illusions*. Princeton, NJ: Princeton University Press.

Chapter 1

Mechanical Trauma and Psychical Trauma

Railway Accidents and Hysteria (1866–1889)

The purpose of this chapter is to trace some historical paths that allow an account of the processes of the "psychologisation of trauma" (Hacking, 1995) that took place in the second half of the nineteenth century. The use of the plural is essential here since, from the old surgical notion of trauma to the modern psychological conception, there has not been a single, natural or expected development. Rather, multiple processes occurred (railway and work accidents, insurance and pensions for injury or disability, the debate on hysteria) that, in different spheres (medical expertise, experimentation with hypnosis) and different intellectual geographies (England, Germany and France), led to dissimilar conceptions about the nature of trauma. However, these had in common the inclusion of certain traits that differed from those attributed to mechanical trauma and that only later would be defined as "psychological" attributes, completely independent of the "organic" kind (the temporal latency between the event and the appearance of symptoms, the participation of representations or affects in the pathogenic process, etc.).

At the same time, this notion of *psychologisation*, to which numerous historians refer (Gauchet & Swain, 2000; Hacking, 1995; Leys, 2000; Micale & Lerner, 2001), is complex and should be problematised. The shift from a completely somatic and mechanical notion of trauma to different versions that included psychical elements cannot be understood as a sudden leap or a total transformation from one sense to the other nor as the result of the emergence of a new psychological discipline that would be fully autonomous in respect to medicine. It is true that towards the end of the nineteenth century, it was possible to observe fundamentally psychical conceptions of trauma in the works of Janet and Freud. However, we should not forget that before this, there had already been authors who, within the general framework of a somatic conception of the disease, began to attribute a psychical nature to some of the elements that made up the trauma.

The complex nature of the historical processes that led to psychologisation can also be seen in certain disagreements which are present in historiographical approaches to the subject. For example, Ian Hacking referred to one of the first extensive works on the topic, written by Esther Fischer-Homberg, entitled *Die traumatische Neurose. Vom somatischen zum sozialen Leiden* [*The Traumatic Neurosis. From Somatic to Social Suffering*]. This author held the idea that the

DOI: 10.4324/9781003380016-2

complete psychologisation of trauma had been produced within the Freudian theory and only after 1897 (Hacking, 1995, p. 183). In his view, Freud had conceived the possibility that "purely psychic events, fantasies of infantile sexuality, could produce neurosis" (Hacking, 1995, p. 183). However, this affirmation is debatable. Not only because, as Hacking correctly points out, "the trauma was already well psychologized in Freud's theory from 1893–1897" (Hacking, 1995, p. 183), but also because that year coincided with the Viennese psychoanalyst's abandonment of his "Seduction theory" and, therefore, with the introduction of the idea that a neurosis could arise from a psychical conflict even if there had not been a traumatic event that caused it.[1]

Furthermore, for Hacking, the full psychologisation of trauma would only have taken place after the publication of Pierre Janet's *Psychological Automatism*, which the former considers "the first work to systematically study the traumatic causes of hysteria" (Hacking, 1995, p. 191). In contrast, Charcot continued to conceive trauma as a physical event rather than a psychological shock (Hacking, 1995, p. 188). This interpretation of the works of the Salpêtrière Doctor still retains the remnants of a traditional partition: the French clinician remained engrossed in neurology, and only his most famous disciples were able to free themselves from the ties to this discipline. Regarding this point, Marcel Gauchet and Gladys Swain's reading is more subtle and precise because, although it recognises that Charcot continued to inscribe his work in the field of neurology, it also traces the psychological elements that were already present in his work (Gauchet & Swain, 2000). Furthermore, as we shall see in the next chapter, it is arguable that Janet's first thesis is a work that systematically studied "the traumatic causes" of hysteria.

Ruth Leys' point of view is different. For this author,

> the term trauma acquired a more psychological meaning when it was employed by J. M. Charcot, Pierre Janet, Alfred Binet, Morton Prince, Josef Breuer, Sigmund Freud, and other turn-of-the century figures to describe the wounding of the mind brought about by sudden, unexpected, emotional shock.
>
> (Leys, 2000, pp. 3–4)

The enumeration of authors makes it possible to avoid the simplest historical hypotheses, which would indicate that the shift from somatic to psychical conceptions occurred as an abrupt and sudden rupture caused by the genius of a single author. Between the absolutely somatic trauma, with verifiable lesions, to which the old notion referred, and the more psychological versions that emerged in the nineteenth-century literature, it would be necessary to locate a series of intermediate links rather than a radical transformation that allowed the automatic transition from one acceptation to the other.[2] However, Ley's book does not deal with this series since it begins directly with Freud and immediately directs its attention to the twentieth century.

For our part, we will try to reflect upon three different but linked moments that successfully highlight the complexity of the historical processes that made it possible for the notion of trauma to acquire a psychological meaning in some areas. First, in 1866, the publication of the book *On Railway and Other Injuries of the Nervous System* (Erichsen, 1866). This book extended the classic anatomical perspective to cases of accidented subjects whose particularity resided in the diffuse nature of their injuries and the "suspicions" of simulation. Second, the criticisms of Erichsen's position, stemming from a new approach to nervous diseases, masterfully exemplified in the book *Injuries of the Spine and Spinal Cord without Apparent Mechanical Lesions, and Nervous Shock, in their surgical and Medico-Legal aspects* (Page, 1883). Lastly, we will shift our attention from England to France, where the problem of accidents was combined with neurological studies on hysteria and controversies around hypnosis. In this context, new hypotheses arose about the role that emotions and ideas could have in the production of nervous symptoms (Charcot, 1889). These three moments seem to delineate a gradual but firm path towards a growing psychologisation. However, we are forced to add a fourth moment because, before the end of the 1880s, the nosographic category of "traumatic neurosis" was coined in Germany (Oppenheim, 1900). Thus, a double movement occurred: on the one hand, the notion of trauma was transformed into a specific nosographic category; on the other hand, the trauma was once again conceived from a somatic point of view.

In other words, the psychologisation of trauma does not refer to a linear or necessary historical process. On the contrary, carefully following the temporal, geographical and conceptual shifts that occurred between the 1860s and 1880s will allow us to reconstruct the sinuous paths that the transformations of this notion took before the emergence of Psychoanalysis. In addition, it will make it possible to understand that these changes cannot be seen as the result of the advancement of knowledge within clinical disciplines; rather, they respond to multiple factors, among which stand out: extra-disciplinary cultural processes (such as the development of the railway and the establishment of insurance policies) and broader epistemic transformations, which were independent of and prior to the specific problem of trauma (such as the development of physiology over anatomy, or the use of hypnosis for experimental purposes).

1.1 Traumatic (Rail)ways

It is impossible to address the psychologisation of trauma historically without referring to the cultural impact of the railway and the economic and legal consequences of its accidents. The invention of the train allowed large masses of people to move daily through urban, suburban and rural centres for a minimum cost and to cover in a few hours distances that previously took days. In a way, it made the region, the entire country, or even the continent become the new village that, without becoming global, increased the number of possible experiences that the average inhabitant could have. In this way, the railway became a paradigmatic example of the hopes aroused by technological progress in Western culture.

However, at the same time, it also became the symbol of horror that technical progress could introduce into everyday life. It is clear that other means of transportation and technological inventions have also generated pain and death. Some, such as the war machines, because they are explicitly designed for these purposes. Others, by leading humankind to dangerous areas, thus leaving it at the mercy of the most fearsome natural inclemencies: such is the case of ships that ventured overseas. However, these dangers were largely restricted to those who participated in armed conflicts or those who decided to set sail towards unknown and dangerous natural territories. On the other hand, a train that derails, collides, overturns, etc., introduces the possibility of sudden catastrophe striking in the places and during the activities of everyday civilian life. This type of catastrophe was no longer due to the inclemency of nature or divine punishment. It was humanity that, by forging their progress, generated the horror.

The fact that habitual existence could be suddenly altered and endangered by a product of human knowledge generated in the common sense an insidious and anticipatory fear of a potential evil whose moment of appearance, magnitude and exact consequences could not be foreseen. The anxieties that arose were reflected and, at the same time, magnified by the press. A fragment of the August 29, 1868, edition of the English newspaper *Saturday Review* is illustrative of the image that was constructed around these accidents: "We are, in the matter of railway travelling, always treading the unknown… All that we know of the future is that it is full of dangers; but what these dangers are we cannot conjecture or anticipate" (Harrington, 2001, p. 33). It did not matter, on this point, that the statistics showed that trains were a safe means of transportation, which increasing numbers of people began to use each year.[3] The fear generated by railway accidents was proportional to the increase in its users, although entirely independent of the number of accidents produced.

The train, marvellous and horrific, and its unpredictable and anxiously awaited accidents appeared as ambiguous figures that gave way to new problems that required novel solutions. Initially, they were one of the main factors that led to the implementation of an insurance system to face potential legal claims that the users of the railway system could make against the railway companies. In Great Britain, the Railway Passengers Assurance Company was established in 1849. As Harrington states, this was an implicit recognition of the public's growing fear regarding railway safety (Harrington, 2001, p. 34). This recognition, far from generating peace of mind, could also function as the acceptance of the expected nature of potentially tragic accidents.

Then, if the injuries caused by a railway accident could imply financial compensation, the discussion about the real or simulated nature of the damages suffered by the plaintiffs took place with great force. Since then, the grounds were set for a medico-legal dispute where the alleged victims and the defenders of the interests of the insurance and railway companies pushed medical experts to rule on particular cases, especially in those cases which could not easily be classified into extreme poles of verifiable injury or frank simulation. In this grey area, new explanations about nervous illness began to be developed that would lead, years later, to new conceptions of the old medical term of trauma.

1.2 Real Damage or Simulation?

Initially, the terms "real damage" and "simulation" were proposed as an exclusive disjunction. This pair of opposites seemed to reproduce both sides of the legal complaint in the expert debate. For railroad and insurer advocate experts, if a case did not present a provable injury, then that person was a simulator trying to extract spurious money from a claim for non-existent damage. On the other hand, the experts defending the alleged victims tried to justify the claim's validity by demonstrating the realness of the symptoms provoked by the accident.

However, this description of the problem in terms of binary opposites is insufficient since it prevents us from seeing the complexity of the debates that arose from the simple questions that a judge could ask an expert in order to determine if there was real damage or if it was a simulation.

As we know from Harrington's research, certain articles in the English newspaper *The Lancet* well illustrated the development of a problematic zone, where the bipartition between reality and simulation had to be abandoned. These publications insisted on distinguishing between the "primary" effects of an accident (such as broken bones, lacerations, burns), which did not present diagnostic or expert difficulties, and the "secondary" effects, whose nature was difficult to conceive and classify, for example, "giddiness, loss of memory, pains in the back and head (…) tingling and numbness of the extremities, local paralysis, paraplegia, functional lesions of the kidney and bladder (…) and even slowly ensuing symptoms of intellectual derangement" (Harrington, 2001, p. 40).[4] It was not strange for "fright" to be mentioned as one of the factors suffered by victims of a railway collision. However, there were no indications in these publications that this emotion could directly produce the disturbances mentioned above. Rather, these were explained as "consequent on the physical jolts and shocks of the accident" in accordance to the firm "somaticist orientation of Victorian medicine" (Harrington, 2001, p. 42).

But a mantle of uncertainty still hung over these cases since it was not clear what kind of somatic condition was at play when no unmistakeable signs of injury could be found anywhere in the body. What type of disturbance would have been produced? What type of body would the accident affect?

The first crucial medical text that attempted to conjecture about the nature of such conditions was written by John Eric Erichsen, a British physician and surgeon, who had written a "highly successful standard surgical textbook" (Harrington, 2001, p. 43). He devoted a series of lectures to the subject of railway accidents and their subsequent illnesses while teaching at University College London. These lectures were presented as the fruit of his labour as an expert in defence of the injured, and six of them were later published in book form in 1866 under the title of *On Railway and Other Injuries of the Nervous System*. This book constituted an excellent example of the new controversies that arose since that time around the category of trauma. It unwittingly and unintentionally served as the starting point for a process of transformation of knowledge and practices that dealt with these issues. In addition, from its publication until at least the 1880s, Erichsen's work constituted an obligatory reference for medical specialists and experts engaged in legal processes. Both those who sought to prove the existence of harm caused by the accidents and those who tried to deny it ended up referring to his ideas as the support to legitimise their arguments or as the main obstacle to overcome in order to win the epistemic or legal disputes.[5]

Most historians and academics who have dealt with the history of trauma have placed Erichsen and his book in a foundational place regarding modern conceptualisations of trauma. However, beyond this specific convergence, many divergences appear in the readings on the work of the British surgeon.

The book *Traumatic Stress: The Effects of Overwhelming Experience on Mind, Body and Society* (Van der Kolk, McFarlane & Weisaeth, 1996), which attempts to account for the "current state of knowledge" about trauma, included a chapter dedicated to history. In it, the series of reference authors began with Erichsen. According to the authors, the surgeon "ascribed the psychological problems of severely injured patients to organic causes (…) physical signs of anxiety then, as now, were easily misdiagnosed as symptoms of organic illness" (Van der Kolk, McFarlane & Weisaeth, 1996, p. 48).

As can be appreciated, Erichsen was the first link in a chain of specialists who contributed to developing knowledge about trauma. However, his ideas about the "organic causes" of his patients' illnesses were placed on a list of errors, of "misdiagnoses" which had to be overcome for it to be discovered that they were "psychological problems" of "anxiety". Evidently, in this book, the focus on the current knowledge of the subject biases the view of the past. In the present day, Erichsen's ideas seem clearly organicist; and his patient's symptoms seem clearly psychical. However, this presentist view runs the risk of occulting the way in which these controversies were posed almost a century and a half ago. At the same time, it simplifies and distorts the epistemic and expert battle that Erichsen sought to win.

Ian Hacking, for his part, maintained that Erichsen dedicated himself to studying the conditions of certain accident victims whose "symptoms did not seem to correspond to any discernible physical injury" although "head injury, together with what he called 'spinal concussion', was at the heart of the problem" (Hacking, 1995, p. 185). This brief reading of Erichsen's ideas got slightly closer to the type of problems that the surgeon had set out to tackle. But immediately, concerned with pointing out that the British doctor was opposed to comparing these cases of injured men with hysterical patients, the Canadian historian stated that "victims of railway spine had no lesions" (Hacking, 1995, p. 186). Erichsen would have thoroughly repudiated this statement since it precisely denies the lesional nature of these cases, which constituted the central hypothesis that the British surgeon intended to demonstrate.

For her part, Nicole Edelman wrote an excellent book focused on the transformations of the notion of hysteria in the French context. There she maintained that "Erichsen's autopsies revealed an inflammation of the cortical membranes and substances" and that, therefore, he "deduced the organic aetiology of these problems, which he considered to be manifestations of hysteria" (Edelman, 2003, p. 152). From the ideas expressed in these sentences, we consider correct only the one referring to the organic aetiology since the British surgeon did not localise the anatomical alteration in the cerebral cortex nor did he consider the cases he studied to be cases of hysteria.

Through this very brief state of the art, we wanted to illustrate the importance attributed to Erichsen and the lack of close readings to which his book has been subjected, with the exception of some of the articles found in the collective book *Traumatic Past: History, Psychiatry and Trauma in the Modern Age, 1870–1930* (Micale & Lerner, 2001). When Erichsen's work is declared foundational, a striking detail is often neglected: the word "trauma" was not mentioned in his book's 103 pages. The term's inclusion in this history can only be understood by the fact that several authors in the 1880s (such as Page, Charcot, and Oppenheim) who criticised the hypotheses defended by Erichsen did indeed make use of the notion of trauma to address railway accident victims. Furthermore, the simple equivalence established between the surgeon's work and the category of railway spine is also questionable. From his perspective, the clinical presentation he referred to was not limited to railway accidents since "the same effects may result from other and more ordinary injuries of civil life" (Erichsen, 1866, p. 22). In any case, from his perspective, the train presented characteristics that could increase the severity of damage to the nervous system, such as "rapidity of the movement", its sudden nature, and the helplessness to which the passenger was subjected.[6] However, these particularities would not constitute a qualitative difference with other accidents, which could be as minor as tripping on the stairs and, nevertheless, be associated with the same syndrome.[7]

Undoubtedly, the title of the book and the diffusion of the term railway spine hindered the possibility of observing these indications made by the surgeon. Nevertheless, for him, this point is crucial: if the cases he studied were to be considered an obscure disease that would only develop in cases of train accidents, his arguments would probably be subject to more suspicion than if it were an illness whose existence and recognition in medical knowledge was prior to and independent of the legal claims regarding railway disasters.[8] In this way, Erichsen differed from many of his contemporary colleagues who, unlike him, believed that these symptoms could not exist outside of these types of accidents.[9]

If this surgeon did not explicitly refer to the category of trauma or railway accidents, why must he be included in this history of trauma? His role was important because of the validity he gave to this series of cases that could not be accused of simulation but that, at the same time, did not present the typical characteristics of organic diseases recognised by the medical knowledge of his time. Cases that, furthermore, were characterised by presenting symptoms that tended to arise late and inexplicably. His ideas attempted to legitimise that grey area between the absence of disease and the most common nervous illnesses (be these lesional, hereditary or what was then called neurosis). At the same time, his proposals were one of the ways the link between events and symptoms became plausible, even when the existence of an anatomical lesion was not so evident.

It is true that Erichsen did not seek to develop a grey area; rather, as we shall see, he intended for his cases to be included within the category of diseases produced by material lesions. It is also true that his conceptualisations became quickly outdated. However, his work allowed for the configuration and legitimation of a new field of diagnostic, aetiological and legal problems. The answers that he was able to give were, undoubtedly, much less important than the questions and debates that his proposals generated.

1.3 The Sought-After Link between Accident, Injury and Symptoms

The lectures reproduced in Erichsen's book were intended to draw attention to

> certain injuries and diseases of the spine arising from accidents, often of a trivial character – from shocks to the body generally, rather than from blows upon the back itself – and to endeavour to trace the train of progressive symptoms and ill effects that often follow such injuries.
>
> (Erichsen, 1866, p. 17)

This phrase, taken from the beginning of the first lecture, includes the three elements that the nineteenth-century doctor intended to link: accidents (which could be trivial), unconventional spinal injuries (without fractures or dislocation of the spinal cord) and symptoms of progressive development. However, achieving this goal was not an easy task, because:

> … the absence often of evidence of outward and direct physical injury, the obscurity of their early symptoms, their very insidious character, the slowly progressive development of the secondary organic lesions, and functional disarrangements entailed by them, and the very uncertain nature of the ultimate issue of the case, they constitute a class of injuries that often tax the diagnostic skill of the surgeon to the very utmost (…) -Thus- it is often difficult to establish a connecting link between them – the particular symptoms – and the accident.
>
> (Erichsen, 1866, pp. 17–18)

If the author himself recognised the difficulties in linking the accident with the symptoms and in locating an organic injury, why defend a somatic hypothesis? Could the nature of disease be better explained by a psychological theory? Perhaps today it seems evident that this grey area could not be readily equated with diseases due to injury, and some authors might point out Erichsen's blindness while they claim the psychological nature of certain pathologies and trauma. However, this presentist reading of the past runs the risk of suffering from a blindness analogous to the one it intends to denounce since it conceals two elements that we consider worthy of highlighting.

First, the clinical picture described by Erichsen did not accurately coincide with the cases studied in the framework of later conceptualisations. The symptoms were not the same as in those patients categorised as being: victims of general nervous shock (Page); sufferers of traumatic neuroses (Oppenheim), hysterics (Charcot), neurotics (Freud); or as cases of post-traumatic stress disorder according to the current nosographic criteria. Therefore, it cannot be understood as a clinical picture that would exist and remain unchanged in all times and places and whose only variation would be the way in which each author conceived it. The symptoms that Erichsen described, the phenomena that he "saw", were in close relation to the conceptual framework[10] from which he approached his patients.

Second, and in close connection with the previous point, this presentist reading would prevent us from perceiving the motives behind why Erichsen not only saw certain symptoms and neglected others but why he also "saw" lesions that were difficult to observe. The reasons for his particular gaze were not to be found in his more or less genius or stubborn qualities but in his theoretical framework. As a surgeon and expert, his practice was guided by the knowledge that pathological anatomy had been producing since the dawn of the nineteenth century. According to this area of knowledge, an illness must be codified in terms of visible signs obtained through clinical observation. These signs must correspond to an anatomical lesion localisable in a specific part of the body, as the autopsies of the corpses of those who, in life, had suffered from the same symptoms confirmed. If this lesion cannot be localised, the presumed disease (and the medical status of the person treating it) might be discredited, as has been illustrated in the history of psychiatry by the hopes and disappointments that progressive general paralysis provoked.

However, strictly speaking, pathological anatomy has little to say regarding aetiology. Even when it is possible to find a lesion whose existence produces the symptoms observable in the clinic, nothing can be said about what generated it. As Foucault lucidly pointed out:

> For Bichat and his successors, the notion of seat is freed from the causal problematic (…); it is directed towards the future of the disease rather than to its past; the seat is the point from which the pathological organization radiates. Not the *final cause*, but the *original site*.
>
> (Foucault, 2003, p. 140; italics in original)

Erichsen's approach ran into two significant obstacles: not only the usual "the absence often of evidence of outward and direct physical injury" (Erichsen, 1866, p. 17) but also uncertainty about the cause of a lesion even when it could be localised. Such uncertainty increased even more when there was a considerable time interval between the accident's date and the onset of symptoms.

Perhaps for this reason, Erichsen decided to begin his argument by referring to patients who had developed symptoms after suffering "a severe degree of external violence applied to the vertebral column" (although the organic injury was not obvious) and, from there, attempt to "understand more clearly the phenomena resulting from the slighter form of injury" (Erichsen, 1866, p. 27). At this point, his exposition moved away from the typical demonstration of pathological anatomy, which placed the cadaver on the operating table. His strategy was, instead, rhetorical: if it was believed that a hard blow to the back could cause an injury despite it being difficult to observe, why is it that the same thing could not occur in more trivial situations? For Erichsen, in all cases, the final cause of the symptoms was an accident that injured the body.

At the same time, the surgeon attempted to demonstrate that the resulting illness was not obscure and new but a clinical picture accepted by certain sectors of neurological knowledge at the time: Concussion of the Spine (Erichsen, 1866, p. 27).[11] It was believed that just as a cerebral concussion could cause damage to the brain despite not fracturing bones, the same could occur with the spinal cord, affecting the peripheral nervous system. We will later see how these ideas were strongly challenged by Page. Erichsen recognised that it was "by no means easy to give a clear and comprehensive definition of the term, 'Concussion of the Spine'":

> ...this phrase, that is generally adopted by surgeons to indicate a certain state of the spinal cord occasioned by external violence; a state that is independent of, and usually, but not necessarily, uncomplicated with any obvious lesion of the vertebral column (...) a condition that is supposed to depend upon a shake or jar received by the cord, in consequence of which its organic structure may be more or less deranged, and by which its functions are certainly greatly disturbed (...).
> (Erichsen, 1866, p. 27)

Erichsen's words, plagued with terms that denote imprecision, showed his intention to consecrate a clinical picture whose existence was still in doubt. Nevertheless, diagnosing it this way allowed him to link cases of railway accidents with other cases of spinal concussion, which "occurred between sixty and seventy years before the first railway was opened" in his country (Erichsen, 1866, p. 24).[12]

In the third lecture, he dealt with cases of "concussion of the spine from slight injury" (Erichsen, 1866, p. 43). These were examples in which the blows were either not violent or had fallen upon parts of the body other than the spine, meaning that "the relation between the injury sustained and the symptoms developed -is- less obvious..." (Erichsen, 1866, p. 43). In addition, these cases were characterised by a longer time interval between the occurrence of the accident and the development of the more serious symptoms, making it "no easy matter to connect the two in the relation of cause and effect" (Erichsen, 1866, p. 43). Time and again, the surgeon seemed to expose the point that could be objected to in his arguments but that he simultaneously intended to resolve in his favour. If other experts could interpret that these symptoms "exist only in the imagination of the patient" or that they would respond to certain conditions of the nervous system not dependent on the alleged accident, he aimed to weave the causal link between the latter and the symptoms (Erichsen, 1866, p. 44).

Case 6 well exemplified the typical evolution of many of the examples described by the British doctor, which are characterised by the insidious and progressive development of symptoms (Erichsen, 1866, pp. 49–52). Following a railway collision, in which he was "suddenly dashed forward and then rebounded violently backwards" (Erichsen, 1866, p. 49), the patient believed he was unhurt and felt well. However, on his return home, he was greatly excited and could not sleep. A few days later, he looked anxious and depressed and suffered from violent pains in the head, loud noises in the ears and confusion of thought. As time passed, his memory became affected, and he confused the names of things and people. Three months later, spasmodic contractions of the muscles and more severe back pain appeared, ending with spinal rigidity and lack of sensitivity and spatial recognition in his lower limbs.

Case 8 took to the extreme the idea of the progressive development of the disease and the equivalence between train accidents and those of everyday life (Erichsen, 1866, pp. 53–55). It described a 26-year-old woman whose sensory and motor symptoms were thought to depend on a spinal injury caused by a fall from her cot at the age of 18 months! We conjecture that these extreme cases were necessary for Erichsen's argumentative strategy. If the reader believed it possible that a minor accident occurring at such an early age could produce symptoms insidiously and progressively for years, then it would be easier to admit that a railway accident could generate spinal concussion, even when the accident was mild or when the pathological signs appeared much later. In addition, this case illustrated the type of treatment that many surgeons of that time practised after arriving at the diagnosis of hysteria. Like many other women, this patient had had her clitoris extirpated without experiencing any therapeutic benefits to her condition. Erichsen, however, was opposed to diagnosing these types of cases as hysteria and criticised that form of practice. Nevertheless, he did not cease to be a man of his time. Towards the end of the book, he raised the need for a differential diagnosis between cases of spinal concussion and hysteria. The surgeon found it

> extraordinary (…) that so great an error of diagnosis could so easily be made" by thinking that "a man advanced in life, of energetic business habits (…) in no way subject to gusty fits of emotion (…) has suddenly become 'hysterical', like a love-sick girl?
>
> (Erichsen, 1866, pp. 92–93)

We believe that this quote demonstrates well the doctor's attempts to separate a clinical picture, which he supposed was caused by an anatomical lesion, from a category that did not yet fit in with the medical rationality of the mid-nineteenth century. As we shall see, hysteria was only conceived as an illness common to both sexes and accepted within neurological knowledge a few years later, within the framework of Charcot's lessons.

Continuing with Erichsen's book, the fourth lecture was devoted to the "concussion of the spine from general shock" (Erichsen, 1866, p. 55). Unlike the functional meaning that the term would acquire in the work of Page and some of his contemporaries in the 1880s, here the term *shock* retained a mechanical meaning: it refers to cases "in which the patient has received no blow or injury upon the head or spine, but in which the whole system has received a severe shake or shock..." (Erichsen, 1866, p. 55). From his perspective, this type of incident leads to an even more insidious development of the disease, and it occurs in train accidents and everyday life. In this lecture, *Case 10* is about a man who was involved in a train collision without receiving any blows, but from which he came out "frightened and shaken" (Erichsen, 1866, p. 57). The "fright" will acquire paramount importance in some of the later conceptual configurations of trauma, but here it had no pathogenic value. Only the "shake" could generate the injury and explain the insidious development of the symptoms. As can be seen, his gaze was always focused on a mechanical action exerted on the spinal cord (neither a physiological action in the strict sense nor a psychological one). At the same time, the insistence on the mechanical nature of the accident that generated the injury necessarily supposed, as its correlate, an anatomical body whose functions would only be affected by a lesion generated in the nervous tissue.[13]

The last two lectures were dedicated to recapitulating the general characteristics of the cases he tried to legitimise and inscribe in the logic of the diseases caused by injuries. One of the most notorious features of the cases would be "the disproportion that exists between the apparently trifling accident (...) and the real and serious mischief that has occurred" (Erichsen, 1866, p. 72). But far from putting his certainties in doubt, the surgeon found arguments in this characteristic to validate the existence of an injury. From his perspective, if the person had suffered bone fractures in their limbs, they might not experience nervous lesions, "as if the violence of the shock expended itself in the production of the fracture or dislocation, and that a jar of the more delicate nervous structures is thus avoided" (Erichsen, 1866, p. 73).

Another common feature of these cases was the slow and progressive development of symptoms that could even include periods of symptomatic remission. Regarding this point, Erichsen leaned towards a restrictive statement, almost axiomatic, which he was not willing to discuss. Despite appearances, in these cases, "*there has never been an interval of complete restoration of health.* There have been remissions, but no complete and perfect intermission in the symptoms" (Erichsen, 1866, p. 83; italics in original). Why so much eagerness in asserting that full recovery never existed? Because if he admitted that possibility, the weak link between a minor event and the ulterior symptoms would be further weakened. If the patient only developed a few pathological signs, to later heal and get sick again, nothing would prevent us from thinking that the second pathological period would respond to causes other than the accident. That is why he affirmed that "it is by this chain of symptoms, which, though fluctuating in intensity, is yet continuous and unbroken, that the injury sustained, and the illness subsequently developed, can be linked together in the relation of cause and effect" (Erichsen, 1866, p. 84).

After considering that he had succeeded in proving the hypothesis that the first and efficient cause of the illness would reside in the accident, Erichsen inquired into "the pathological conditions (…) that are the direct causes" or the mechanism of formation "of these phenomena" (Erichsen, 1866, p. 84).[14] For him, the cases of concussion of the spine resulting from direct and violent blows upon the back find their pathological condition in an injury to the spinal cord caused by the extravasation of blood within the spinal canal, or by the rupture, inflammation, or softening of the cord itself. In the cases of shock or sprain, the symptoms depend on a "less directly obvious character than those above mentioned. They *doubtless* consist mainly of chronic and subacute inflammatory action in the spinal membranes, and in chronic myelitis, with those changes in the structure of the cord", as demonstrated by "the *only case*" described from post-mortem examination (Erichsen, 1866, p. 84; italics added). As can be seen, the scarcity of autopsies and evidence contrasted with the robustness of the certainties with which he argued that the pathological mechanism depended on an injury.

Therefore, we disagree with Harrington, who argued that Erichsen's attitude was "ambiguous" and that, given the lack of evidence of injury in the majority of cases, the surgeon was forced to "distinguish 'mental' or 'emotional' shock from 'physical' shock and to accept, if only implicitly, the causative role of the former in provoking the disorders associated with railway spine" (Harrington, 2001, p. 44).[15] If one thing is clear after a careful reading of the book, it is that the British doctor believed in the existence of an injury even though there was no convincing evidence to prove it. The entire text was oriented towards weaving causal links between the accident, the injury and the symptoms. In this framework, the fear or the emotional disturbances resulting from a train accident could only take on two roles: either that of the description of a superfluous detail of the subjective experience of the accident or that of a secondary consequence of the anatomical affection generated by the mechanical action of the collision. The influence of pathological anatomy as a framework for interpreting experience was so great in Erichsen's work that it did not allow the consideration of the morbid impact of other factors, such as those that we would now call psychological. Strictly speaking, there is no hint of psychologisation here: the trauma was still considered a mechanical action against an anatomical body. The only novelty introduced by Erichsen was the establishment of a new problematic zone, in which the cases did not so easily fit into the category of frank simulation or into the category of traditional illnesses caused by injuries.

Because of the preceding, it could be affirmed that in Erichsen's work, pathological anatomy did not function as a systematic practice of articulation between what was perceived in the cadavers and the clinic. Instead, it operated as a *model* that determined the field of the thinkable and the visible. What Erichsen could or could not perceive did not depend on a supposed personal blindness but on the framework of thought from which he approached experience, which made him "see" lesions even when the cadavers did not bear them.

For this surgeon, an event (in itself, or better yet, due to its mechanical and objective characteristics) could cause such alterations in a body that would absolutely determine the future illness. In this conception, the person was seen as a completely passive victim in the face of an event that was wholly external and decisive. In other words, the victim's subjective particularities would not play any role in the genesis of the illnesses: neither their past traits (some type of antecedent or predisposition) nor their current attitudes (for example, the subjective position adopted during or after the accident) would have a minor effect on the result. The totality of their suffering was determined by an objective and current experience, which was lived passively.

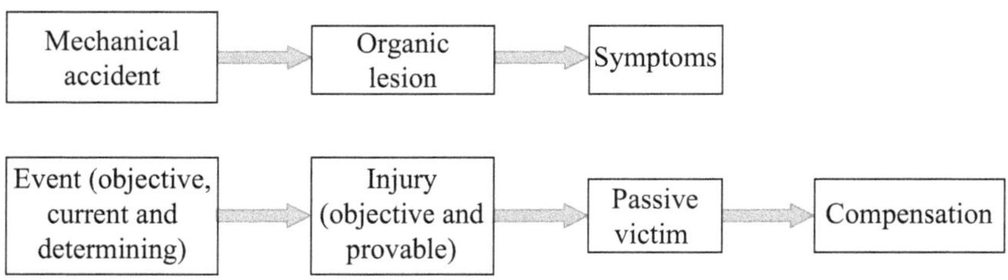

Therefore, it is not surprising that in his famous book, the section dedicated to possible treatments took up only three pages, nor is it surprising that the surgeon recognised that he did not have "much to say (...) about the treatment of these injuries" beyond suggesting the importance of rest (Erichsen, 1866, p. 100). In contrast, after presenting each case of railway accidents, and after demonstrating the realness of their illness, the monetary sum that was awarded to the injured person in the judicial process appeared. Faced with a totally external and determining event that impacted a completely passive victim, the only possible treatment seemed to be compensation for the damages suffered.

As we will see below, the clinical picture of spinal concussion was called into question a few years later. It was accused of containing inaccuracies and of leaving many phenomena unexplained. Nevertheless, this configuration, which linked a contingent event with a victim's suffering in a relationship of linear causality, did not disappear. Rather, it lives on today in many contemporary conceptions of trauma.

1.4 When the Injury Was Not a Sufficient Explanation

Despite the acceptance that Erichsen's ideas had for two decades, it did not take long for different hypotheses to emerge. Although these admitted that mechanical shock could cause damage to the spinal cord, such as the British doctor suggested, they emphasised more and more the role that emotions could play in the development of later disturbances. Such is the case of Le Gros Clark, who, between 1868 and 1869, published a series of lectures in the British Medical Journal, which were released as a book one year later. This surgeon considered that many of the symptoms arising after a railway collision

> may be referred to what we are accustomed to regard as concussion of the spine, but many also are due to general rather than special nervous shock (…) I am, therefore, disposed to regard these cases of so-called railway spinal concussion as, generally, instances of universal nervous shock, rather than of special injury to the spinal cord.
>
> (Le Gros Clark, 1870, pp. 151–152)

The illness continued to affect the nervous system. However, two things were beginning to change. On the one hand, to the possibility of damage to the cord (which was searched for and supposedly confirmed in numerous cases and autopsies), a disorder in the nervous system as a whole was added, whose nature and location were not made explicit. The most immediate symptoms seemed to depend more on the first factor; the later ones on the second. On the other hand, this disorder was not generated by a mechanical action but by "emotional shock" (Le Gros Clark, 1870, pp. 151–152).[16]

In any case, this did not mean that the illness and the trauma were considered disturbances of a psychical nature. The emotions generated in a railway accident (fear, fright, terror, helplessness) altered the normal functioning of the nervous system in conjunction with the spinal injury, which continued to be sought for. It was more about considering another dimension of the experience than questioning the nervous and anatomical nature of the illness. Furthermore, in these texts, emotions did not belong to an independent psychical sphere but were considered functions of the nervous system. Nevertheless, although some authors continued to cling to the guidelines of pathological anatomy, a new epistemic framework gradually emerged from which to approach these phenomena.

What appeared in the works of Le Gros Clark and other physicians, such as J. Jordan or R. Hodges, as a complement to the anatomical point of view (Caplan, 2001, p. 61; Harrington, 2001, p. 49), became independent and consolidated with Herbert Page's book entitled *Injuries of the Spine and Spinal Cord without Apparent Mechanical Lesions, and Nervous Shock, in their surgical and Medico-Legal aspects* (Page, 1883). While Erichsen worked as a medical expert in cases of accident victims, Page worked as a surgeon at the London and Western Railway Companies. He was also respected outside the field of expertise, receiving the Boylston Medical Prize from Harvard University in 1881 for a preliminary version of the book published in 1883.[17]

Unlike many of his colleagues who worked for railway companies, Page did not consider simulation the only alternative to the allegedly real and lesional nature of post-train accident symptoms. Instead, this doctor attempted to construct an alternative explanation for both options. He considered these disturbances true and of a nervous nature, although no longer dependent on anatomical damage to the spine. That is why the title of the book is somewhat misleading. In his view, in the field of railway disasters, a conjunction between injuries of the spine and nervous shock did not exist. Instead, these two options constituted an exclusive disjunction:

either the injured victims suffered spinal damage, as Erichsen proposed, or their illness depended on a nervous shock without injury. Moreover, throughout the entire book, he attempts to prove that the first proposition is not true.

To further his purpose, Page first took it upon himself to analyse in detail the diagnosis of spinal concussion (Chapter 1) and Erichsen's use of this category (Chapter 2). He insistently tried to point out the imprecision of the term in medical writings, as well as the hastiness with which the ambiguous aspects of many clinical observations and autopsies were considered evidence of direct damage to the spinal cord, when from his point of view they must be interpreted in another manner.[18] Furthermore, the relevance of the nosographic category of spinal concussion depended on the validity of its analogy to cerebral concussion. From the perspective of this neurologist, a simple shake of the cerebral mass could generate a transient symptom (the momentary loss of consciousness) without it implying bone or vascular damage (Page, 1883, pp. 21–28). In contrast, it would not be possible for direct damage to the spinal cord to produce some kind of transient symptom equivalent to unconsciousness (for example, rapidly remitting paralysis). Pathological signs associated with the cord would arise only as a consequence of an external injury to it, in the spine or the vascular system, and in those cases, the symptoms would never be transient. To substantiate his claims, Page resorted to anatomical arguments: the bones and ligaments surrounding the spinal cord would constitute much stronger protection than those containing the brain mass (Page, 1883, pp. 29, 49). For this reason, it would be impossible to generate a spinal injury directly from a blow, jolt or twist, and it seems "highly improbable that it -the spinal canal- should be especially liable to suffer injury in any single kind of accident such as railway collisions" (Page, 1883, p. 50).

When specifically addressing Erichsen's book, he again criticised the breadth and imprecision of the term spinal concussion. Erichsen, in his book, applied the term to mild and fatal cases with immediate and insidious symptom development, which produced effects on parts of the body associated with the peripheral nervous system as well as psychical pathological signs linked to the brain. In addition, Page stopped to analyse in detail many of the patients presented in that vital text. From this, he pointed out the outdated nature of the methodology used in the autopsies, the lack of conclusive evidence on the injury, and the incompatibility of certain symptoms with a spinal injury. In particular, he was interested in separating

> those symptoms which we must have recognised are much *more cerebral or psychical*,[19] from those which can only find an explanation in some actual lesion of the spinal cord or of the nerves which are given off from them.
>
> (Page, 1883, p. 83; italics added)

As he himself acknowledges, one of the objectives of his work was to demonstrate that in the majority of cases of railway accidents, the spinal cord would remain unharmed without thereby being able to doubt the honesty of those who claimed to be ill (Page, 1883, p. 90). The disturbance would lie in another ("cerebral or psychical") sphere, to which he devoted the rest of the book. In this way, Page was disposed to "regard these cases of so-called railway spinal concussion as, *generally, instances of universal nervous shock, rather than of special injury to the spinal cord*" (Page, 1883, p. 101; italics in original).

1.5 From the Anatomical Lesion to General Nervous Shock: The Functional Disturbance

"General nervous shock" was a term whose

> lack of precision -according to his own words- appears suitable to describe the class of cases -in which- (…) the course, history, and general symptoms indicate some *functional disturbance* of the whole nervous balance or tone rather than *structural damage* to any organ of the body.
>
> (Page, 1883, p. 143; italics added)

This passage indicates a complete change of position, not only because the doctor was putting forward an alternative interpretation of railway accidents but also because he was beginning to adopt a new *conceptual framework* from which to approach them.

As we have seen, pathological anatomy only recognises as medically legitimate those illnesses based on a localisable lesion in the organism. In order to be able to conceive a merely functional disturbance and, at the same time, for it to be considered true by medical knowledge, it was necessary to resort to another *framework*: that of *experimental physiology*, which had been gaining ground since the mid-nineteenth century in France, Germany and England.

Traditionally, physiology had been nothing more than an *anatomia animata.* As a discipline, it was subordinated to the latter (Barona, 1991, p. 40). For this reason, the vital functions were only studied in reference to the structure. "The body was a static hierarchy of organs, each with its characteristic function" (Danziger, 1990, p. 25). Later, the systematisation of experimental practice in physiology allowed for not only the independence of this branch of knowledge from anatomy but also the possibility of constituting vital functions as "abstract objects of investigation that might involve several organs as well as invisible processes" (Danziger, 1990, p. 25). From this perspective, an illness could develop from processes that would not leave any type of visible mark on the organism other than the alteration of the function.

The way in which Page adhered to the functional perspective did not, however, imply the beginning of an experimental research practice. Physiology acted for him as a conceptual matrix that made conceivable, on the one hand, a purely functional illness and, on the other hand, a body as a conglomerate of functions (rather than a static hierarchy of organs).[20]

At the same time, his book illustrated a semantic shift in the terms common to the medical studies of these illnesses. In Erichsen's text, the word shock referred to a mechanical impact on the organism that, although not always implying a direct blow to the back, would affect the structure of the spinal cord. In Page's book, the anatomical reference did not seem to disappear altogether when he stated that "We are all familiar with the term 'shock' as synonymous with the 'collapse' which is a concomitant of all profound and sudden injuries, whether inflicted upon the head or upon some other part of the body" (Page, 1883, p. 143). However, just a few pages later, we learn that:

> (…) fright may of itself conduce to the condition recognised as shock (…) And medical literature abounds with cases where the gravest disturbances of function, and even death or the annihilation of function, have been produced by fright and by fright alone (…) The suddenness of the accident, which comes without warning, or with a warning which only reveals the utter helplessness of the traveller, the loud noise, the hopeless confusion, the cries of those who are injured; these in themselves, and more especially if they occur at night or in the dark, are surely adequate to produce a profound impression upon the nervous system.
>
> (Page, 1883, p. 147)

As can be seen, these ideas admit more psychological terms than those of Erichsen but, nevertheless, do not constitute a complete psychologisation. Neither the fright nor the other characteristics of the scene of the accident disturbed an ontologically or methodologically independent psyche but instead produced "a profound impression upon the nervous system" (Page, 1883, p. 147). The intensity of the emotion experienced by the subject operates, in any case, in an analogous way to an electrical current applied to the living substance. Using experiences with electricity as a model, it became conceivable that elements such as affects could modify the functioning of the nerves even if they did not damage their structure.

Understood in this way, the conception outlined by Page was completely compatible with the physiological knowledge of the turn of the century. For this reason, it could include psychology as a dimension that accounts for the highest functions of the nervous system. At best, it can only be said a posteriori that the inclusion of psychological terms in these physiological texts laid the groundwork for a purely psychical explanation of trauma to be thinkable at some point… but not yet. Therefore, we cannot agree with Harrington when he states that Page constructed "a new psychological model of post-traumatic nervous disruption" (Harrington, 2001, p. 51). We prefer to say that he constructed a new *physiological* schema of the nervous disturbance that emotion could generate in a traumatic situation.

In this schema, introducing the element of fright made it possible to relativise the importance given to the mechanical action in the previous conceptual configuration.

For Page, it would not be the accident itself but the emotion generated by it that caused the symptoms (or rather, that aroused the mechanisms that produce the latter).

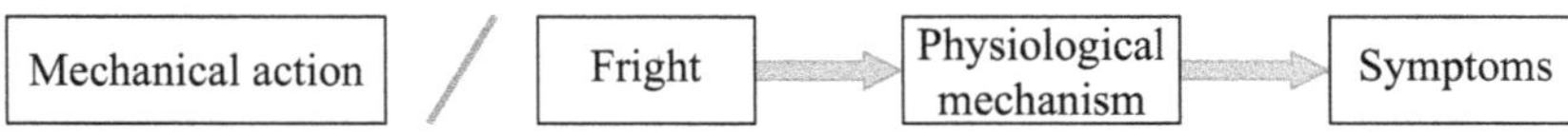

By introducing this affective dimension between the accident and the pathogenic processes, an element was added that seemed to depend both on the objective conditions of the experience and on the subjective particularities of the person who fell ill. It is true that many people could experience fright from a railway collision, but not all of them did so with such intensity that it could generate illness. If an accident acted by its mechanical force, the degree of violence of the blow received and the affected part of the body could be enough to explain why some people remained healthy while others fell ill, without the need to consider the personal attributes of each one. The same did not occur in the conceptual configuration outlined by Page since the (pathogenic or innocuous) incidence of "alarm (…) must be measured" by two factors: "the events of the accident itself", that is, by its intrinsic and current characteristics, "and by the temperament of the individual who has been affected", that is, by a subjective element which was present prior to the experience (Page, 1883, p. 149). In this way, the doctor introduced an element of *predisposition* absent in Erichsen's thinking. The temperament of the individual functioned as a zero point: it did not cause the illness, since the latter required the accident (and the fear generated by it) for the pathological mechanism to function, but it did generate its conditions of possibility.

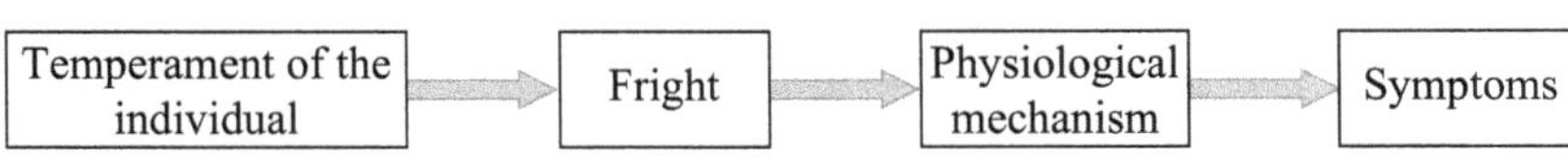

In Chapter 5 of the book, which was presented as a continuation of the theme of general nervous shock, two other elements appeared on the scene that also did not have a place in Erichsen's conception but that we will find again when dealing with Charcot's ideas about trauma. First, the comparison of the state of nervous shock (in both sexes) with *hysteria*. Almost simultaneously with (or even before) the attempt to legitimise male hysteria carried out by the French clinician, Page began to bring the symptomatic effects of railway accidents closer to hysterical disturbances, regardless of the gender of the sufferer. Some sentences illustrate this moment of transition, thanks to which hysteria ceased to be a feminine and gynaecological disease, and trauma ceased to be thought of solely in mechanical and anatomical terms.

> For even if in every-day life women more commonly than men show signs of being emotional, excitable, and hysterical, it is nevertheless true that, as a direct outcome of the nervous shock of a railway collision, men become no less emotional and hysterical than they.
>
> (Page, 1883, p. 172)

This meaning of "hysteria" was relatively lax and seemed like a pseudo-scientific synonym for the layman's term "nervous". However, the author tried to give it a more precise meaning, allowing us to elucidate better his conception of the neurological mechanism at play in these illnesses.

> The "hysterical" condition (…) is essentially one in which there is loss of control and enfeeblement of the power of the will (…) there is loss of the habitual power to suppress and keep in due subjection the sensations which are doubtless associated with the various functions of the organic life of the individual.
>
> (Page, 1883, p. 175)

As was common to medical thought at the time, Page's physiological schema of the role of emotions in the nervous system also included evolutionist ideas about the development of nervous functions.

> In the process of evolution towards a higher state of intellectual activity (…) man (…) has become more and more unconscious of the sensations which of necessity accompany the functional activity of the various organs and structures of his body.
>
> (Page, 1883, p. 175)

Without citing him explicitly, the ideas of Jackson, the founder of clinical neurology, functioned here as an explanatory conceptual framework. Pathology proceeded in the opposite direction to evolution. The emotion generated by the accident was thought to inhibit the higher functions of the nervous system and produce the irruption of a more reflexive and emotional (more automatic and unconscious) functioning.

The second of the two elements common to the thoughts of Page and Charcot was the comparison of the pathological mechanism with hypnosis. According to historian Eric Caplan,

> In suggesting that something akin to a hypnotic state explained not only the persistence of (…) symptoms but also their disappearance (…), Page had provided one of the first exclusively psychological explanations for both the cause and the cure of trauma-engendred symptoms.
>
> (Caplan, 2001, p. 62)

We cannot agree with this affirmation, since it denies the progressive and heterogeneous development of the psychologisation of trauma. It also anticipates events that would only take place a few years later. A psychological explanation of the causes of these pathologies, the functioning of hypnosis, and the constitution of a purely psychical treatment could only be found in the works of Janet and Freud at the beginning of the following decade. Instead, both Page and Charcot explained shock, hysteria and hypnosis in neurophysiological terms, even as they began to include more and more psychological notions in their vocabulary.[21] In the words of the British physician, "the primary seat of functional disturbance" of these clinical pictures "lies in the brain itself" (and not in a psyche that could be approached independently of its organic substratum); in turn, both in shock and "in the hypnotic state induced by a profound mental impression, there is a temporary arrest in the function of that part of the sensorium which presides over and controls the movements and sensations of the periphery" (Page, 1883, p. 189). Definitively, Page intended to inscribe his ideas in a field of neurology capable of conceiving antagonistic functions that had to find a balance (Page, 1883, p. 190).

In short, in a railway accident or any other traumatic situation, an emotion such as fear seemed capable of generating a disturbance in the higher functions of the nervous system (at least in predisposed people). Through this physiological pathway, the intense emotion would allow nervous automatisms to erupt in the form of pathological symptoms.

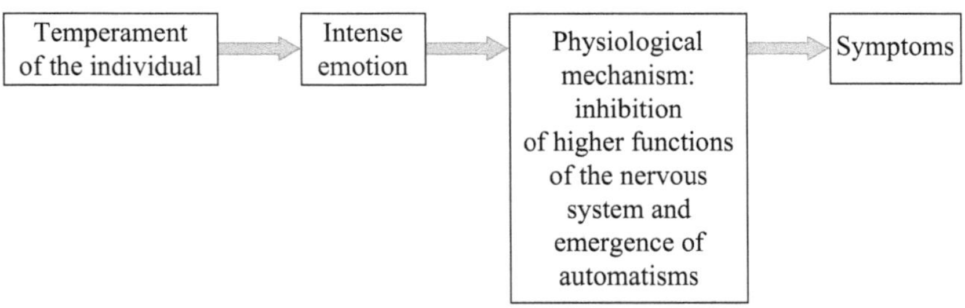

To conclude with the presentation of Page's ideas, we would like to point out the reference that this doctor made to Paget's (1875) concept of "neuromimesis". This notion attempted to explain how the symptoms could "mimic those which are due to undoubted pathological change" (Page, 1883, p. 194). In such cases, it would not be the person but the illness affecting them that "simulated" the organic disease, so it was not possible to question the patient's good faith or find any anatomical lesion in them. For Paget, "the worst cases of nervous mimicry occur in members of families in which mental insanity has been frequent" (Page, 1883, pp. 196–197). Page also admitted that in such severe cases, it was possible to

> find some evidence, either of mental disorder in the previous history of the patient himself, or that he comes of a stock in which mental or emotional disturbances and peculiarities (…) have been recognised as prominent in the family record.
> (Page, 1883, p. 197)

However, in those cases in which a predisposition of this kind did not exist, Page believed he could find in the shock caused by the accident an "adequate cause" for the appearance of these nervous disturbances (Page, 1883, p. 197).

In these lines, a conceptual configuration of trauma was delineated in which a current element (the intensity of the accident) and a past element (the severity of the predisposition) jointly participated in the production of the illness. In each particular case, the importance attributed to either element would vary. Thus, the trauma was located between the recent event and the past history. In any case, the *image* of the traumatised subject continued to be that of a passive victim: either determined as such by the accident or tied to a history for which their lineage would be held responsible. Unlike what Erichsen stated, here, the individual's particularities counted, but much more because of the burden of family predisposition than because of the subjective position adopted by the individual.

The only instance of the factor mentioned above of subjective position coming into play was circumscribed around the expectation of receiving a future pecuniary compensation that, according to Page, "in addition to the worries and anxieties of litigation and dispute", could operate as a "very potent cause for continuance of the symptoms" (1883, p. 182). With these words, a narrow margin of responsibility seemed to open up for the traumatised individual, which would also suppose a very slight possibility of doing something so that the effects of trauma would not be so serious. In this way, Page's conception tied together the past personal and family history, the present of the accident and the expectation of future compensation. All three temporal dimensions seemed to work together in shaping the trauma and developing an illness.

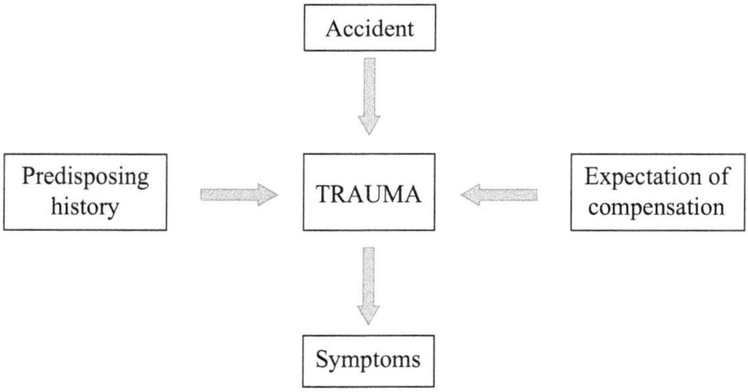

Undoubtedly, the hypothesis about the pathological impact of the individual's interest in obtaining financial reparation (or any other type of benefit for the damage suffered) introduced a heterogeneous element with respect to the rest of the conceptual framework. This idea did not follow on from a physiological model analogous to experiences with electricity nor from a model of evolutionary neurology such as the one established by Jackson; it did not fit as well into a nervous functional schema as an emotion such as fear did. Instead, it could be considered an important shift in the processes of psychologisation, even though Page did not develop it in depth, nor did he make these individual intentions a key concept in his thinking. What is certain is that this hypothesis can lead to a moral consideration of the victim: no longer being merely a passive victim but now actively interested in obtaining benefits. This moral interpretation of the compensation expectations, plus the reference to a hereditary predisposition, could tip the scales of the litigations in the opposite direction to that which Erichsen indicated.

Perhaps for this reason, Page's texts were published in the United States and were widely distributed among the members of the "National Association of Railway Surgeons" (Caplan, 2001, p. 69). This association was created in 1888 to unify the doctors who worked for railway companies and acted as experts in the litigations that these companies had to face. After years of Erichsen's ideas influencing North American courts, which tilted judgments in favour of plaintiffs, the NARS set itself a goal to "provide its members with information and material that they could employ when testifying" in order to defend the interests of the companies for which they work (Caplan, 2001, p. 69). If the simple accusation of malicious simulation ended up being inverted and transformed into accusations of the partiality of these railway professionals (Caplan, 2001, p. 70), the affirmation of the "psychical nature of railway spine" seemed more likely to twist public opinion and the outcome of the litigation (Caplan, 2001, p. 71). Therefore, the physicians stopped accusing the victims of malingery: now only trying to prove that they suffered from a psychical disorder, much milder and much more *curable* than was supposed when they were diagnosed as cases of concussion of the spine. In this way, the railway companies could avoid paying costly compensations while the physicians preserved their professional integrity by offering psychotherapeutic treatment to the victims (Caplan, 2001, pp. 72–73). Caplan's analysis is very lucid on this point:

> One of the great ironies in the development of psychotherapy in the United States concerns this vital role played by economically and culturally conservative railway surgeons. It was these surgeons – not liberal psychiatrists or even progressive neurologists – who were the leading exemplars not only of a revised psychogenic paradigm but of a crude form of psychotherapy itself.
>
> (Caplan, 2001, p. 73)

Caplan exemplified his argument with a railway surgeon from Iowa, J.H. Greene, who would have been "one of the earliest American physicians to recognize the role of so-called suggestion in fomenting traumatic neuroses" and to cite the works of Charcot and Bernheim on the topic (Caplan, 2001, p. 73). We will deal with these authors in the following sections.

1.6 Trauma and Hysteria at the Salpêtrière

In the lectures during 1885 at the Salpêtrière, Charcot never tired of repeating that certain accident patients that were difficult to diagnose could not only be comparable to but *were* cases of hysteria. Such an affirmation was carried out within the context of his endeavour that sought to turn this old category of dubious prestige into a genuine neurological disease. Until then, hysteria was characterised by its symptomatic irregularity and connection with simulation, femininity and sexuality (Foucault, 2006, p. 354). The French master aimed to separate the notion from these four features that made it difficult to include it in the medical rationality of the end of the nineteenth century. Furthermore, he found in traumatised men a propitious terrain to carry out his objective: to convert hysteria into a neurological disease whose veracity was not in doubt, which was common to both sexes and had regular and characteristic signs. At the same time, his clinical work focused on semiology and differential diagnosis, as well as some of his hypotheses about the mechanism of hysterical symptoms, pushed the notion of trauma to the frontiers of psychology, probably more than his contemporaries' ideas ever had.

To understand these transformations, we believe it is convenient to remember that Charcot's first conceptions of trauma were far from the psychological field. Having managed to obtain the position of doctor at the Salpêtrière in 1862, he attempted to turn that site into a place of training and research. In this context, he quickly started giving public lectures focused on clinical work and on pathological anatomy, which would only be recognised by the University of Paris in 1882, the year in which the "Clinical Chair of Diseases of the Nervous System" was created (Edelman, 2003, p. 138; Gauchet & Swain, 2000, p. 22).

One of the first classes devoted to investigating the influence of trauma in the development of hysteria began with a reference to

> certain diseases, which are pathologically dependent on a diathesis, are sometimes developed at the instance of a traumatic lesion. It is usual for these diseases to localise themselves at first in parts where the wound, the contusion, or the sprain is produced. It is so in articular rheumatism for example, and in gout.
> (Charcot, 1892, pp. 32–33)

Immediately, Charcot affirmed that "certain local phenomena of hysteria (…) manifest themselves sometimes in the same way…" (Charcot, 1892, p. 33). In that class (from December 1877), hysteria was considered similar to certain bodily illnesses and understood from a point of view that reflected medical thought before the discoveries of pathological anatomy. The old notion of diathesis seemed doomed to remain in the medical history books. However, it was revived by Charcot and some of his colleagues to resolve specific issues that anatomy could not explain. As Gladys Swain states, diathesis is "the opposite of a localised lesion; it is a kind of terrain, of general disposition to disease that has to do with 'constitution' or heredity" (Gauchet & Swain, 2000, p. 84). Faced with the absence of visible material damage, Charcot, following his predecessor Brodie and his contemporary Verneuil, allowed himself to assume that a mechanical action (the physical trauma), even if *slight* in nature, could unleash a latent predisposition, even when no trace of injury could be found in the organism (Charcot, 1892, pp. 449–451).

We would like to underline two points. First is the reference to the trauma's characteristic of being of a *slight* nature. We have seen that, in Erichsen's book, the attention was not centred on the most spectacular (and obvious) cases of strong blows and localised injuries but on those in which an apparently *harmless* action produced material damage to the spinal cord. According to Page, most of the alleged cases of railway spine were not those of serious physical trauma but those that could generate intense fear, even if they were *mild* in their mechanical nature. In this passage from Charcot's work, the focus once again shifted away from serious trauma. Contrary to certain forms of common knowledge, very widespread today, which associate traumatic experiences with events of spectacular dimensions, the notion of trauma seems to have been greater developed, transformed and problematised as a result of experiences whose consequences were more serious than (and that developed much later than) the event that generated them.

Second, in that class, a schema of hysteria was already plotted out, one that the French master would never abandon. According to this schema, which was based on the old model of diathesis, the trauma would not be the ultimate cause of the illness but, rather, an *agent provocateur*, which could only produce effects in predisposed individuals.

However, his ambition to adapt the study of hysteria to certain characteristics of the framework of pathological anatomy was still present; initially, since the locationist dimension was never wholly abandoned. Trauma could generate both a local symptom in the same area affected by the blow (for example, a localised disturbance of movement or sensation) as well as a general disturbance radiating from that site (as occurred when a hysterical attack was produced from the excitation of a "hysterogenic zone"). In both cases, the trauma itself continued to be a mechanical process (such as a blow or pressure) located in a precise place in the organism, even though the marks it left could only be read through its symptomatic effects and not through a material injury. If, as Swain stated, "diathesis is a kind of non-localisable lesion" (Gauchet & Swain, 2000, p. 84), the trauma would be a kind of localised action without a lesion.

Five years later, in the inaugural class of the Clinical Chair of Diseases of the Nervous System, Charcot's yearning to place hysteria and all illnesses of the nervous system under the umbrella of pathological anatomy was still evident. Despite this, he could not fail to recognise the existence of morbid states in the nervous system, such as epilepsy, chorea and hysteria, which "leave in the dead body no material trace that can be discovered" (Charcot, 1889, p. 12). It could therefore be believed that these pathologies could not be approached from the same clinical and pathological anatomic prism with which other diseases were approached. This was clearly not Charcot's stance. Pathological anatomy still offered him the matrix from which to think about these neuroses and delineate their pathological mechanism, thus implying that he still subordinated the functional alterations to a localisation of the maladies.

Charcot's reasoning began with the clinical and semiological data and hoped to reach a hypothesis about the mechanism. In 1882, he still maintained that the symptomatology of these clinical pictures "approaches, (...) to that which belongs to maladies having organic lesions" (Charcot, 1889, p. 14). If the pathological phenomena were the same, then he thought it logical also to equate the mechanisms.

> [...] besides the similarity in the group of symptoms, [the pathologist] perceives a similarity in the anatomical seat, and *mutatis mutandis*, localises the dynamic lesion from the data furnished by an examination of the corresponding organic one.
> (Charcot, 1889, p. 14).

This *dynamic* or *functional lesion* operated as a poorly formed hybrid between an anatomy with a locationist orientation and a physiology concerned with functioning. Unlike Erichsen, who needed to assume that the lesion existed materially even if it was not visible, Charcot admitted that the substrate might not be disturbed even when a specific area was affected in its functional capacity. Unlike Page, for whom the nervous shock was not spinal but cerebral, but also non-specific in its location, Charcot assumed that the disturbance could be located in a specific region of the nervous system, as occurred in diseases due to injury.

It was only during the classes of 1885, entirely devoted to traumatic hysteria, that this anatomical matrix began to relinquish its hegemony, allowing the development of new hypotheses about trauma and the pathological mechanism of hysteria. These hypotheses were full of new "psychological" terms, even though the author continued to maintain a strong monist and materialist position (Gauchet & Swain, 2000, p. 87). To understand this shift, it is necessary to focus on the increasingly systematic use of hypnosis and suggestion within the Salpêtrière.

1.7 Hypnosis as a Research Technique and as a Thought Model

The use and research of the effects of certain metals and electricity in the Salpêtrière began in 1876 (Gauchet & Swain, 2000, pp. 86–94, 103–117), within the context of the efforts to inscribe these phenomena in a scientific, materialistic and neurological framework. Hypnosis appeared on the scene two years later, linked to a double expectation. On the one hand, it seemed to favour the explanation of these strange phenomena as physiological anomalies typical of hysteria or other neuroses (Edelman, 2003, p. 181; Gauchet & Swain, 2000, pp. 125, 129). Hypnotism would consist of a series of pathological and momentary disturbances of consciousness and will, which could be induced by different means or occur spontaneously, but only in nervous patients. While this abnormal state lasted, the body's physiological state would be modified, and the possibility of suggesting the hypnotised individual would increase. If the alteration of consciousness took the form of catalepsy, the body would remain immobile and be able to sustain the postures that the hypnotist imprinted on it. In the case of lethargy, the muscles would be put in a state of hyperexcitability from which contractures could be induced. Finally, in the case of somnambulism, the state of hyperexcitability would persist, but the possibility of carrying out the orders suggested by the hypnotist was introduced (Gauchet & Swain, 2000, p. 127).

On the other hand, this suspension of consciousness and will and the increased capacity to be suggested were at the base of the second great expectation placed on hypnosis. If during these physiological states, the patient was transformed into a kind of automaton in the hands of the hypnotist, then the use of the technique would open up the possibility of artificially reproducing not only the clouding of consciousness but also typically hysterical pathological phenomena (Carroy, 1991, pp. 2–3, 6; Gauchet & Swain, 2000, p. 126). Contractures, paralysis, blindness and even other disorders belonging to the higher spheres of the nervous system could be studied through an instrument that would bring the investigation closer to the conditions of variable control typical of an experiment. This method would also allow the study of these pathological phenomena without resorting to animal vivisections or autopsies on corpses.

As is known, the Parisian's hopes soon collided with Nancy's criticism (Carroy, 1991, pp. 6–9; Edelman, 2003, pp. 196–197). For this school, hypnotism was not a particular pathological state but an extreme degree of a property common to all human beings: suggestibility. The influence that one human being could exert over another could, on occasion, reach the point of total submission without it being necessary to see this as an anomalous physiological process since, according to Bernheim, anyone could potentially be hypnotised *thanks to* suggestion. Hypnosis, therefore, would be only one of the poles of the gradient of a broader cultural fact, that is, of suggestion, defined as "the influence caused by an idea suggested and accepted by the brain" (Bernheim, 1884, p. 73).

This interpretation not only supposed the subordination of hypnotic phenomena to suggestive activity but also an alteration of the order in which both elements were put into practice in the Salpêtrière's investigations. For the Parisian school, hypnotic states were not induced by suggestion but by different physical elements (such as a shiny object, a tuning fork or a magnet) or by the doctor's gaze and voice (which Charcot regarded as natural objects). They did not interpret that the relationship of the hypnotised person with the hypnotiser intervened in any way (Edelman, 2003, p. 194; Gauchet & Swain, 2000, p. 132). Suggestion only came about in a second moment, *after* reaching the hypnotic state or some other disposition of consciousness that facilitated the suggestive effect. In addition, the suggestion could be verbal; in this case, it basically consisted of a command the hypnotist gave. However, it could also exclude words and be limited to a gesture. Such was the case when the patient was placed in a certain position or when a blow was applied that "suggested" an affection in that specific part of the body (Edelman, 2003, pp. 194–195).

We are interested in underlining these characteristics of how the Parisian clinician conceived the hypnotic procedure and the mechanism of its action. By doing so, as we delve into the lectures of 1885, we will be able to verify that this schema, in which hypnosis precedes suggestion, will serve as a *model* to think differently about the process of formation of hysterical symptoms and about trauma.

1.8 The Role of Ideas

In the school year of 1885, the lectures began with the presentation of six cases of male hysteria. From the beginning, Charcot was wholly determined to put an end to the exclusive link of this illness with the female sex and to demonstrate "the identity of this great neurosis in the two sexes" (Charcot, 1889, p. 220), not only with respect to "young effeminate" men but also in relation to the "vigorous artisan" and the "stoker of an engine", who after an accident could "become hysterical for the same reason as a woman" (Charcot, 1889, p. xxiii).

Traumatised subjects became the royal road to achieving a greater de-feminisation and neurologisation of hysteria.[22] They were also used to reinterpret the controversial cases of railway spine as cases of hysteria.[23] The structure of the presentations of the patients was characterised by including at the beginning of each case a reference to the family history, which always made it possible to find a father with "nervous attacks" or "alcoholism", brothers with "nervous ailments" (Charcot, 1889, p. 227), a "dissipated" grandfather "of a very violent character", a mother with "hysterical attacks" (Charcot, 1889, p. 245) or with "rheumatism" (Charcot, 1889, p. 252), etc. In other words, there was never a lack of signs to confirm the presence of similar or dissimilar heredity in the family history. This hereditary factor was considered to generate the *predisposition* to acquire a nervous disease and explain the triggering of the symptoms from the accident or another provoking agent (poisoning, organic disease, etc.)

Afterwards, he would commonly begin with a description of the symptoms and the development of the current illness. Case I is that of a "big (…), strong and well developed" cooper (Charcot, 1889, p. 227), who in 1882 suffered a cut on his left hand after the cord that held the barrel of wine he was transporting broke. At that moment, he feared for his life. However, he immediately thought that he was not seriously injured (a characteristic that will be repeated in most of the cases) and was able to go and wash the wound. Five minutes later, he had a loss of consciousness (another trait common to many presentations) that lasted 20 minutes. As the days went by, various symptoms appeared successively: weakness in the legs, nightmares about the accident, hystero-epileptic attacks, visions and hallucinations, hemianaesthesia, and a retraction of the field of vision (Charcot, 1889, pp. 227–230).

When explaining the case, Charcot wonders if the trauma (that is, the wound on the finger) was enough to generate a nervous disturb (Charcot, 1889, p. 231). The negative answer to this question paved the way for considering the role of a *psychical* element: the *fright* caused by the accident (Charcot, 1889, p. 231). This reference to fright forces us to make three comments.

First, it becomes necessary to discuss Ian Hacking's position, who argued that in Charcot's male cases, the trauma was still considered a physical event (Hacking,

1995, p. 188). This affirmation seems to ignore the shift that displaced the traumatic element from the mechanical action to the emotion (and, as we shall see, to the ideas) that would arise during the experience.

Second, the class given by the doctor of the Salpêtrière should not be seen as the first time in France that fright or other emotions were given a role in the genesis of disturbances and illnesses. Rather, there were two traditions, distant from modern neurological research, which had already postulated the importance of affective elements. On the one hand, a tradition of political philosophy linked to the Revolution had theorised the latter's role in the radical alteration of the established order. Long before trauma was psychologised, the Jacobins had conceived that *terror* could generate panic, disintegration, and disruption of normal functioning. However, if it were organised, it could also lead to the desired transformation. This tradition, apparently distant from psychological problems, was taken up as the source of the first investigations of group psychology, such as those carried out by Gustave Le Bon very few years after the work of Charcot (Bodei, 1995, p. 321). On the other hand, a tradition linked to alienism, which from the beginning of the nineteenth century conceived the passions as the cause of mental alienation. Charcot could obviously not ignore these hypotheses that were widespread in French medicine and culture. However, the French neurologist acted like these two traditions never existed. This was probably because he was trying to base his ideas on a new framework, that of nervous physiology (which was very different from the conceptual framework of alienism), while at the same time disputing with certain psychiatrists the control of the university chairs and the management of the services of the Salpêtrière (Edelman, 2003).

Third, and in close connection with the preceding, in the conceptual configuration outlined by Charcot, the fright was not linked to a mental illness but to a functional disturbance of the nervous system, analogous to that conceived by Page. The French doctor believed that he could extend this hypothesis to a large part of the cases of traumatic hysteria. In his words,

> this same circumstance of the development of hysterical phenomena, following, and in consequence of, a 'shock', with or without injury, but where emotion plays a great part, you will find again, gentlemen, in the other cases which will now be brought before you.
>
> (Charcot, 1889, p. 232)

Let us observe in this sentence the organisation of the semantic field: "injury" still referred to physical damage, to bodily harm, while "shock" was associated with an emotion such as fright, and played the prominent role in the activation of the symptom-producing mechanism. It would take a few years for the term "trauma" to apply mainly to non-somatic damage. However, it was already notable that, despite heredity being the first cause, the leading role in the production of the illness was given to a psychical element while still being inserted in a physiological conceptual matrix.

In any case, the permanence of an anatomical and locationist framework continued to be clear, at least in the insistence of the hypothesis of a non-material injury in the same area where a wound could be found in similar cases. In Case V, he stated that it would be natural to think that

> the monoplegia in question is due to a cortical cerebral lesion, principally localised in the motor zone of the arm, but it is not of the nature of a gross material alteration. The lesion is purely "dynamic", sine materia, of the nature, in short, of those whose existence we hypothetically suppose.
>
> (Charcot, 1889, p. 252)

The quote clearly shows the hypothetical character of this mysterious dynamic lesion, which remained the only explanation Charcot could imagine to understand the mechanism of hysterical symptoms once an accident (and the emotion aroused by it) triggered it.

However, it is enough to read the following lectures to discover that the clinician was constructing another hypothesis, shaped by the characteristics of the hypnotic procedure and no longer on pathological anatomy, which introduced another psychical element different from emotion. "On Two Cases of Hysterical Brachial Monoplegia in the Male, of Traumatic Origin – Hystero-Traumatic Monoplegia" was the extensive title given to the three lectures that followed the six cases of male hysteria. Two cases were discussed in them, Porcz. and Pin., who were characterised for presenting, following an accident, a highly localised paralysis in one limb, without atrophy and with alterations in sensitivity and the muscular sense, whose diagnosis presented difficulties. After thoroughly describing the development of the symptoms and the semiological characteristics of the condition suffered by Porcz., Charcot asked himself about the nature of this monoplegia and compared the case to that of a patient with a material injury. For the first time, the clinical characteristics of the suspected case of hysteria maintained a similarity with the organic pathologies (an issue that justified the need to undertake the task of differential diagnosis). However, they *were not identical* to the semiological characteristics of these. Let us remember that the functional lesion hypothesis was based on the clinical identity of the symptoms of organic diseases with those of hysteria. If the semiological features were different, would the mechanisms be analogous? The French master seemed to hesitate but initially insisted on his previous thoughts:

> There is without doubt a lesion of the nervous centres (…) But certainly it is not of the nature of a circumscribed organic lesion of a destructive nature. We have here unquestionably one of those lesions which escape our present means of anatomical investigation, and which, for want of a better term, we designate *dynamic* or *functional* lesions.
>
> (Charcot, 1889, p. 278)

As can be seen, Charcot once again relied on the dynamic lesion hypothesis, even when he no longer had the support of a clinical identity with organic diseases. An alternative explanation immediately arose when, after having studied Pin. in the same terms (and concluding that it was also a case of traumatic hysterical monoplegia), he wondered about the appropriate *therapeutic approach*. This question played a very marginal role in the authors seen up to here. In Erichsen's and Page's books, the validation of the illnesses in the grey area between indubitable injuries and the simulation had only led to the need for a medical recognition of the disease and a pecuniary compensation for the damages suffered after an accident. Whether it was regarding an organic lesion or a functional nervous shock, the question of a possible cure had not yet been raised in depth. By identifying these cases as hysteria, Charcot recognised that the prognosis was better in these cases than in those with organic lesions. However, the therapeutics proposed until then for hysteria were based solely on empirical measures "appropriate to rousing vital energies (…); -such as- the repeated application of aestheogenic means, and in particular static electricity, prolonged hydrotherapeutic appliances, etc." (Charcot, 1889, p. 288). The French master longed to go further:

> our interference will show itself with more effect if, instead of relying on empirical notions, it can be founded on a *physiological basis*; if, for example, we can recognise, at least in part, *the mechanism of the production of traumatic hysterical paralysis*.
>
> (Charcot, 1889, p. 288; italics added)

Moved by questions regarding therapeutic approaches, the French clinician began to study the mechanisms of hysterical symptoms in a way that sought to be more physiological and less anatomical than the hypothesis of a dynamic lesion.

To do so, he proposed to return to a topic that he had already dealt with: that of the paralyses "depending on idea, paralyses by imagination" (Charcot, 1889, p. 289), which had been studied for the first time by Russell Reynolds in 1869. At this point, the use of hypnosis appeared with great force. Charcot used it as an instrument that allowed him to study paralysis experimentally. Nevertheless, hypnosis also functioned as a model for conceiving a new hypothesis about the mechanism of hysterical phenomena.

These two sentences seem to condense the core of the argument that Charcot intended to develop:

> We know that in subjects in a state of hypnotic sleep it is possible (…) to originate by the method of suggestion (…) an idea, or a coherent group of associated ideas, which possess the individual, and remain isolated, and manifest themselves by corresponding motor phenomena. If this be so, we know that if the idea suggested be one of paralysis, a real paralysis virtually ensues….
>
> (Charcot, 1889, p. 289)

If a subject were placed in a *hypnotic* state, it would be possible to *suggest* ideas that they, lacking the power of their consciousness and will, could not remove. These imposed ideas would find themselves isolated or (to use a term that will later be consecrated) *split* from "the *ego*" (Charcot, 1889, p. 290; italics in original).

Armed with the instrument and the conceptual matrix provided by hypnosis and suggestion, Charcot returned to Porcz.'s and Pin.'s analyses. After making some preliminary remarks, he introduced Greuz., a hysterical young woman whom he hypnotised and suggested that her arm was paralysed. The semiological characteristics of the anomaly produced by suggestion were different from those of illnesses due to lesions and identical to those of both accident victims, for which Charcot was led to affirm that it had been possible "*to obtain artificially in our hypnotised patient by means of suggestion, a perfect imitation of the monoplegia caused in our two other patients by a process apparently very different, the action of traumatism*" (Charcot, 1889, p. 302; italics in original). He later repeated the experience with a second hysteric, Mesl., with the same clinical results. So, he went one step further: from the phenomenical equivalence to the identity of the mechanism. "This difference" in the mode of production of symptoms, "can be made to disappear" (Charcot, 1889, p. 304). To achieve this, in the hypnotic state, he used a nonverbal suggestion: he gently hit one of the hysterical patients in the same part of the body where the two injured men had received the impact. Again, the clinical results were equated and formed the basis for a deeper identification around both elements of the research procedure: the hypnotic state and suggestion.

Regarding the first element, it is clear that:

> the Nervous Shock experienced at the moment of the accident (...), is (...) equivalent in a certain measure (...) to the cerebral condition which is determined in 'hysterics' by hypnotism.
>
> (Charcot, 1889, p. 305)

In this sentence, we again come across a conceptual configuration analogous to the one we are trying to reconstruct in relation to Page's text. In an accident, such as a railway collision,[24] it would be possible for the intensity of the emotion to generate a disturbance in the functioning of the nervous system in such a way that the higher functions, and in particular consciousness and will, are left out of play. The subject would thus enter a state equivalent to that brought about by hypnosis.

However, a suggestion was also at work. Neither in the case of hypnotised hysterics nor accident victims was it the mechanical action of the blow that had provoked the symptoms. Instead, in both cases, the sensation in the body has "originated (...) the idea of motor paralysis of the member", which "because of the annihilation of the ego (...) acquires sufficient domination to realise itself objectively in the form of paralysis. The sensation, in question, therefore, in both the cases plays the part of a veritable suggestion" (Charcot, 1889, p. 305). As can be seen, the trauma no longer operated there as a physical blow but as a suggestion, which introduced an idea behind consciousness' back. Under those particular conditions, it was capable of generating a symptom. As if to confirm this semantic and conceptual shift, in the same lecture, the great clinician qualified this process as a "*traumatic suggestion*" (Charcot, 1889, p. 307), being probably the first time the term traumatic was used explicitly to designate something other than an impact on the organism.

Here, we have two psychical elements, emotions and ideas, playing an essential role in the mechanism of hysterical symptoms, in the context of an investigation that sought to remain neurological. With these elements playing a central role, the psychologisation of trauma deepened: the material shock and the mechanical action no longer determined the illness; the accident merely aroused emotions that, due to their intensity, could disturb nervous functioning and introduce representations capable of imposing themselves beyond consciousness. Also, the current event alone did not explain the pathology: a prior disposition was required. Therefore, the deterministic power that Erichsen had granted exclusively to the present situation (to the accident) was here quite limited, although not eliminated.

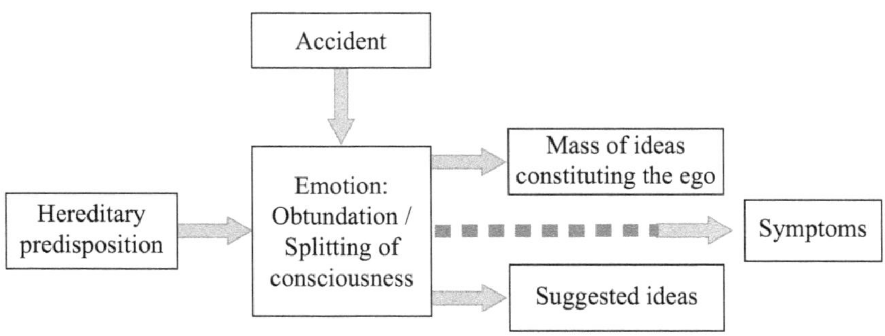

This new conceptual configuration of trauma and of the mechanism of symptoms generated in Charcot the hope of a new type of treatment. Even though the attempts to hypnotise Porcz. and Pin. had failed, it would still be possible to suggest to them,[25] "affirming in a positive manner (…) that their paralysis (…) is not incurable…" (Charcot, 1889, p. 308), and in this way attempt to cure the symptom by relying on the same suggestive pathway that had generated it. The French physician also proposed a particular form of gymnastics: they were repeatedly to squeeze a dynamometer with all their strength and, in each experience, attempt to increase their mark. What could be believed to be a simple mechanical exercise was based on the same principles as the new hypothesis on the pathological mechanism:

> Here we act *psychically*. It is well known, unless I am mistaken, that the production of an image, or of a mental representation (…) of the movement to be executed, is an indispensable preliminary condition to the execution of that movement. (…) We can readily conceive that the repetition of the dynamometric

> exercise would tend to revive in the centres the motor representation, which is a necessary preliminary to the voluntary movement.
>
> (Charcot, 1889, pp. 309–310; italics in original)

This quote on therapeutic approaches most likely illustrates better than others how Charcot conceived the psychical dimension. This dimension did not constitute an independent sphere of physiology, not even in ontological or explanatory terms. The fixed idea of motor weakness would not act upon a mind separated from the brain but on the "cortical motor centres". It would, therefore, operate as a physiological process of inhibiting voluntary movement. On that account, we agree with the lucid description of Marcel Gauchet, who defined the French clinician as a "frontier-man: not the one who crosses the frontier but the one who indicates that there is a frontier to be crossed" between the physiological and the psychical dimensions (Gauchet & Swain, 2000, p. 163).[26] Until the end of his days, the Salpêtrière master continued to think that psychology was nothing more than a way to denominate some of the superior functions of a certain part of the brain.

However, the French clinician's frontierlike thinking should not hide the fact that the vocabulary used in his explanations had been filled with psychological terms. Although these do not entirely affirm the existence of a purely psychical trauma, they allow us to think that emotions and representations may have a pathogenic role, even in the absence of an organic wound. Therefore, we cannot fully agree with Caplan when he states:

> Like most physicians of his day, Charcot saw little reason to challenge the sanctity of the somatic paradigm and the prevailing medical wisdom concerning the physiological foundation of all diseases. His investigation of hysteria was resolutely somatic in its orientation.
>
> (Caplan, 2001, p. 64)

For all the above reasons, we prefer to say that, within the framework of a neurological orientation, Charcot contributed to install the hypothesis that emotions and ideas could have a *traumatic* efficacy. This supposition was not an accidental change of direction in his teaching. Instead, from that moment on, it appeared insistently each time he tried to construct hypotheses about the mechanism of hysterical symptoms.[27] Furthermore, this psychologisation (which never abandoned its physiological framework) deepened over time. As Gauchet (2000, pp. 160–163) and Micale (2001, pp. 124–125) point out, the Le Log. Case (or Le Logeais), presented in 1886, implied a further step in that direction. Le Log. was the victim of an accident in which the carriage he was in was hit by another carriage, which caused him to be violently thrown to the ground, losing consciousness, but without the horses or the carriage directly impacting his body. Nevertheless, the patient "*has made out a long history of the accident* in which he firmly believes, and of which the circumstances appear to him from time to time *in his dreams*" (Charcot,

1889, p. 375; italics in original). According to the victim's recount, the carriage had indeed passed over his body, in the same place where later, after a period of "incubation", he developed paralysis (Charcot, 1889, p. 385). The *difference between the objective event and its subjective representation* (or between *the fact and its narration*) led Charcot to the following reasoning:

> ...this conviction, which has even appeared to him in his dreams, is absolutely erroneous (...) But (...) the consequences of this local shock (...) have determined the auto-suggestion whence results the paraplegia. It is worthy of remark that in the case of Le Log- as in others of the same kind, the paralysis was not produced at the very moment of the accident, but it was only after an interval of several days, after a sort of incubation stage of unconscious mental elaboration.
>
> (Charcot, 1889, pp. 386–387)

In Charcot's analysis, the reference to a local mechanical shock was still present, but it did not act by its physical force but as a source of autosuggestion. In addition, the symptomatology had not developed according to how the accident occurred but according to how the subject represented it during a process of elaboration of ideas that took place behind their consciousness' back. In this conceptual configuration, the subjective representation of the experience ended up being more important than the objective data, with the exception of the fact that the accident had indeed occurred and was not the product of an utterly illusory phantasy or a lie.

The footnote introduced after the quote served to specify that the process involved a cerebral unconscious and physiological (not psychical) mechanisms that were produced automatically "by reason of the easy dissociation of the mental unity of the *ego*" suffered by the subject, as a result of the emotion produced by the shock (Charcot, 1889, p. 387, n. 1). However, his reasoning outlined the bases of a schema (accident/emotion/splitting/idea/symptom) that we will come across again almost identically in the first works of Janet and Freud, although they did not feel compelled to quickly translate these processes to the locationist language based on the cortical centres. In other words, the way in which the elements are related in this conceptual configuration remained valid for some years, even when the somatic reference tended to disappear.

At the same time, the fact that the psychologisation of trauma has been accentuated in the framework of Charcot's teaching (by making it conceivable that ideas could have traumatic efficacy) did not lead to the elimination of the trait of passivity in the *image* of the traumatised individual. It is clear that the injured/hysterical patients described by Charcot were not determined as such solely by the current accident, since their pathological circumstances were considered much more determined by past heredity (a condition that Charcot thought was necessary for an *agent provocateur* to be able to trigger the disease that had been latent until then). Due to this double determination, the traumatised patient was more comparable to an automaton or an organism subjected to automatic physiological processes than to a subject fully responsible for their actions. Even conceiving the possibility of a therapeutic approach for their symptoms did nothing more than confirm the passive position in which they were put. If the key to a successful treatment resided in the use of suggestion when in a state of obtundation, the traumatised subject continued to be conceived as a being permeable to ideas that are imposed on them from the outside; without any participation of their consciousness, will, or agency that would have made them a participant in the healing process. Precisely, much of the development that the then-novel psychotherapies and psychoanalysis acquired, very shortly afterwards, had as their starting point the critique of and the attempt to separate the automatic and passive nature of the intervention by suggestion.

It is necessary to point out two more issues regarding these processes of psychologisation. First, until the final decade of the nineteenth century, the transformations of the notion of trauma did not imply any reference to an element that today is inseparable from that category: the question of memory. The different authors we studied admitted that the accident (either due to the physical blow or due to the functional alteration generated by the emotion) was capable of causing amnesia. However, that it aroused a problem *in* (an individual's) memory did not imply that the pathological process or the nature of trauma were thought of as a problem *of* memory. Only after the work of Janet and Freud did it become possible, and even common, to conceive that a memory, even if forgotten by consciousness, could make itself present not only as an evocation of the past but also as a current source of some sort of illness or malaise. In the next chapter, we will deal with this historical process of the *memorialisation* of trauma.

However, before that, we would like to highlight a second issue. The paths of psychologisation, which linked the modern problem of accidents with the history of hysteria, did not constitute a single track, which would necessarily lead from anatomy to psychology, as if it were the unfolding of a truth that was at hand, awaiting its discoverers. The nascent psychical explanations, rather, always coexisted with tendencies towards somatisation, such as the hypotheses defended by Hermann Oppenheim that we will analyse below.

1.9 Trauma as a Specific Nosographic Category

In 1884, legislation on accident insurance was established in the German State, which seemed to respond to the demands of the working class to the same extent that it hindered the possibility of radical changes by transforming the political proclamations for working conditions into an expert technical problem: that of the work accident (Eghigian, 2001; Lerner, 2001; Lerner & Micale, 2001; Schäffner, 2001). At the same time, this legislation gave doctors the role of "'surveyors' who must establish whether an accident was an 'adequate cause' of an injury and then assess its impact on the victim and the insurance company" (Schäffner, 2001, p. 81). Five years later, the Imperial Insurance Office recognised "traumatic neuroses" (Lerner, 2001, p. 149) as one of the pathological conditions that merited pecuniary compensation. Hermann Oppenheim forged this nosographic category after six years of clinical work at the Charité Berlin University of Medicine, which depends on the University of Berlin. During this period, he had dealt with neuroses, particularly with pathological clinical pictures linked to accidents. His 1889 monograph, *Die traumatischen Neurosen nach den in der Nervenklinik der Charité in den 5 Jahren 1883–1888 gesammelten Beobachtungen*, allowed for the institutional recognition of his notion, but, at the same time, generated great controversy and strong opposition from a good part of the German medical field. Even more so when, after 1890, Oppenheim and his notion were held responsible for a "nervous epidemic" or "a virtual epidemic of 'pension hysteria'" (Lerner, 2001, p. 150; Lerner & Micale, 2001, p. 13), that is to say, for an unusual number of compensation claims and job or military desertions due to alleged cases of traumatic neuroses. These claims generated suspicions about the truthfulness of the reported disability and from many sectors, these neurotics (and the doctors who diagnosed them) were accused of threatening the nation's economy and morals (Lerner, 2001, pp. 145–150).

The greatest originality of Oppenheim's conception (and one of its most criticised features) was proposing a specific clinical entity for trauma. As we have seen, traditionally, this term did not designate any disease in particular. Instead, it referred to a process characterised by its mechanical action on the organism and by its production of lesions which generated different illnesses (depending, above all, on the place where the wound was located). At the same time, the term *neurosis* (even before the investigations carried out at the Salpêtrière) was frequently utilised in relation to a group of diffuse disturbances of nervous functioning, which were characterised, precisely, by not presenting an obvious sign of anatomical damage. By combining both notions under the category of *traumatic neurosis*, Oppenheim was uniting two terms that were usually antipodes of medical thought: illnesses acquired by injury and suspected functional diseases whose only clear sign seemed to be hereditary aetiology. At this point, the move made by this German physician was comparable to that made by Charcot in introducing the reference to traumatic hysteria. However, while the combination of trauma and hysterical illness enabled the French clinician to make the role of ideas in the production of symptoms thinkable, Oppenheim leaned again towards somatic hypotheses and the objective and current qualities of the traumatic experience.

For the German physician, certain accidents could generate a specific type of nervous illness independent of personal or family history and, above all, independent of the affected individual's interests in claiming a pension. That is why he affirmed that "a neuropathic and toxic diathesis" could merely favour "the onset of these neuroses" (Oppenheim, 1900, p. 733), but never truly cause them because "the traumatic neuroses are the result of psychic and physical shock. Both act mostly upon the cerebrum and evoke molecular alterations in the same areas which govern the higher psychic and motor and sensory functions and those of the special senses" (Oppenheim, 1900, p. 741).

By considering the possibility that, in some instances, "psychic shock – fear or excitement – " may be the sole cause of the problem, his conception seemed to approach Page's. However, from his perspective, the cause of the disease "is almost always a trauma – in the traditional sense of an impact on the organism – which is accompanied by a pronounced – mechanical – shock of the affected part of the body or with a severe psychic shock" (Oppenheim, 1900, p. 734). In other words, the aetiology of the clinical picture, whose legitimacy he was attempting to defend, was centred on mechanical trauma; all other elements, including shocks of a psychical nature, were secondary and superfluous. Therefore, we consider that Wolfgang Schäffner exaggerates when interpreting Oppenheim's theory in terms of "psychic trauma". Schäffner bases his view on a quote from Oppenheim on the traumatic neuroses, in which the German doctor differentiated his nosographic category from *railway spine* because, in the latter, the site of the disease was found in the spinal cord and, in the former, "the principle place of the illness is the brain, the *psyche*, wherever the trauma may have attacked" (Schäffner, 2001, p. 83; italics added). From our perspective, in this sentence, the German physician used the term *psyche* in a sense common to the neurological field of the end of the nineteenth century: a synonym for the higher functions of the nervous system based in the brain. Therefore, we believe that he was not proposing that this illness was psychological but that it was *cerebral* (unlike railway spine), even if the impact had affected a part of the body other than the head.

Of course, we consider it evident that Oppenheim's conceptual configuration was more complex than Erichsen's and that it included elements that were not taken into consideration by his British colleague. Nevertheless, his conception tended towards anatomy and somatisation. The ultimate material base of the pathology resided in "finer material lesions" that, despite not being observable by the instruments of analysis of the time, were "present, and form the basis of some phenomena" (Oppenheim, 1900, p. 741). This last idea, combined with the persistence of the mechanical nature of the trauma, and with having attributed to the accident a determining and causal power (which relativised the role of the individual's antecedents and expectations), distanced his conception from that of contemporary authors, such as Page or Charcot. For this reason, he did not hesitate when making explicit that his theory was opposed to that of his French colleague, "who regarded traumatic hysteria to be due to autosuggestion", as well as when seeking to clarify that although "the desire for money" or the claims for the individual's violated "supposed rights" could cause depression and irritability, he could not "agree that symptoms arise in this way" (Oppenheim, 1900, p. 741).

That said, criticism of this conception soon multiplied in the German territory. The primary opponents of his category of traumatic neurosis were not fringe figures in the medical world but those who held academic and managerial positions in universities and hospitals, with predominantly working-class patients (Lerner, 2001, p. 147). Oppenheim, who lost his academic position[28] shortly after publishing his monograph on the work carried out at the Charité hospital, settled in at a private polyclinic in Berlin, despite which he acquired an international reputation for his work as a clinical neurologist. Undoubtedly, most of the patients who attended his new workplace were from the middle class (Lerner, 2001, p. 147).

At the Berlin Medical Congress held in 1890, Oppenheim was criticised not only for underestimating the possibility of simulation in pursuit of economic gain but also for ignoring the role that predisposition and "wish complexes" would have in certain cases (Lerner, 2001, pp. 151–152). For the medical establishment, it was necessary to consider the hereditary background of the individual *before* the accident, as well as certain psychological factors that could appear *after* the accident when facing the possibility of receiving a pension. According to these doctors who critiqued Oppenheim's views, "it was not the accident, but actually the insurance itself that caused psychic injuries" (Schäffner, 2001, p. 82). As can be seen, the greatest role in the production of the illness was given to subjective particularities (past or present) and not to the objective conditions of the traumatic experience. Furthermore, the recognition of the pathogenic influence of certain elements of a psychical nature (such as *Begehrungsvorstellungen* – "imaginative desires/wish complexes" – according to the term proposed by Strümpell in 1895) was a characteristic of certain sectors that were opposed to legitimising the idea that a traumatic situation (on its own) could generate symptoms (Lerner, 2001, p. 14). Therefore, one can hardly speak here of the psychologisation of trauma; rather, the first term was clearly opposed to the second: if the pathological processes were psychical, then the trauma did not play any role in the production of the disease.

In summary, the notion of traumatic neurosis, which introduced the idea that certain neurotic clinical pictures were caused solely by somatic processes generated by a traumatic experience, ended up fuelling contrary positions, which led to the institutionalisation of psychological conceptions of neuroses and the questioning of the category of trauma. Several years later, the First World War gave Oppenheim a new opportunity to promote his nosographic category and his deterministic and somatic conception of the illness. However, this event ended up being an opportunity for his detractors to finish burying the relevance of his ideas and to manage to impose the diagnosis of hysteria on those same cases. We will more extensively work on the German debate during the Great War in Chapter 4 of this book. However, before this, we will address the historical processes that allowed trauma and memory to be combined, starting from the first works of Pierre Janet and Sigmund Freud.

Notes

1 We will work on this problem in depth in Chapter 3.

2 Furthermore, we must not forget that the possibility of conceiving trauma in somatic terms was never eliminated, as is palpable even today, with the boom in neurobiological research revolving around the clinical category of PTSD. As occurs with many notions and problems that are part of the "psy" territory, regarding the notion of trauma, the tendencies towards "psychologisation" coexist and permanently dispute with the tendencies towards "somatisation".

3 Concerning this, Harrington presented some eloquent data, for example, that in 1861, there were 49 cases of death due to railway accidents in England out of a total of 163 million passenger trips; this being a particularly bad year (Harrington, 2001, p. 33).
4 Harrington cited an article of *The Lancet* from February 8, 1862 (pp. 156–157).
5 The historian Eric Caplan collects an illustrative series of medical testimonies (especially from those professionals who worked for the railway companies on both sides of the Atlantic), through which it is possible to observe the weight that Erichsen's proposals continued to have even at the beginning of the following century. For example, Doctor Harold Moyer, who worked in North America for the railroad companies, seemed to complain bitterly in 1901 that "[The] term spinal concussion as used by Erichsen nearly forty years ago, has served as a foundation for an extraordinary superstructure and one that has maintained itself decade after decade in spite of the advances in our knowledge of neural pathology" (Moyer, 1901–1902, p. 151; cited in Caplan, 2001, p. 59). The quote is illustrative of the importance that Erichsen's hypotheses acquired, as well as the ability of certain scientific ideas to persist in different areas of the collective imagination despite having lost legitimacy in the field of knowledge where they were coined.
6 A few pages later, Erichsen insisted on the fact that "there is in reality nothing special in railway injuries, except in the severity of the accident by which they are occasioned" (Erichsen, 1866, pp. 44–45).
7 As in case number 9 of the book (Erichsen, 1866, pp. 55–57).
8 As we will see, an author such as Oppenheim carried out the opposite strategy since he sought to defend the existence of a new clinical picture that would be specific to traumatic situations.
9 His ideas were also far from the common sense of many professionals and laymen who even today consider certain events, such as train accidents, wars or sexual abuse to be traumatic by nature and in all cases.
10 By "conceptual (or epistemic) framework (or matrix)" (which for the purposes of this article we will consider synonyms), we understand the web of concepts with which experience is approached and that delimit the field of the thinkable and the visible.
11 Erichsen's teacher, the surgeon Benjamin Brodie, had been one of the people responsible for the recognition of said clinical picture in the 1830s (Harrington, 2001, p. 42).
12 In the first lecture, he had presented a case of spinal concussion from the eighteenth century, the consequence of an overturned carriage, which he considered important "for it is identical in its course and symptoms with many" railway accidents (Erichsen, 1866, p. 24).
13 Even though this idea may seem strange, an analogous reasoning, although sustained in a very different conceptual framework, would appear many years later in relation to those affected by neuroses during the First World War. From the perspective of Freud and other authors, soldiers that suffered physical injuries on the battlefield had fewer chances of developing a war neurosis than those who remained unharmed.
14 It is necessary to retain this distinction between aetiology and the mechanism of symptoms as we will find it again in subsequent conceptual configurations. That which, in each one of the latter, is considered the "traumatic element" can be placed, either in the category of aetiology (the final cause of the disease) or in the category of the mechanism (direct or material cause of the disease).
15 It is striking that on this important point, Harrington was unable to include any explicit citations of Erichsen, as he did in the rest of his article.
16 Harrington made a similar statement and also included a reference from 1873. In that year, the physician John Furneaux Jordan stated that "the principal feature in railway injuries is the combination of the psychical and corporeal elements in the causation of shock" (Harrington, 2001, p. 49).

17 The almost simultaneous publication of Erichsen's and Page's book in England and the United States shows the enormous interest these issues had on both sides of the Atlantic.
18 For example, if in the case of having verified an injury, the symptoms developed slowly, then it would be more probable that their mechanism corresponded to a haemorrhage that only secondarily affected the spinal cord, than in direct damage to it (Page, 1883, p. 9). Erichen's broad use of the term led him to include haemorrhagic injuries within the category of spinal concussion, while Page opposed this inclusion. From his perspective, this term could only be used in reference to injuries that were directly produced by a mechanical shock, without mediating any other type of anatomical damage (fractures, dislocations, haemorrhages, etc.).
19 We believe that it is necessary to pay attention to this disjunction, which here is clearly not exclusive. Rather, it seems to indicate that in his thinking an equivalence was established between both terms. Or more so, a subordination of what today we consider to be psychical, to the functions of the brain.
20 As it did for Erichsen, pathological anatomy functioned as a conceptual framework and not as a research practice.
21 In turn, their successors were able to eliminate more and more of these types of references to the nervous system, even though in their psychological conceptions, they retained a good part of the logical framework that tied the concepts into these physiological schemas.
22 Edelman's reading of male hysteria allows us to understand that, despite the attempt to defeminise the pathology, certain differences between both sexes remained. The hysterical man was almost never characterised by the overwhelms and excesses that were present in the presentations of hysterical attacks in women. The former was more "sombre, depressive, very often neurasthenic, while the woman more closely resembled the child and its airiness" (Edelman, 2003, p. 149).
23 In the first of the lectures dedicated to the six cases of masculine hysteria, which was the eighteenth class of volume III of his "Lectures", there were explicit references to Page and to the American physicians Putnam and Walton who had dealt with the effects of railway accidents. These doctors had made it possible to liken post-traumatic symptoms to hysterical symptoms and to shift the attention from the spinal cord to the brain. Charcot also mentioned certain French colleagues who were willing like him to admit the existence of male hysteria, which until then had been almost unthinkable (Charcot, 1889), and criticised Oppenheim for not interpreting his cases as hysteria (Charcot, 1889).
24 Following Charcot's sentence quoted above, a footnote suggested that a mechanism of this kind (where emotion would generate a shock or hypnotic state) was at work in cases of railway spine (Charcot, 1889, p. 305, n. 1).
25 This implied a certain flexibility in the procedure, although the difference with Nancy remained: not everyone could be put under the effects of suggestion, but only those who were predisposed to nervous pathology, in whom: "most of the manifestations of hypnotism, both psychic and somatic, may be encountered in the waking state, without the necessary intervention of hypnotic practices. It appears that the hypnotic condition which in the case of others is an artificial state, may be for those singular beings an ordinary one, their normal condition. These individuals sleep, if you will allow the term, while they appear perfectly awake" (Charcot, 1889, p. 306).
26 Micale made a similar interpretation by stating that, in the historical process of the psychologisation of trauma, "Charcot was a transitional figure: While working within the reigning neurophysiological paradigm of his time, with its emphasis on the anatomy and biology of heredity, he granted greater causal latitude to the role of the emotions -and of the ideas, we would add- than earlier medical writers" (Micale, 2001, p. 123).

27 For example, in the 24th lecture, when faced with a case of hysterical coxalgia, Charcot stated that: "just as there are psychical paralyses produced by what has been called in former lectures *traumatic suggestion*, so also there are spasmodic coxalgia due to the same mechanism" (Charcot, 1889, p. 336; italics in original). In the 25th lecture, when dealing with a case of spasmodic contracture in a man, he again stated that paralysis could be artificially produced by applying a moderate blow to one of the limbs of the hypnotised patient. Thus, "the sensations of weight, of absence of the limb (…) which occurred after a blow on the limb in these cases (as in those where the phenomena are produced independent of hypnotism), would be the point of departure of the 'suggestion', which has the effect of developing the paralysis (…) Such was the theory, as I proposed it to you, in order to interpret facts of this nature" (Charcot, 1889, p. 344).

28 Lerner suggests that his Jewish status may have contributed to the rejection of his candidacy for the position of Extraordinary Professor, in a context of growing anti-Semitism at the University (Lerner, 2001, p. 146).

References

Barona, J. (1991). *La fisiología: Origen histórico de una ciencia experimental.* Madrid: Akal.

Bernheim, H. (1884). *De la suggestion dans l'etat hypnotique et dans l'etat de veille*. Paris: Doin.

Bodei, R. (1995). *Geometría de las Pasiones. Miedo, esperanza y felicidad: filosofía y uso político*. México, DF: Fondo de Cultura Económica.

Caplan, E. (2001). Trains and trauma in the American Gilded age. In M. Micale & P. Lerner (Eds.), *Traumatic Pasts. History, Psychiatry, and Trauma in the Modern Age, 1870–1930* (pp. 57–80). Cambridge: Cambridge University Press.

Carroy, J. (1991). L'invention d'un sujet expérimental: hypnose, suggestion et expérimentation. In J. Carroy (Ed.), *Hypnose, suggestion et psychologie. L'invention des sujets* (pp. 157–178). París: PUF.

Charcot, J.-M. (1889). *Clinical Lectures on Diseases of the Nervous System*, Volume III. London and New York: Routledge (2014).

Charcot, J.-M. (1892). *Leçons sur les maladies du système nerveux. Tome premier.* En *Ouvres complètes de J. M. Charcot.* Paris: Bureaux du Progrès Mèdical.

Danziger, K. (1990). *Constructing the Subject. Historial Origins of Psychological Research.* Cambridge: Cambridge University Press.

Edelman, N. (2003). *Les métamorphoses de l'histérique. Du debut du XIX siècle à la Grande Guerre.* Paris: La Découverte.

Eghigian, G. (2001). The German welfare state as a discourse of trauma. In M. Micale & P. Lerner (Eds.), *Traumatic Pasts. History, Psychiatry, and Trauma in the Modern Age, 1870–1930* (pp. 92–114). Cambridge: Cambridge University Press.

Erichsen, J.E. (1866). *On Railway and Other Injuries of the Nervous System.* Philadelphia, PA: Henry C. Lea.

Foucault, M. (2003). *The Birth of the Clinic*. London: Routledge.

Foucault, M. (2006). *Psychiatric Power. Lecture at the Collège de France, 1973–1974.* New York: Palgrave Macmillian.

Gauchet, M. & Swain, G. (2000). *El verdadero Charcot.* Buenos Aires: Nueva Visión.

Hacking, J. (1995). *Rewriting the Soul: Multiple Personality and the Sciences of Memory.* Princeton, NJ: Princeton University Press.

Harrington, R. (2001). The railway accident: Trains, trauma, and technological crisis in nineteenth-century Britain. In M. Micale & P. Lerner (Eds.), *Traumatic Pasts. History, Psychiatry, and Trauma in the Modern Age, 1870–1930* (pp. 31–56). Cambridge: Cambridge University Press.

Le Gros Clark, F. (1870). *Lectures on the Principles of Surgical Diagnosis: Especially in Relation to Shock and Visceral Lesions.* London: John Churchill and Sons.

Lerner, P. (2001). From traumatic neurosis to male hysteria: The decline and fall of hermann oppenheim, 1889–1919. In M. Micale & P. Lerner (Eds.), *Traumatic Pasts. History, Psychiatry, and Trauma in the Modern Age, 1870–1930* (pp. 140–171). Cambridge: Cambridge University Press.

Lerner, P. & Micale, M. (2001). Trauma, psychiatry and history: A conceptual and historiographical introduction. In M. Micale & P. Lerner (Eds.), *Traumatic Pasts. History, Psychiatry, and Trauma in the Modern Age, 1870–1930* (pp. 1–30). Cambridge: Cambridge University Press.

Leys, R. (2000). *Trauma. A Genealogy.* Chicago, IL: The University of Chicago Press.

Micale, M. (2001). Jean-Martin Charcot and *les névroses traumatiques*: From medicine to culture in French trauma theory of the late nineteenth century. In M. Micale & P. Lerner (Eds.), *Traumatic Pasts. History, Psychiatry, and Trauma in the Modern Age, 1870–1930* (pp. 115–139). Cambridge: Cambridge University Press.

Moyer, H. (1901–1902). The so-called traumatic neurosis. In *The Railway Surgeon 8*. Cited in Caplan, 2001.

Oppenheim, H. (1900). *Diseases of the Nervous System.* Philadelphia, PA and London: J. B. Lippincott Company.

Page, H. (1883). *Injuries of the Spine and Spinal Cord without Apparent Mechanical Lesions, and Nervous Shock, in Their Surgical and Medico-Legal Aspects.* Philadelphia, PA: P. Blakiston, Son & Co.

Paget, J. (1875). Nervous mimicry. In J. Paget (Ed.), *Clinical Lectures and Essays*, Volume 2 (pp. 172–251). London: Logmans, Greens and Co.

Schäffner, W. (2001). Event, series, trauma: The probabilistic revolution of the mind in the late nineteenth and early twentieth centuries. In M. Micale & P. Lerner (Eds.), *Traumatic Pasts: History, Psychiatry, and Trauma in the Modern Age, 1870–1930* (pp. 81–91). Cambridge: Cambridge University Press.

Van der Kolk, B., McFarlane, A. & Weisaeth, L. (Eds.). (1996). *Traumatic Stress: The Effects of Overwhelming Experiences on Mind.* New York: The Guilford Press.

Chapter 2

Trauma and Memory

The Janet-Freud Debate, 1889–1895/1913–1914[1]

After having analysed the different ways the notion of trauma, still in medical territory, began to enter the psychological domain, we now intend to study a period in which this category was combined with the question of memory. Before the 1890s, the trauma had not been thought of as a problem of a mnemic nature. The anatomical, physiological and hypnotic *models* that we attempted to reconstruct made it possible to think of the trauma as a lesion in the living tissue (Erichsen), as a molecular modification in the brain (Oppenheim), as a functional disturbance caused by a nervous shock (Page) or as a physiological mechanism, analogous to hypnosis and suggestion, where emotions and ideas played a central role (Charcot). Within this plurality of conceptions, we have pointed out a shift from the event considered a mechanical action to the problem of its representation, even though the somatic orientations had never been completely abandoned.

The novelty introduced in the last decade of the nineteenth century was mainly provided by Janet and Freud, who began to understand trauma in terms of the interplay between memory and amnesia. Very broadly speaking, a trauma was not for them a mechanical blow nor was it an emotion or an idea, but rather it was the memory of an experience that, despite having been "forgotten" by the subject, acted upon them outside the control of their consciousness and will.

The importance acquired by the mnemic function in this small field linked to trauma should be placed in relation to a broader context: the problematisation of memory towards the end of the nineteenth century. As Ian Hacking has pointed out, for centuries, a wide range of *arts of memory* or mnemotechnics swarmed Western Culture, aimed at increasing the individual's ability to remember in the absence of easily accessible forms of records or of material archives (above all, before the invention of the printing press). After these techniques became increasingly unnecessary, different *sciences of memory* appeared simultaneously, making memory an object to be studied and no longer a capacity to be developed (Hacking, 1995, pp. 198–209). The new scientific approaches to memory were: "(a) the neurological studies of the location of different types of memory; (b) experimental studies of recall; and (c) what might be called the psychodynamics of memory", where the two authors that we will address in this chapter would be found (Hacking, 1995, p. 199). To these three approaches pointed out by Hacking, the hereditarian tradition

DOI: 10.4324/9781003380016-3

should be added. It was an approach of great influence in the field of the clinic of the neuroses, which supposed the existence of a biological memory whose traces could be transmitted from generation to generation.

Furthermore, we consider that this development of systematic research on memory cannot be explained solely by the disappearance of the mnemotechnic arts and the spread of technologies that facilitated the material record of the past. Towards the end of the nineteenth century, the consequences of other changes were also becoming more noticeable. Although these are more difficult to delimit within a limited time period, they were very important over the long term in Western culture. We refer fundamentally to the modern process of acceleration in the pace of transformations (technological, cultural, social, political, etc.) that could occur within a lifetime, which contrasted enormously with the relatively static nature of ancient regimes. Modifications in the political system, new means of transportation, transformations in working conditions, urban life and variations in the social position of the genders constitute some of these processes of change. These transformations made tradition, understood as the teachings that past generations could leave as a legacy to their successors in order to face experience, increasingly insufficient for structuring modern life (Hartog, 2003; Koselleck, 1993). The changing and uncertain framework served as the terrain for the development of systematic studies of heredity and memory, as if scientifically studying what remains of the past tried to compensate for the insufficient nature of ancestral transmission.

Focusing, again, on the more limited field of trauma, we would like to point out the existence of abundant recent literature whose authors are linked to the field of neuroscience, which dwells upon this same time period and starts a new debate on the works of Freud and Janet. These historical works not only attempt to influence the field of psychopathology and psychotherapies but are also taken up in some contemporary studies on social memory. In the book *Trauma: Explorations in Memory* (Caruth, 1995), which aims to address the problems of memory in different dimensions of Western culture, we find a paragraph written by Bessel van de Kolk and Onno van der Hart that nicely illustrates the terms in which the historiographical controversies about the role of Janet and Freud are currently framed:

> Using only careful clinical observations, these early psychologists, particularly Janet, developed a comprehensive formulation about the effects of traumatic memories on consciousness. Even though Janet's views were well known during the early part of this century (…) and though he accurately *anticipated* the developments in the neurosciences in the 1970s and 1980s, his monumental legacy was *crowded out by psychoanalysis*, and largely forgotten, until Henri Ellenberger rescued him from total obscurity in *The Discovery of the Unconscious*. For the past seventy-five years, psychoanalysis, *the study of repressed wishes and instincts* (…) *virtually ignored the fact that actual memories* may form the nucleus of psychopathology and continue to exert their influence on current experience by means of the process of dissociation.
>
> (Van der Kolk & Van der Hart, 1995, p. 159; italics added)

This passage has the virtue of pointing out the need to rethink the ideas of the great French physician and philosopher, which for much of the twentieth century remained under the shadow of Freudism. However, this passage also presents many features that stain the past with the colour of present battles, in which psychoanalysis, once capable of "crowding out" Janet's work, appears as the direct target of attack. This approach incurs a paradox: the historical reconstruction uses the same conceptual schema propitiated by the theory it intends to denounce. It considers that the texts of the Collège de France professor would contain a truth that had been "forgotten by repression" until its later return. Furthermore, Janet and his complex thinking are reduced to the figure of the "pioneer" who "anticipates", with the discovery of unproblematic "facts", the investigations that today are considered true. In short, this perspective conceives the histories of trauma and psychology as the linear development of a truth anticipated by pioneers and definitively established by current authors, which had been occulted by the pressure psychoanalysis exerted.

In some of these works, it is possible to read that "Janet distinguished narrative memory from the automatic integration of new information without much conscious attention to what is happening" (Van der Kolk & Van der Hart, 1995, p. 160); that he was "repeatedly and mistakenly quoted as emphasizing hereditary factors in hysteria" when he "emphasized most forcefully, however, the role of vehement emotions such as terror in response to traumatic events" (Van der Hart & Horst, 1989, p. 403); that he was "the first to show clearly and systematically how it – dissociation – is the most direct psychological defence against overwhelming traumatic experiences" (Van der Kolk & Van der Hart, 1989, p. 397); and finally, that his "therapeutic approach to traumatized patients was the first attempt to create a systematic, phase-oriented treatment of post-traumatic stress" (Van der Kolk & Horst, 1989, p. 403). Whoever reads these types of articles might be convinced that the brilliant French philosopher and physician constructed a theoretical and therapeutic system centred on trauma, in which the cause of the illness would not be found in heredity but rather in traumatic experiences. The latter would, in themselves, produce a dissociation of consciousness and impede the normal functioning of narrative memory, thus constituting a "literal" memory of the event. Moreover, his Viennese colleague is presented as someone clouded by his theory about the repression of desires and instincts, someone who did not see (and did not make it possible to see) the role that lived events could have in the production of the illnesses (Van der Kolk & Van der Hart, 1995, p. 159). At the same time, very few textual citations of both figures appear in these works, which seems to facilitate the substitution of the original terms by a more contemporary vocabulary, which brings Janet's ideas even closer to contemporary developments in neuroscience.

Faced with this panorama, we wish to transform each of these affirmations into questions. Did Janet actually construct a theoretical and therapeutic system focused on trauma? Did heredity, in his works, play a marginal role with regard to traumatic experiences? Was dissociation, for him, a "defence" against trauma?

Was his conceptualisation of the mnemic function based centrally on an opposition between two types of memory, one narrative and the other literal or traumatic? Moreover, did Freudian theory actually ignore the role that certain events could have in producing pathological phenomena? Were his ideas about repression and defence completely opposed to Janet's, and did they apply only to elements (such as desires and drives) that were considered completely "internal" and independent of lived events?

In this chapter, we will aim to address these questions by studying two brief but fundamental periods in Janet's and Freud's works (1892–1895/1913–1914). As opposed to that kind of biased reconstruction, we argue that, in fact, Freud's works gave much more importance than Janet's to the relationship between trauma, memory and pathology. Furthermore, we reconstruct the paths that led them to the field of neuroses and two essential parts of their debate: the discussion about the relevance of hereditary and accidental factors, and the one about the function of memory within the framework of treatment. We believe that these issues are important not only for the history of psychoanalysis but also for current psychoanalytic practice. Finally, as bibliographic sources, we use theoretical and clinical works, allowing for a better appreciation of the relationship between trauma and memory in both authors' theories and practices.

2.1 Janet and Psychological Automatism (1889)

Pierre Janet was born on May 30, 1859, into a Parisian bourgeois family.[2] His uncle, Paul, was a professor of philosophy at the *Sorbonne*, while his brother Jules worked as a doctor. Pierre's intellectual trajectory led him to combine both professions. After finishing his studies at the *École Normale Supérieure*, he had to move to Le Havre at the age of 23, for having obtained the position of associate professor of philosophy at that small city's Lycee. At that site, he alternated secondary school teaching with philosophical research, whose main data source was provided by a series of pathological cases studied through hypnosis and suggestion. After six years of work, he finally defended and published the first of his great works entitled *Psychological Automatism: Essay of Experimental Psychology on the Lower Forms of Human Activity* (1889).

Many authors working from a historical perspective have pointed out the importance of Pierre Janet's first doctoral thesis (Dagfal, 2013; Ellenberger, 1970; Hacking, 1995; Leys, 2000).[3] According to Ian Hacking, this dissertation constituted "the first systematic work to study the traumatic causes of hysteria" (Hacking, 1995, p. 191). However, neither trauma nor hysteria seems to have been the explicit focus of that work. For its author, the object of study was "human activity in its simplest, most rudimentary forms" (Janet, 1889, p. 1). With this phrase, he was referring to the automatic activities of the spirit that, in an evolutionary framework, would be older than the superior and complex functions. These activities would also be characterised by being regular and responding to determinism but without being completely exempt from consciousness (Janet, 1889, p. 2). For Janet, sick individuals were those "who thus present to an exceptional degree a phenomenon or a characteristic which will be hardly apparent in a normal man" (Janet, 1889, p. 5). However, this distinction was only quantitative since the French philosopher followed the principle established by Claude Bernard, according to which "the laws of disease are the same as those of health" (Janet, 1889, p. 5). Therefore, hysteria and the neuroses were not his objects of study, but rather the royal road to investigating certain automatic psychological phenomena common to all human beings, since they provided "the field most favorable to the experimental studies of psychology and especially to the studies on automatism" (Janet, 1889, p. 8). The inscription of his research within the framework of a doctorate in letters and his lack of a medical degree allow us to understand better why there are no references to therapeutics in the extensive published work.

This nuanced distinction between the object of study and the area where it is most frequently found should not be forgotten if one intends not to subsume Janet's ideas to current interests centred on trauma. The author's purpose and the novelty he introduced did not lie in the affirmation that an idea could have a traumatic impact (a hypothesis that, as we have seen, had already been held by other authors), but rather, in the attempt to shift the study of the automatic activity of the human being from the field of physiology to that of philosophy. Janet sought to show that all of these phenomena have some degree of consciousness, even when the ego (the "personality") was unaware of them (Janet, 1889, pp. 39, 117 and 314).

During the second half of the nineteenth century, certain involuntary and automatic phenomena, such as somnambulism, hypnotic suggestion, paralysis and anaesthesia, had begun to be explained from a physiological *model* based on reflex actions. This model followed Laycock and Carpenter's work, who conjectured the identity of the functioning of the entire nervous system and, therefore, the existence of unconscious brain processes (Gauchet, 1994). In the previous chapter, we pointed out that Charcot, after admitting that emotions and ideas can produce symptoms, hastily emphasised that these psychological terms refer only to the higher functions of the nervous system (Charcot, 1889; Gauchet & Swain, 2000, pp. 160–163). In 1889, the small step taken by Janet implied a leap from the cerebral unconscious to a new territory, in which automatisms could be explained *entirely* in psychological terms, even though much of his reasoning had been constructed in the field of neurophysiology.

At the same time, in order to define these phenomena which remained outside the scope of the ego, Janet used the term "unconscious"[4] in the first pages but later preferred to replace it with "subconscious". As Alejandro Dagfal (2013) has already pointed out, the French philosopher explained this change in the following way:

> This expression -the unconsciousness of certain acts-, applied to the preceding facts, hardly has any more meaning: what is an unconscious judgement, an unconscious multiplication. (…) These phenomena seem to belong to a particular consciousness below the normal consciousness of the individual. (…) and we

> will only summarize these observations by henceforth calling these acts subconscious facts, having a consciousness below normal consciousness.
>
> (Janet, 1889, p. 168)

This terminological clarification aimed to separate his ideas from the neurophysiological tradition of the cerebral unconscious as well as from the romantic unconscious (Dagfal, 2013, pp. 371–372, n.2). At the same time, he established between subconscious acts and normal consciousness a difference of degree rather than a radical opposition. In order for a psychical event to form part of the ego or the conscious personality (that is, for a subject to be able to say, "I am the one who feels or remembers this phenomenon"), according to Janet, two successive operations would be required:

1 A first operation during which "primitive conscious phenomena" would coexist "simultaneously and in isolation", such as sensations, memories or images, which could come "from a current impression made on the senses" or by "the automatic play of association" (Janet, 1889, p. 307). These phenomena could be "tactile (…) such as T T' T", muscular like M M' M", visual like V V' V", auditory like A A' A"" (Janet, 1889, p. 306).

   T T' T" M M' M" V V' V" A A' A"

   We have here "phenomena -which is- conscious but not attributed to a personality" (Janet, 1889, p. 306), sensations or memories that would suppose a psychical record even though it was still not possible for the subject to say "I see, I feel", since this apparently simple act, would require the following condition:
2 An active and actual operation of synthesis by which these sensations are linked to each other, aggregate, merge, merge into a single state "forming a" new phenomenon (…) perception P. (Janet, 1889, p. 307).

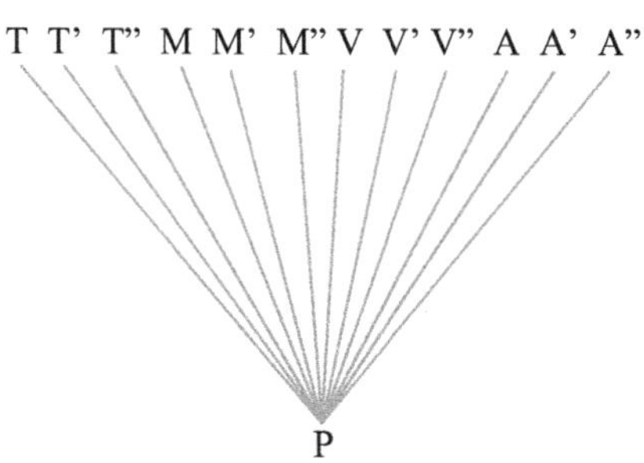

This activity of synthesis, at work during every moment in life, would allow the isolated sensations to be linked to "the group of images and previous judgments constituting the ego or the personality" (Janet, 1889, p. 306). Janet aimed to differentiate said synthesis from the automatic association of ideas. While the former brings together past memories and current sensations, isolated phenomena and the (complex) idea of the *moi* (Janet, 1889, p. 117), the automatic association "is not a current activity, it is the result of an old activity which formerly synthesised some phenomena into a single emotion or perception and which left them with a tendency to occur again in the same order" (Janet, 1889, p. 192).

In other words, we consider it necessary to make two distinctions. On the one hand, the synthesis differed from simple psychical phenomena due to its complex and agglutinating nature, allowing the latter to be brought together to form a "personal" perception. On the other hand, it differed from the automatic association due to its ability to bring together the past and the present in new orders of increasing complexity. In contrast, the automatic play of ideas would suppose a conservative activity that asserted the past and disregarded the current situation (Janet, 1889, pp. 484–485).

According to this schema, the simple elements endowed with consciousness and the past tendencies, remnants of previous syntheses, always coexisted with the current activities of synthesis, even if a changing balance was established between them. Pathological automatisms occurred when the capacity for "creative" synthesis decreased or ceased (Janet, 1889, p. 487). Therefore, two different but related situations could take place. On the one hand, many of the simple phenomena would be recorded but *split off* from the current personality. To the extent that this situation was repeated, these elements could end up inducing the splitting of the personality or the formation of a "second existence", alien to the self (Janet, 1889, pp. 131, 354 and 359).

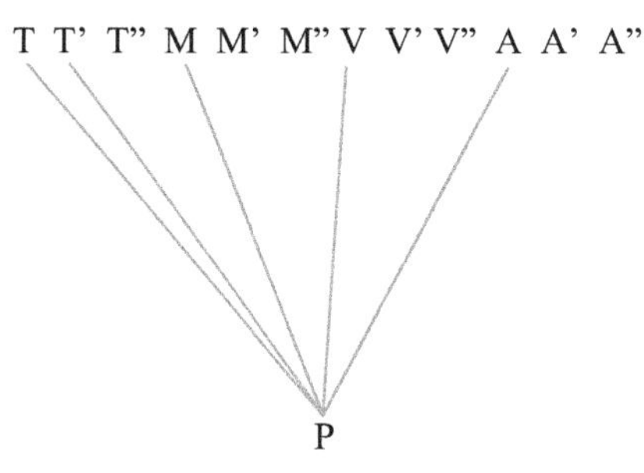

Furthermore, the automatisms would end up imposing themselves: the complex acts would no longer arise as the result of a new synthesis, which would integrate the simple elements with each other and with the self, but as a consequence of the reappearance of tendencies constructed in the past and repeated in the present (Janet, 1889, pp. 485–487).

The axis of Janetian ideas was centred on the subject's greater or lesser ability to group new experiences with the previous ones, the simple elements with the complex ones, and to integrate them into the self or the personality. Illness would occur due to "a weakness in psychological synthesis" (Janet, 1889, p. 364) or, in other words, due to a "narrowing of the field of consciousness" (Janet, 1889, p. 310), understanding the latter as "the largest number of simple or relatively simple phenomena that can occur at the same time in the same consciousness" (Janet, 1889, p. 194).[5] Therefore, for the French philosopher, dissociation was not a mechanism (much less, a "defense", as Van der Hart and Horst proposed) but *the result of this deficient capacity to synthesise.*

This conceptual configuration served Janet to approach the different automatic phenomena mentioned in his book. In the first part, he analysed experimentally (that is, with the use of hypnosis and suggestion) three forms of total automatism, catalepsy, somnambulism and suggestion, phenomena during which normal consciousness and volition seemed to be completely abolished.[6] In all the cases, Janet verified a weakness in the capacity to synthesise simple phenomena into the conscious personality.

But, what provoked these alterations? What was the cause of this disturbance that prevented the synthesis of the past images with the current ones found in the self? Could it caused by a trauma? One of the cases presented in this book could suggest this hypothesis. When Janet questioned Lucie in the third differentiated state of somnambulism ("Lucie 3"), certain childhood memories surfaced that Lucie 1 seemed completely unaware of. Before the age of nine, she experienced great fear when "men hid in the curtains and suddenly jumped on her, an emotion which will form the main scene of all hysterical crises" (Janet, 1889, p. 106). Everything seemed to affirm that the mnemic content that Lucie did not remember but that she repeated in her crises was dissociated from her normal consciousness *due to* the fear or the unpleasure that she felt during the experience....

However, Janet never managed to make a statement of that kind. In those pages, her situation interested him as an example of amnesia linked to muscular anaesthesia that, if overcome, for example, through electrical stimulation, allowed the recovery of the forgotten memories. Nowhere in the book is it possible to find the idea that a trauma could cause a split in consciousness. It was not even given the role of *agent provocateur*. In the subsequent analyses of each of the automatisms, we can find some form of dissociation of consciousness and weakness in synthesis, but without the author establishing a judgement regarding aetiology.

Regarding suggestion, Janet criticised the amplitude that this term had acquired with the Nancy School and restricted its definition to "that influence of one man over another which is exercised without the intermediary of voluntary consent" (Janet, 1889, p. 140), that is to say, without the ego being aware of having approved the influence. In his opinion, if words are addressed to suggestible individuals,[7] they understand them. However, they cannot prevent that they "always determine, without the consent of the person, acts and hallucinations" (Janet, 1889, p. 146). Those words would remain split off from the conscious personality and without the ego being able to intervene.

The same split or disaggregation of the personality was found in his approach to partial automatisms: subconscious acts, anaesthesias, paralysis and amnesias. These phenomena were considered "*as a lesion, a weakening, not of sensation*", which remained intact (whether it was a current sensation or the mnemic image of a past sensation), "*but of the faculty of synthesizing sensations in personal perception, which brings about a real disintegration of psychological phenomena*" (Janet, 1889, p. 314; italics in original). Hysterical patients could often present these phenomena since the "essential characteristic of their illness" would be none other than "the narrowing of the field of consciousness, the diminution of the power of perceptual synthesis" (Janet, 1889, p. 310).

In short, the almost 500 pages of the book constructed a detailed description of automatic psychological phenomena. They outlined an explanation of the mechanism that would determine the latter: the weakness in psychological synthesis, leading to the disintegration of the psyche. However, in no part of the book is the cause of this weakness specified nor does the author mention if a trauma could be involved (as an aetiological factor or, at least, as an *agent provocateur* of a prior disposition). It will only be possible to find some sort of definition in this regard in the period close to the presentation of his medical thesis. At that time, he presented aetiological hypotheses and therapeutic proposals. However, before analysing these topics, we would like to dwell upon Freud's first writings about the neuroses.

2.2 Freud and the Clinic of the Neuroses (1886–1892)

Sigmund Freud was born in Freiberg, Moravia, on May 6, 1856, into a Jewish family.[8] Between 1876 and 1882, he worked in the physiological laboratory of Ernst Brücke.[9] Graduated as a doctor in 1881, he left the laboratory and entered the General Hospital, although most of his work was then concentrated on the study of the nervous system at the Institute of Brain Anatomy. In 1885, he received a scholarship to rotate through Paris and Berlin. That trip greatly contributed to a shift in his career path. The young doctor participated in the activities of the Salpêtrière between October 13, 1885, and February 28, 1886, a period in which Charcot, as we have seen, was working in-depth on hysteria, trauma and the role of emotions and ideas in symptom production. Trained in anatomical research and still interested in such problems, he found himself disappointed by a disorganised laboratory (Freud, 1886a, p. 8), although surprised and, at first, fascinated by the teaching of the French clinician.[10] However, his first works on the neuroses, with undoubtedly Charcotian roots, did not include the novel hypotheses about the mechanisms of symptom formation. Perhaps, for someone trained with Brücke in the strictest locationist discipline, it was not easy to assimilate that "functional" perspective. Even more so, if we bear in mind that Charcot's hypotheses were modelled on a technique, hypnosis, whose inclusion in the field of the sciences was not as common in German-speaking areas as it was beginning to be in France.

In the report presented after that study trip, Freud underlined the prejudices that Charcot had managed to overcome (Freud, 1886a, pp. 10–11). The young Viennese doctor sought to highlight certain aspects of the French clinician's endeavour, some of which we have pointed out in the previous chapter. He especially emphasised the possibility of hysteria occurring in men (Freud, 1886a, p. 11), as well as the establishment of pathognomonic symptoms governed by laws that allowed for a differential diagnosis between organic conditions and simulation (Freud, 1886a, p. 12). As a simultaneous observer of the French and German schools of neuropathology, he pointed out the controversy between the Salpêtrière and certain German physicians, such as Thomsen and Oppenheim (whom he visited on the same trip). In the face of this controversy revolving around "the proposal to regard neuroses arising from trauma ('railway spine') as hysteria", he leaned towards the Parisian view, according to which these clinical pictures did not constitute a specific traumatic illness but should instead be included in the old nosographic category (Freud, 1886a, p. 12).

That same year, Freud presented a monograph (the text of which has not been preserved) and a case entitled "Observation of a Severe Case of Hemi-Anaesthesia in a Hysterical Male" (Freud, 1886b) to the *Gesellschaft der Aerzte* (Society of Medicine). The focus of both texts was the issue of male hysteria. The poor reception of the paper and the lack of interest in the case were interpreted by Freud many years later as an effect of his colleagues' refusal to conceive of hysteria in men (Freud, 1925, p. 15). Frank Sulloway presented an alternative interpretation in this regard: to Freud's superiors, Charcot's ideas, defended by the young doctor in both presentations, were not inconceivable but rather unoriginal (Sulloway, 1979, p. 38). As we have seen in the preceding chapter, many German-speaking physicians were inclined to conceive of post-traumatic symptoms as neurotic and not as the result of somatic illness.

Beyond this historiographic controversy, we are interested in emphasising that the case presented by Freud was organised according to the same sequence followed by his teacher: it began with the family history to later delve into the detailed description of the symptoms and the possibility of diagnostic confirmation. At this point, the paper concluded before discussing any hypothesis about the mechanism that led to the development of the symptoms.

This absence of explanatory hypotheses about the nature of the disturbance-producing process began to be modified in a short encyclopaedia article entitled "Hysteria", published in 1888. The beginning of the text characterised Freud as someone willing to: "be content meanwhile to define the neurosis in a purely nosographical fashion by the totality of symptoms occurring in it", given that it had not yet been possible to find the "physio-pathological formula" that explained the alterations that were at its base (Freud, 1888a, p. 41). It is true that most of the paper emphasised describing in detail the symptoms that were pathognomonic of the disease and that allowed for a differential diagnosis. However, the author was also beginning to test hypotheses about the disease's pathological mechanism and aetiology.

We will begin with the question of the mechanism. Since hysterical symptomatology does "not in any way present a copy of the anatomical conditions of the nervous system" (Freud, 1888a, p. 49),[11] Freud considered it necessary to "dismiss the thought that some possible organic disorder lies at the root of hysteria" (Freud, 1888a, p. 49). Even so, the nature of the pathology was nevertheless nervous: "hysteria is an anomaly of the nervous system which is based on a different distribution of excitations, probably accompanied by a surplus of stimuli in the organ of the mind" (Freud, 1888a, p. 57). This surplus "manifests itself, now as an inhibitor, now as an irritant" of different nervous functions "and is displaced within the nervous system with great freedom" by means of "cerebral" activity, which is "unconscious, automatic" (Freud, 1888a, pp. 49–50). The idea of unconscious brain processes was common in the late nineteenth century, following the works of Laycock, Carpenter, Griesinger and Jackson. At the same time that Janet began to address psychological automatisms without the need to localise them somewhere in the nervous system, Freud seemed to continue to be part of the tradition of the cerebral unconscious. However, this did not exclude (as in the work of Page and Charcot) the possibility of conceiving the role of ideas and emotions in nervous functioning. In this direction, the Viennese doctor maintained that the "conscious or unconscious ideas" distributed the surplus of stimuli that characterised hysteria (Freud, 1888a, p. 57). These hypotheses probably constituted one of the first occasions in which the two basic elements of the Freudian edifice appeared related: certain *ideas*, which would be in charge of displacing, distributing and processing *sums of excitation.*

These two elements were not radically new: the way in which Freud conceived them was familiar to certain physiological schemas that we worked on in the previous chapter. Furthermore, the idea of automatic and unconscious nervous activity was, at that point, common in the field of clinical neurology. Furthermore, as we have seen, the advances in nineteenth-century physiology depended, to a large extent, on the use of electrical energy as an experimental technique and as a model that generated analogies, which allowed emotions to be conceived as "excitations". However, it was not so common to make the distribution of excitations the key to understanding a disease such as hysteria.[12] The same point made it possible to explain spontaneous cures and the therapeutic approaches: "Anything that alters the distribution of the excitations in the nervous system may cure hysterical disorders" (Freud, 1888a, p. 57). A psychical motive (such as the impulse to attack an opponent with a hitherto paralysed hand), an emotion (such as fright) or a convulsive attack could cure the symptoms of hysteria by altering the excitatory distribution. The same principle was valid for explaining seemingly different therapeutic methods. Both Weir Mitchell's procedure (Freud, 1887, p. 55), which combined rest, isolation, massages and faradisation and Josef Breuer's,[13] which consisted in leading "the patient under hypnosis back to the psychical prehistory of the ailment and compel him to acknowledge the psychical occasion on which the disorder in question originated" (Freud, 1888a, p. 56), seemed to depend on the redistribution of energy. This energetic or "*economic*"[14] point of view will remain present in most of the Viennese doctor's work, albeit alternating its preeminence with the "topographical" and "dynamic" points of view.

We would now like to turn to the questions of aetiology and trauma, also addressed in the article from 1888. Although the mechanism of hysteria was explained by energy imbalances, deep down said illness continued to be for Freud what it was for Charcot: "a *status*, a nervous diathesis, which produces outbreaks from time to time. The aetiology of the *status hystericus* is to be looked for entirely in heredity" (Freud, 1888a, p. 50). Only in the presence of heredity, as the only necessary condition and primary cause of the illness, could trauma play the role of an "incidental cause" (Freud, 1888a, p. 51).

The nature of trauma in that text remained ambivalent, as is illustrated by the following sentence: "a hitherto unobserved hysterical dispositing being aroused by a powerful physical trauma, which is accompanied by fright and momentary loss of consciousness" (Freud, 1888a, p. 51). A "physical" trauma seemed to be anatomical, even more so when he immediately added that "the part of the body affected by the trauma" could become "the seat of a local hysteria" (Freud, 1888a, p. 51). Conversely, the affect "fright" suggested the consideration of a psychical dimension; or, at least, it could allow us to think of the role of emotions in a physiological mechanism that also provokes the "momentary loss of consciousness", like in the cases of railway accidents which are "regarded as hysteria by Charcot" (Freud, 1888a, p. 51). At the same time, if the ideas could modify the distribution of the surplus of stimuli, they could also be traumatic or, at least, have a role in the constitution of a traumatic situation.

Be that as it may, two issues were evident in this text: on the one hand, trauma could only cause symptoms if there was a prior hereditary predisposition; on the other hand, there was no connection between trauma and memory, nor was this function prominent in any aspect of hysteria. Nor did the idea of a "sexual" trauma appear in this article. That is to say, Freud considered it necessary to admit "that conditions related *functionally* to sexual life play a great part in the aetiology of hysteria (as of all neuroses),[15] and they do so on account of the high psychical significance of this function" (Freud, 1888a, p. 51; italics in original). It is not entirely clear what the author meant by "conditions related *functionally*" to sexuality: were they ideas of sexual content? Could some type of sexual energy or the participation of sexuality in the production of the energy surpluses typical of hysteria be supposed here? In any case, the "functional" dimension was opposed to the anatomical consideration of the sexual organs, whose role in the development of hysteria is "as a rule over-estimated" according to Freud (Freud, 1888a, p. 50). However, this functional dimension of the sexual sphere was not yet described as "traumatic", nor did the reference to sexuality appear when the author addressed the topic of trauma. Instead, it seemed that the functional conditions of sexuality and certain traumas could operate as *different* provoking agents or incidental causes of hysteria.

In the years to come, Freud alternated neurological works with writings on hypnosis and suggestion. On this subject, although he celebrated the extension of the hypnotic technique, typical of Nancy's supporters, he did not wholly abandon his Charcotian roots. The Viennese doctor found "two opposing camps": those who, like Bernheim, assumed that the hypnotic state would depend on a suggested idea and that, therefore, it would be an entirely psychical phenomenon and those who maintained that hypnosis "is based upon physiological changes -that is, upon displacements of excitability in the nervous system" (Freud, 1888b, p. 77). Freud deduced that if Nancy's partisans were correct, then all the phenomena described in La Salpêtrière would be psychical and products of suggestion, idea that he was not willing to admit since he considered that in hypnosis and hysteria, there were "objective, physiological phenomena" (Freud, 1888b, p. 79). The similarity of the Freudian ideas with the neurophysiology of his time contradicts the theses of Kenneth Levin, who sought to demonstrate the Viennese doctor's early interest in psychology and affirmed that his conceptual schemas would derive exclusively from the psychological thought of Herbart and not from the neurology that founded the cerebral unconscious (Levin, 1985, pp. 82, 107–108).

It was not until the following decade that the Freudian texts gradually delved into the psychological territory and began systematically testing hypotheses about the mechanism at the root of hysterical symptoms. From then on, the notion of trauma acquired in his works an exclusively psychical character and was closely linked to memory.

For example, in the notes he added to his German translation of his teacher's *Leçons du Mardi* (published between 1892 and 1894), Freud argued that: "The core of a hysterical attack (…) is a *memory*, the hallucinatory reliving of a scene which is significant for the onset of the illness" (Freud, 1892–1894, p. 137; italics in original). In other words, the attack was not reduced to the motor, physiological discharge but was organised around the *traces of a past scene*, which had been preserved in memory and which, instead of being evoked via a narrative about the past, were *repeated* in the present in a hallucinatory manner. "The *content of the memory* -Freud continued- is as a rule (…) a psychical *trauma*", which could be defined as "an *accretion of excitation* in the nervous system, *which the latter has been unable to dispose of adequately by motor reaction*" (Freud, 1892–1894, p. 137; italics in original). As is clear from these quotes, the trauma did not act through a mechanical action on a part of the organism but by generating a quantitative surplus and leaving a mnemic mark that was relived in a hallucinatory manner. The quote was short and condensed. Nevertheless, it introduced a series of problems that will remain in force throughout our entire development: What is the nature of the traces left by trauma? How are the memories of a scene and the quantitative excess related to trauma linked? Why would a traumatic memory be accessed via repetition and not through recollection?

In 1893, Freud published an article in French with notable Charcotian roots, which also included one of the first references to the works of Pierre Janet. We refer to the comparative work between organic and hysterical paralyses (Freud, 1893a). After following in his teacher's footsteps and semiologically differentiating both types of paralyses, he began interrogating the nature of the lesion at the root of the hysterical symptoms. We have already seen how Charcot had gone from the idea of the "dynamic lesion" (based on an anatomical model) to that of "traumatic suggestion" (a hypothesis based on hypnosis). Some time later, Janet affirmed that the "lesion" of the hysterical paralyses and other psychological automatisms did not consist in an anatomical alteration but in a disturbance "of the faculty of synthesising sensations in personal perception" (Janet, 1889, p. 314). The Viennese doctor later followed this same path. At times, the text seems to suggest that Charcot – or at least "many who read" his works – continued to believe that a "dynamic lesion is indeed a lesion, but one of which no trace is found after death" that, nevertheless, operated in the same anatomical centre as the "corresponding organic syndrome" (Freud, 1893a, p. 168). However, neither is this statement entirely true (because, as we saw, Charcot also had other hypotheses regarding the mechanism) nor was Freud's position completely original. He was, rather, part of a broader process of conceptual transformation, whereby the idea of a lesion and the nature of hysteria moved further and further away from the anatomy of the nervous system. As he himself acknowledged, some of his ideas were based on Janet's most recent hypotheses, published in the *Archives de Neurologie* (a journal edited by Charcot). Above all, the statement that said hysteria "takes the organs in the ordinary, popular sense of the names they bear" (Freud, 1893a, p. 169) had already been made by his French colleague (Janet, 1892a).[16]

In short, Janet and Freud were attempting to "move into the sphere of (…) psychology" (Freud, 1893a, p. 171) much more clearly than the great clinician of the Salpêtrière. But the Austrian physician did not go much further than his master or his contemporary colleague when he stated that the lesion in hysterical paralyses consisted in "the abolition of the associative accessibility of the conception of the arm" or, in other words, that the idea of that part of the body could not "enter into association with the other ideas constituting the ego" (Freud, 1893a, p. 170). In one and the other, the problem of the dissociation or splitting of the field of ideas was central; a mechanism that led to certain ideas remaining outside the ego, thus operating pathologically outside the subject's consciousness and will.

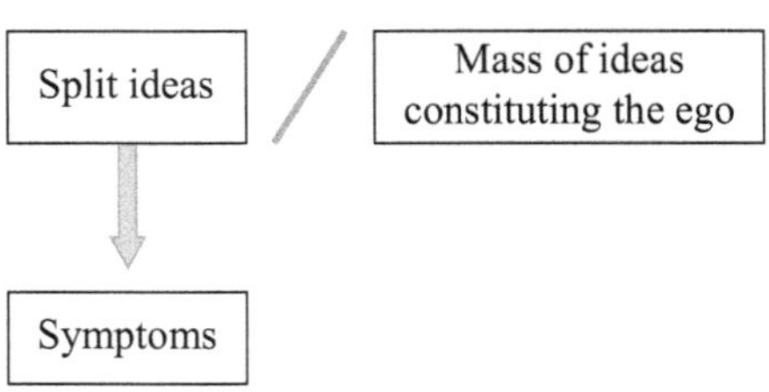

The nuanced distinction between the different authors only appeared in their given reasons for why the association of ideas was impeded. For Charcot, as we pointed out, the emotion caused by the accident generated a state analogous to the hypnotic state, and the ideas introduced in said state could operate as suggestions (or autosuggestions) that could not be opposed by will. For Janet, the splitting was the product of a deficit in the ability for synthesis, whose ultimate causes were not made explicit in his first thesis. In Freud's text, the dissociation of an idea such as that of the arm would be due to the fact that said conception would find itself involved "*in a subconscious association which is provided with a large quota of*

affect" and he added that "*it can be shown that the arm is liberated as soon as this quota is wiped out*" (Freud, 1893a, p. 171; italics in original).

In order to better understand these ideas, the author himself referred to his joint work with Josef Breuer, entitled "On the Psychical Mechanism of Hysterical Phenomena: Preliminary Communication" (Breuer & Freud, 1893).[17] This text, originally published in the Berlin journal *Neurologisches Zentralblatt* and later included in *Studies on Hysteria* (Breuer & Freud, 1895), is central to understanding the first Freudian conceptualisations of trauma, as well as his nascent controversies with Janet.

From the beginning, the authors were willing to extend the Charcotian notion of "traumatic hysteria" (Breuer & Freud, 1893, p. 5). By affirming that all hysterical symptoms had a traumatic origin, the authors shifted their attention from "major trauma" (Breuer & Freud, 1893, p. 6), whose pathognomonic model was undoubtedly the railway accident, and placed it on more insignificant situations, albeit capable of arousing "distressing affects -such as those of fright, anxiety, shame or physical pain" (Breuer & Freud, 1893, p. 6). In general, these situations did not operate in isolation but acquired a traumatic effect by "summation", by forming a "group" that seems to constitute the "components of a single *story of suffering*" (Breuer & Freud, 1893, p. 6; italics added). The trauma was, therefore, not reduced to an exceptional and strange event in the subject's life. Instead, it was constructed around the *plot of a story* whose past milestones were not available to consciousness, even when those memories forgotten by the subject continued to be "actually operative" long after having occurred (Breuer & Freud, 1893, p. 6). The famous phrase "*hysterics suffer mainly from reminiscences*" (Breuer & Freud, 1893, p. 7; italics in original)[18] seems to crown the close *relationship* established between *trauma, history, memory and current suffering.*

However, this relationship was not linear or unidirectional. Although it is clear that the authors assumed a "causal relation between the determining psychical trauma -past- and the hysterical phenomenon -current-" (Breuer & Freud, 1893, p. 6), the event did not determine the symptom on its own. The traumatic effect also depended on the *response* that the subject gave to that experience that aroused the affect. The memories that were at the core of the hysterical symptoms continued to have efficacy long after the event had occurred and did not give in to "the wearing away process to which, after all, we see all our memories succumb" (Breuer & Freud, 1893, p. 8) just because the subject was unable to produce a "reaction" to the experience in such a way that allowed for the affects to be discharged (Breuer & Freud, 1893, p. 8).

For the authors, an adequate reaction (which would allow health to be preserved) implied carrying out *an action*; for example, responding with revenge when faced with an insult. In this way, "a completely 'cathartic' effect" was achieved, which allowed for an affect to be "'abreacted'" or eliminated (Breuer & Freud, 1893, p. 8). However, they also conceived the possibility that *words*, or even the *association* of the memory that arouses affects with other ideas "which may contradict it" could function as substitutes for the motor action and allowed for the discharge of the affects (Breuer & Freud, 1893, pp. 8–9).[19]

In contrast, when "the reaction -through action or its substitutes- is suppressed, the affect remains attached to the memory" (Breuer & Freud, 1893, p. 8), and therefore "we have the possibility of the event in question remaining a psychical trauma" (Freud, 1893b, p. 37). If the equivalence established between action, word and association of ideas is considered, it is more clearly understood why "these experiences are completely absent from the patient's memory when they are in a normal psychical state" (Breuer & Freud, 1893, p. 9): memory and affect remained connected to each other but without being able to be associated with the rest of the ideas. In other words, they would be *split off* from the ego. Therefore, if the idea of the arm (to return to the example of the text on paralyses to which we referred) remained associated with this split idea, then the ego would not be able to make use of that body part at will, and a motor or sensibility symptom would arise. As can be seen, the splitting of consciousness, present in the works of many French doctors, once again played a central role in the mechanism of hysterical symptoms. The authors themselves admitted to agreeing with "Binet and the two Janets" when they made the following observation:

> *the splitting of consciousness which is so striking in the well-know classical cases under the form of* 'double conscience' *is present to a rudimentary degree in every hysteria.*
>
> (Breuer & Freud, 1893, p. 12; italics in original)

Regarding the motives that prevented individuals from reacting adequately to an affect-tinged experience, the authors assumed two series of reasons. First, reasons that were linked to the content of the memories: ideas that made the trauma "irreparable" (Breuer & Freud, 1893, p. 10) or "so great" (Freud, 1893b, p. 38); "ideas to which reaction was impossible for social reasons" (Freud, 1893b, p. 38); ideas that "the patient wished to forget, and therefore intentionally repressed from his conscious thought" (Breuer & Freud, 1893, p. 10). Second, reasons that had nothing to do with the content but with the particular moment in which said ideas, even if they were insignificant, appeared: at that time the subject would find themself in a "hypnoid" state of modified consciousness. In both cases, a "splitting-off of groups of ideas" would come into play, regardless of whether it arose spontaneously due to the existence of a *predisposition* to dissociate or whether it was *acquired* following an accident whose content prevented the reaction and produced the splitting of consciousness (Breuer & Freud, 1893, p. 12). As can be seen, revolving around the axis of the splitting of consciousness, a *tension* began to appear *between the hereditary factors and the accidental factors*, which shortly led to a differentiation of Freud and Breuer's views, on the one hand, and Janet and Freud's, on the other hand, as we will analyse in the next section.

To summarise the ideas expressed in the "Preliminary Communication", we wish to return to the different elements found in this conceptual schema. First, it is clear that the trauma did not operate as a mechanical action that impacted the organism, but it did so due to the memory of the event and the affects aroused. In turn, the traumatic effect depended not only on the experience but also on the absence of a response that would have allowed the generated affects to be discharged[20] and the idea to be associated to the dominant mass of ideas constituting the ego. Although this consideration of the subjective response in the production of the trauma did not completely eliminate the determinism to which the individual experiencing the traumatic situation was subjected, it did introduce a dimension of responsibility (because if they had reacted, the symptoms would not have been produced). It also gave way to the possibility of rectifying the pathogenic effects if the reaction could be provoked afterwards. Therefore, the complete experience of the trauma included both the event's characteristics and the subjective response to it. Finally, this lack of reaction to an affect-tinged idea left the memory separated from consciousness and introduced the symptom in the place of the absent memory.

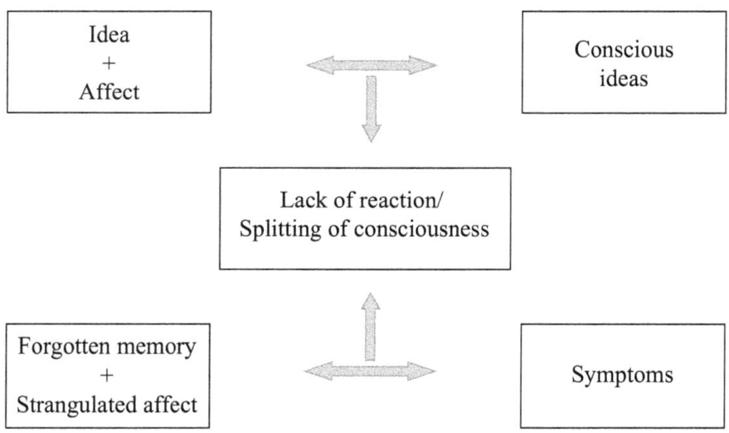

At the same time, the article we have been analysing is highly significant because it included a detailed presentation of a therapeutic approach for treating hysterical symptoms: the "cathartic method" invented by Josef Breuer. Freud had already announced the existence of this method five years prior. However, it had not been considered the treatment of choice even in a paper such as "A Case of Successful Treatment by Hypnotism" (Freud, 1892–1893), published very shortly before the "Preliminary Communication". In this case, Freud resorted only to suggestive commands during hypnosis in order to cure the inhibition of breastfeeding suffered by a parturient woman. The novelty introduced in this article written together with Breuer was not only that cathartic therapy came to be considered the best therapeutic method but also that it was presented as if it had been constructed in close relation to the mechanism of symptoms. The treatment worked by "abreaction"

because it encouraged the patient who experienced a psychical trauma "without reacting to it sufficiently" to "*experience* it a second time, but under hypnosis", forcing them to "complete his reaction to it" which had been absent in the original experience (Freud, 1893b, p. 39; italics added). For both authors, through this procedure, the patient "can then get rid of the idea's affect, which was so to say 'strangulated', and when this is done the operation of the idea is brought to an end" (Freud, 1893b, p. 39).

The method involved the use of memory in the therapeutic process. If the origin of the symptom escaped conscious remembrance because it was split off from the ego, it was only possible to eliminate the pathological disturbance if:

> *we had succeeded in bringing clearly to light the memory of the event by which it was provoked and in arousing its accompanying affect, and when the patient had described that event in the greatest possible detail and had put the affect into words* (...) The psychical process which originally took place must be repeated as vividly as possible.
>
> (Breuer & Freud, 1893, p. 32; italics in original)

That being said, this procedure was different from the act of remembering. If recalling past experiences generally involves a differentiation between the moments of the story and the event, this distinction would seem to be erased during the cathartic process. Many of the terms used in the description of the method underlined that it would be a question of the subject, regarding the psychical process which originally took place, having to, literally, "experience it a second time"; of it being "repeated as vividly as possible".

At the same time, despite the central role given to the splitting of consciousness in the explanation of the pathological mechanism, the therapy seemed to be more focused on the discharge of the affects.[21] When again explaining how the technique worked, the authors argued that the method:

> ...brings to an end the operative force of the idea which was not abreacted in the first instance, by allowing its strangulated affect to fund a way out through speech; and it subjects it to associative correction by introducing it into normal consciousness (under light hypnosis) or by removing it though the physician's suggestion, as is done in somnambulism accompanied by amnesia.
>
> (Breuer & Freud, 1893, p. 42)

As can be deduced from the quoted fragment, the elimination of the affects seemed to be guaranteed; not so much the association of the forgotten idea with the rest of the ideas. This is because, when a memory was recovered during the state of deep hypnosis, its connection with the waking ego (and, therefore, the overcoming of amnesia and dissociation) was not always achieved. Here, we seem to find the reason behind why the possibility of using "the physician's suggestion" remained in this text; its use being intended to eliminate the pathogenic efficacy of an idea by ordering its suppression during the state of somnambulism (as in the case from 1892 to which we referred).

In other words, recovering the forgotten memory did not seem to be the focus of this method, which proposed the repetition of the traumatic situation to enable the discharge of the affects. But also, the presentation of the procedure did not allow an understanding of if it could enable the reaction that had been absent on the first occasion. On the one hand, if the subject had not been able to respond to the affect-tinged experience because they were in a hypnoid state, what guarantees that they could do so in a second hypnoid state, artificially created by the doctor? Would this possible response in the induced hypnoid state be due to the doctor's request for them to react, even though the authors did not refer to this type of suggestion? On the other hand, if the reasons that made the subjective response impossible had to do with the content of the idea (content that made the idea "so great", "irreparable" or that it was one the subject "wished to forget"), how could the reaction be guaranteed during therapy if no attempt was made to modify how the person conceived said content? Would it not be necessary to work on modifying the relationship that had been established between said idea and the ego (or, in other words, work on transforming the subjective position adopted in relation to that idea)?

The problem of repression was addressed by Freud in 1894. When doing so, the tone of the references to Janet was noticeably modified. If, until now, we have seen how the Vienesse physician recognised the similarity of his ideas on the pathogenic mechanism and therapy with those previously held by his French colleague, we will soon be able to observe the beginning of a debate between both authors, which fundamentally dealt with heredity and acquired factors in hysteria and with the way to conceive an effective therapy for hysterical symptoms. This controversy will allow for a better appreciation of their respective conceptions of trauma and memory.

2.3 The Conceptual Debate between Janet and Freud (1892–1894): Weakness or Defence?/Heredity or Trauma?

In 1892, Pierre Janet gave three conferences on hysteria at the Salpêtrière hospital (Janet, 1892a, 1892b, 1892c), which Freud soon commented on in his article on paralyses (Freud, 1893). Those conferences were published the same year in *Archives de neurologie*, a journal directed by Charcot, and were reprinted in 1893, as part of a book called "*L'Etat mental des hysteriques: Les stigmates mentaux*" (Janet, 1893c).[22] In these conferences, Janet mentioned anaesthesia, amnesia and suggestions (diseases of sensibility, memory and will, respectively). Together, they make up the stigmata, or mental states of hysteria that, in contrast to accidents (such as subconscious acts, fixed ideas and somnambulism), should be present in all cases of that illness. In many parts, Janet's intention to present his most innovative ideas in continuity with the thought of Charcot is noticeable. Charcot was not only the director of the Hospital Service where he gave the conferences, but also of the doctoral thesis he was about to present and defend.

Regarding hysterical anaesthesia, Janet argued that these could be systematised, localised or general (1892a, p. 327). He searched for a mechanism common to all of its forms. To this end, Janet used a framework outlined in his first thesis (Janet, 1889) in which sensibility, or the possibility of saying "I feel" (of articulating a new sensation with the "ego"), would imply a "two-moment operation" (Janet 1892a, p. 34). As we have seen, the first moment was characterised by "elementary sensations, affect states (...), subconscious phenomena (...) that are simple, psychological facts, without the intervention of a concept such as that of personality" (Janet, 1892a, p. 341). The second moment entailed a process by which "a grouping was carried out, a synthesis of all the interrelated, elemental phenomena that, in turn, combined with the vast and precursory notion of personality" (Janet, 1892a, p. 341). For Janet, this synthesis was not a "defense mechanism", because he did not believe in the existence of a psychological conflict to resolve. Rather, the synthesis consisted of a normal psychological process that allowed integrating each element to "the groups of previous images and judgments that form the ego or personality" (Janet, 1889, p. 306). From this viewpoint, hysterical anaesthesia did not imply a failure of the first operation ("elementary sensations persist"), but of the second one ("disappearance of personal perception"), due to the "narrowing of the field of consciousness" that would be typical of hysteria (Janet, 1892a, pp. 344–345). This failure made elementary sensations (or elementary memories) remain isolated from consciousness, becoming potentially pathological. Thus, for Janet, "hysterical anesthesia is not (...) an organic disease" but "a disease of the personality" (Janet, 1892a, p. 352).[23]

Concerning memory disorders, Janet stated that "amnesia is very important in hysteria, it is one of the cardinal symptoms of that condition" (Janet, 1892b, p. 30). From his perspective, memory problems constituted "the main factor that intervened, to a greater or lesser degree, in all the other symptoms", such as paralyses, mutism, crises, delusions and somnambulism (Janet, 1892b, p. 30). In other words, memory is not only a function that can be altered by a particular illness, but it is also a factor central to the characterisation of all psychological phenomena. Janet identified two functions of the memory: the "conservation of memories" and the "reproduction–albeit diminished–of [pre-existing] images" (Janet, 1892b, p. 38). Specific amnesias could alter each of these functions. In the case of hysterias, however, neither of these functions was completely compromised. In these illnesses, loss of memory was understood as a problem of the capacity to synthesis. According to Janet, "there is no concrete destruction of elemental psychological phenomena, sensations or images; instead, there is always an impotence, an insufficiency of the synthesizing ability", of the ability to incorporate a past image to the rest of personality. This insufficiency is the reason for which an element is dissociated from a subject's consciousness and can only be reproduced in certain circumstances characterised by automatisms, such as dreams, automatic writing and somnambulism (Janet, 1892b, p. 54).

Janet presented the weakening of the ability to synthesise in his third conference, as a part of an analysis on the use of suggestion in hysteria. The underlying condition that makes the subject vulnerable to suggestion is "of the same nature as anaesthesia and hysterical amnesias" (Janet, 1892c, p. 469). Thus, the failure of the capacity to integrate an elementary sensation from the present, or to integrate an elementary image from the past (stored in the memory) to the group of ideas that make up the ego, leads to a negative phenomenon: the *absence* from personal consciousness of a sensation or a memory. In the case of suggestion, however, the inability to synthesise causes a positive phenomenon: the presence of an idea whose constituting elements (visual, tactile, olfactory, motor, etc.) are present in a manner completely independent from a subject's will. For example, during a hysteric attack, the person not only does not remember a past event in a faithful manner but also "repeats, (…) with extraordinary precision an occurrence, an accident, or an idea" (Janet, 1892c, p. 449). Alternatively, in certain artificially induced suggestions, it could be seen that "some ideas take on enormous importance, repeat themselves, last, manifest themselves through real acts, via objective images of true hallucinations" (Janet, 1892c, p. 452). Through the use of examples such as these, Janet defines suggestion as, "the automatic development of all the elements contained in an idea, development that is produced without the participation of the will or the personality, unrelated to present circumstances" (Janet, 1892c, p. 457). In other words, suggestion depends on a "specific problem of the will", on an "abulia" (Janet, 1892c, p. 469). That is, a weakness of the synthesising power that makes it unable to stop the automatism of associations, since it can no longer integrate pre-existing ideas with the personality nor with the demands of the present situation. As a result, the hysterical subject cannot conduct their behaviour voluntarily but repeats the past. Strictly speaking, there would not be a conflict between past and present,[24] but the former would prevail unmodified because the latter has become powerless to integrate it.

The structuring of all phenomena of the illness around the weakness in synthesis was even more explicit in the article entitled "*Quelques définitions récentes de l'hysterie*" (Janet, 1893a, 1893b). After definitively refuting that all hysterical phenomena could be defined by the mere influence of representations – as upheld by Möebius and Strümpell (Janet, 1893a, pp. 421–423) – Janet introduces a second group of definitions of hysteria that had in common the belief that the most essential feature of the illness was "the splitting of the personality" (Janet, 1893a, p. 426). From this perspective, ideas that emerged during a state of altered consciousness were dissociated from regular consciousness and acquired the strength needed to develop symptoms (Janet, 1893a, p. 435). According to this perspective, the ideas themselves were not central to the production of the pathogenic phenomena since "the strength of these ideas depends on their being isolated" (Janet, 1893a, p. 435). The splitting was the cause that certain ideas became pathologic (as we shall see further on, soon after, Freud would change this principle by stating that the defence against certain ideas would cause the splitting). Finally, Janet included a fragment of his first thesis, where he declared that "the essential trait of this dissociative illness is the emergence, within consciousness, of two groups of phenomena, one that makes up the regular personality, and another one that has a tendency towards (…) the development of an abnormal personality" (Janet, 1889, p. 367, 1893a, p. 436).

Freud's name appeared for the first time in Janet's works in connection with these ideas. For the latter, the "Preliminary Communication" (Breuer & Freud, 1893) was "a text essential to confirm our earliest studies", since the Viennese authors considered that the disposition towards dissociation was a fundamental feature of pathological hysteria (Janet, 1893c,d, pp. 437–438). Janet's first reference to Breuer and Freud's work set the tone for the numerous references that would follow (Dagfal, 2013). At first, the French doctor emphasised that his own ideas on the subject preceded those of Breuer and Freud and, secondly, he sustained that what his colleagues upheld as essential, general or universal only explained some elements of the illness but not all of them. From Janet's perspective, by considering the splitting of the personality as the oldest and most fundamental phenomenon of hysteria, Freud and Breuer were ignoring two factors: on the one hand, that stigmas could not be explained by the dissociation of an idea from the ego (Janet, 1893b, p. 1) and that, on the other hand, the cause of this dissociation continued to remain unknown. For Janet, this dissociation was based on a weakness, "the impotence presented by the subject… to gather and condense his psychological phenomena so as to assimilate them to his personality" (Janet, 1893b, p. 7). "The splitting of the personality" would be "the immediate consequence of this psychological weakness in the ability to synthesize", of this "narrowing of the field of consciousness", that would constitute the primary and most essential element of hysteria, present in all cases and capable of providing an explanation for all accidental phenomena (Janet, 1893b, p. 10).

The central role given by Janet to the weakness in the ability to synthesise allowed him to liken hysteria to another type of illness: psychasthenia (Janet, 1893b, p. 22). Although presenting different symptoms, such as "the delirium posed by doubt, (…) obsessions, impulses, phobias, etc." (Janet, 1893b, p. 22), both hysterias and psychasthenias, shared the same "mechanism", the same psychological "diminished integrative activity" (Janet, 1893b, p. 24). One year before his Viennese colleague, Janet introduced an innovation in traditional nosographic classifications by uniting two semiologically very different pathologies that, nevertheless, share the same pathogenic mechanism.

However, the question remains as to the origin of this weakness preventing the integration of certain psychological phenomena to the rest of the personality. If a traumatic event could cause it, then it is true that Janet was the clinician who "emphasized most forcefully (…) the role of vehement emotions such as terror in response to traumatic events" (Van der Hart & Horst, 1989, p. 403). However, the text quoted above, which summarises Janet's ideas on the subject, as well as those of his contemporaries, stresses the heredodegenerative aspect of the illness:

> Pathogenic inheritance plays in hysteria, as in other mental illnesses, an absolutely fundamental role… we can state that this pathology is a "degenerative

> illness." A great number of circumstances play the role of "provoking agent" and manifest, by means of a series of accidents, this latent predisposition. These are: haemorrhages, anaemic and chronic illnesses, infectious diseases, typhoid fever, organic illnesses of the nervous system, diverse intoxications, physical and moral shocks, shameful emotions and, above all, a series of emotions of this kind.
>
> (Janet, 1893a, p. 27, emphasis added)

Psychological trauma held a tiny place in this long list of provoking agents that manifested a "psychological unfitness" of a hereditary nature (Janet, 1893a, p. 28). Janet, like his predecessors, continued to consider the aetiological question in *hereditary terms. Thus, contemporary authors' claim that the concept of trauma was central to Janet's work is far-fetched.*

Our hypothesis is that Freud, during the same period, followed exactly the opposite path. The time he had spent in Paris during the previous decade had influenced his first works, showing that he was a faithful and dedicated student of Charcot's. Charcot's work attempted to trace the semiological boundaries of hysteria and to find a physiological explanation for the production of symptoms. However, as Freud advanced in his exploration of a pathogenic mechanism and aetiology, the breach between him and his French colleagues widened. At this time, trauma became the privileged means to establish a possible accidental origin of the illness instead of hereditary factors.

The first text where the dispute became evident was "The Neuro-Psychoses of Defence. (An Attempt at a Psychological Theory of Acquired Hysteria, of Many Phobias and Obsessions and of Certain Hallucinatory Psychoses)" (Freud, 1894). Like the "Preliminary Communication", this article was published in the Berlin journal *Neurologisches Zentralblatt.* From its title, we can observe two questions. On the one hand, like Janet, Freud had the intention to liken hysteria with obsessive and phobic disorders, in an attempt to present a psychological mechanism common to both illnesses (even though he did not agree with Janet that what was at stake was a weakness in the ability for synthesis). On the other hand, Freud put forth the possibility that hysteria was an acquired illness and that the "splitting of consciousness" was not a "primary feature of the mental change of hysteria" which was "based on an innate weakness of the capacity for psychical synthesis" (Freud, 1894, p. 46).

The greatest novelty presented in the text was introduced through a new form of the old illness: *defence hysteria.* In this case, the splitting of consciousness would be produced as a "*result of an act of will on the part of the patient*" that comes about when "*an occurrence of incompatibility took place in their ideational life*" (Freud, 1894, pp. 46–47; italics in original). In other words, it would occur to a patient when

> their ego was faced with an experience, an idea or a feeling which aroused such a distressing affect that the subject decided to forget about it because he had no

> confidence in his power to resolve the contradiction between that incompatible idea and his ego by means of thought-activity.
>
> (Freud, 1894, p. 47)

What was then elevated to the status of a particular class of hysteria was insinuated in the "Preliminary Communication" when analysing the reasons why a reaction would be impeded in the face of an experience that aroused intense affects. The authors then said that the lack of response could be due to "things which the patient wished to forget, and therefore intentionally repressed" (Breuer & Freud, 1893, p. 10). One year later, Freud introduced other elements that made it possible to specify the direction his thinking would follow from then on. The "distressing" character of the situation which led the person to "forget about it", was undoubtedly due to an increase in the amount of affect, in the quantities of excitation, which would go against the principle of constancy that Freud assumed governed the functioning of the system. However, it was also due to the "incompatible" nature of the idea whose appearance produced the increment of affect, that is, due to the "contradiction" that this idea introduced with respect to the set of ideas that made up part of the ego. This contradiction caused the pathological mechanism of "defence" to be set in motion.

In this way, Freud introduced something that was not present in his previous writings. The splitting of consciousness to which he often referred assumed the existence of two separate "spaces" that ideas could inhabit: the ego and a second "psychical group" (Freud, 1894, p. 49).[25] By considering the existence of "psychical spaces", Freud gave birth to the point of view usually classified as *topographical*, even when not referring to any anatomical location. The development of an *economic* point of view implies the existence of affects whose increment would be unpleasant and that the psychical apparatus aimed to discharge. What was also added at this time was the *dynamic* point of view, the one that takes the "conflict" into account. This point of view addresses the contradiction that could take place in the field of ideas and the interplay between differentiated psychical agencies).

As an example of these cases of "incompatibility", Freud mentioned the ideas arising "on the soil of sexual experience and sensation", that "chiefly" caused the person's "efforts at defence": the intention of "pushing the thing away, of not thinking of it, of suppressing it" (Freud, 1894, p. 47). In this way, sexuality began to play a more significant role in the Freudian conceptualisation of the neuroses. Moreover, it did so in a particular way: by constituting the attribute, content and quality of certain ideas. By being "sexual", these ideas came into conflict with the ego.[26]

We have seen that the hypothesis about the splitting of consciousness belongs to the French clinical tradition and that the hypothesis about displaceable and dischargeable affects can be linked to neurophysiological research and energy models. What would be the origin of the hypothesis of a psychical conflict? For Paul-Laurent Assoun, "the Freudian dynamic feeds ultimately on a model that was built on a tradition of German psychology that goes back to the early nineteenth century, to (Johann Friedrich) Herbart" (Assoun, 1981, p. 129).[27] The same author summarised some of the main characteristics of the ideas of Herbart, who had proposed a psychology far removed from the traditional psychology of the faculties of the mind. For him, ideas are like elementary atoms of the psyche that imply the constitution of a field of forces (Assoun, 1981, p. 130). "However, the result of this conflict could not be the annihilation of incompatible ideas"; on the contrary: "there is the observable possibility that this or that idea be *repressed* by another" (Assoun, 1981, p. 131; italics in original). Assoun himself specified that Herbart utilised the terms *verdrängen* and *verdrängung*, which would later be used by Freud to define the main defence mechanism. Furthermore, the ideas of this author were quite widespread in Austrian enlightened circles, thanks to the fact that the psychology textbook then used in secondary schools was based on the ideas of Herbart (Assoun, 1981, p. 113; Sulloway, 1979, p. 67). Furthermore, although there is no evidence that Freud had read Herbart directly, many of the latter's hypotheses were taken up and used by German physiologists and psychiatrists, such as Müller and Griesinger, whom Freud read, or Meynert, with whom he worked (Assoun, 1981, p. 134; Sulloway, 1979, p. 67). For all these reasons, it becomes necessary to admit a close relationship between the ideas of Herbart and those of Freud. The former would have functioned as a condition of possibility so that the latter could conceive the idea of a psychical conflict at the base of the neuroses.

We wish to now dell upon the analysis of the pathogenic mechanism of "defence", as outlined by Freud at the time. Faced with an incompatible idea, the ego in "its defensive attitude" aims to treat it as "*non arrivée*": but would fail in its attempt because "the memory-trace and the affect which is attached to the idea are there once and for all and cannot be eradicated" (Freud, 1894, p. 48). The ego would then settle for weakening the intense idea by separating it from its affect. In this case, the idea was not eliminated: it had only been "repressed" or, in other words, split off from the set of ideas of the ego (Freud, 1894, p. 49). From then on, the incompatible idea formed the nucleus of a "second psychical group", making it impossible to be consciously remembered (Freud, 1894, p. 49).[28] And also, "the sum of excitation which has been detached from it must be put to another use" (Freud, 1894, p. 49). In the case of hysteria, it is transformed into something somatic through a process that the author names "conversion" (Freud, 1894, p. 49). In the case of what was later called "obsessional neurosis" (Freud, 1896a), the freed affect attaches itself to other ideas by means of a "false connection", which in turn become obsessional ideas (Freud, 1894, p. 53). In both cases, the pathological phenomenon emerged in the place of repressed ideas and acted as a mnemic symbol of what had been forgotten. The symptom was consequently a pathological way to remember what consciousness attempted to forget.

Moreover, in this text, Freud defined the "traumatic moment" as the instant at which the appearance of an idea incompatible with the ego caused the splitting of consciousness (Freud, 1894, p. 47). This raises the question regarding what the author means by trauma, since his argument places memory in such a central role. One may come to the conclusion that the source of trauma does not depend either on the event or on the intrinsic traits of the idea that is to be repressed. Neither does it depend on a supposed weakness of the subject that experienced the situation. Instead, it would depend on the relationship of incompatibility established between an idea and the group of ideas that make up the ego. If the nature of trauma depends on a relationship, then it is possible to understand why the same situation can be traumatic for some (if it is incompatible with their ego) and harmless for others (for whom the idea is not contradictory). Moreover, this "relational" character of trauma allows us to understand why certain events are often traumatic for many members of the same community, who share the same common ideas.

Finally, as in the "Preliminary Communication", the response given by the subject to the traumatic element was still important. Not all cases led to a "defence" that produced symptoms. In fact, symptoms only appeared in those cases where "the subject decided to forget about it because he had no confidence in his power to resolve the contradiction between that incompatible idea and his ego by means of thought-activity" (Freud, 1894, p. 47). The possible answers were two: forgetting the incompatible idea (which led to neurosis) and trying to solve the contradiction. The German term used by Freud for this second option is *Denkarbeit*, or in other words, thought-*activity* (or even, *mental work*).

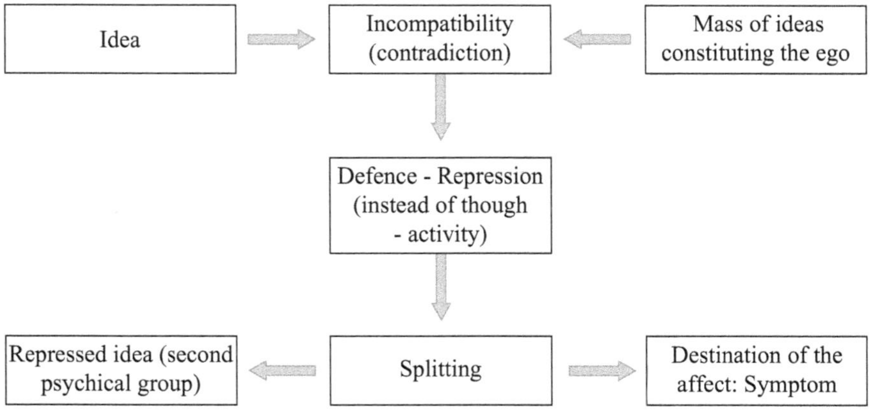

Despite the fact that Freud maintained that the splitting was the consequence of an "act of will"[29] of a person who had "decided" to forget about a contradiction, there are other passages of the text that made the nature of that act more complex. On the one hand, he recognised that it was not possible for him to affirm that "an effort of will to thrust things of this kind out of one's thoughts is a pathological act" (Freud, 1894, p. 48). On the other hand, there were people who "under the same psychical influences, remain healthy" (Freud, 1894, p. 48). What, then, ultimately determines health or illness? "The ability to bring about one of these -anomalous- states (…) is to be regarded – Freud recognised – as the manifestation of a pathological disposition, although such a disposition is not necessarily identical with individual or hereditary 'degeneracy'" (Freud, 1894, p. 48). This paragraph denoted the difficulties Freud encountered when arguing against Janet and the hereditary tradition. To maintain that the splitting of consciousness did not depend directly on an innate weakness but on an act of will only shifted the problem of predisposition and of the ultimate cause of the illness but did not solve it. When faced with a contradiction, the reason why some fell ill and others remained healthy was not a matter of will. There would be a previous condition capable of determining one result or the other. For the time being, Freud was unable to specify that condition.

In the following chapter, we will analyse the theory that Freud presented in 1896 as an alternative to hereditarian theories. However, before that, we would like to study another debate between Charcot and Freud. Thus far, we have only analysed some works where both physicians presented a conceptual exposition of their hypothesis on the neuroses. However, it is also necessary to consider other works that give an outline of their clinical practice, presenting their views on the therapeutic effects of their own practices.

2.4 The Therapeutic Debate between Janet and Freud (1894–1895): When Remembering Is Not Enough

In 1894, Pierre Janet published an article that clearly illustrated certain general clinical headlines that were part of his work throughout his lifetime, despite his constant openness to methodological transformations.[30] The "History of a Fixed Idea" appeared in the *Revue Philosophique de la France et de l'Etranger*, directed by Théodule Ribot. In this paper, Janet presented the treatment of Justine, a 40-year-old woman in whom the fear of cholera appeared as a fixed idea that made her daily life extremely difficult (Janet, 1894b, pp. 121–122). Justine suffered hysterical attacks every time that any reference, albeit remote, was made to something that could be related to the idea of cholera. These attacks included contortions and expressions of terror, followed by amnesia, which could last for hours. Janet considered that, since she was consumed by this idea, Justine was "unable to perceive conscious phenomena nor conserve her memory of them" (Janet, 1894b, p. 124). The clinician decided to "enter, so to speak, in the dream". When Justine says "the cholera, it's going to take a hold of me", I – Janet – reply: "Yes, it took a hold of your right leg" and the patient, who seemed completely dazed and unable to respond to stimuli outside the delirium she was in, violently withdrew her right leg" (Janet, 1894b, p. 124)

By entering the delirium acted out during the attack, Janet was able to "provoke certain responses" and to "slowly direct the spirit towards other subjects", even though upon regaining consciousness the amnesia also relapsed in the conversation (Janet, 1894b, p. 124). In this way, the doctor took advantage of the convulsive and delirious episode to recreate a state of somnambulism (Janet, 1894b, p. 125). He had to be careful when questioning her about cholera "because this question tends to reproduce the state of delirium", but doing so also made it possible to "obtain all the information" he was looking for.

For Janet, during Justine's attacks, the fixed idea of "cholera" was excessively developed the moment that Justine lost consciousness (Janet, 1894b, p. 122). This idea had its origin in the impact generated on her by seeing two cholera-ridden corpses at the age of 17. When asked about how to cure a patient of this fixed idea, Janet used the opportunity to criticise Breuer and Freud's proposals. He stated that they had merely, "Reproduced (…) previous studies of ours on subconscious fixed ideas" (Janet, 1894b, p. 127). According to Janet, the German-speaking authors had concluded that the problem with these ideas was that they had not been sufficiently expressed by the patient and, thus, "in order to cure the patient, the outward expression of these fixed ideas had to be facilitated" (Janet, 1894b, p. 127). In this way, the cathartic method was equated to a "curious need to confess" (Janet, 1894b, p. 127). According to Janet, the effort to get the patient to express their fixed idea was only

> the first and simplest part of the work; a fixed idea is not cured by means of its expression – in fact, quite the opposite. Do Justine's countless attacks not sufficiently express her fixed idea of cholera? (…) could this new expression, this new attack, be considered a cure?
>
> (Janet, 1894b, p. 127)

Thus, it was not enough for the patient to express a remembrance (even less so when this expression took on the form of a symptomatic repetition). Something else was necessary.[31] Could this "something else" be the use of suggestion? Like his Viennese colleagues in "Preliminary Communication", he argued that "proper suggestion, the pure and simple interdiction, can certainly be of service (to us)" (Janet, 1894b, p. 127). Nevertheless, he acknowledged that "the automatic idea of cholera remained stronger than his suggestions" (Janet, 1894b, p. 128). For this reason, he proposed a different procedure that was "slower, indirect, but perhaps more powerful" (Janet, 1894b, p. 128). This procedure made Janet's practice more complex and thus disputed the assumption that his practice consisted of merely recovering a remembrance by converting a "traumatic memory" into a "narrative memory". As Ruth Leys points out, contemporary analyses of Janet's work by authors such as Van der Kolk, Van der Hart or Judith Hermann, which highlighted the importance of remembrance in his work, seemed to ignore an element that Janet considered to be at the heart of his practice: to "make the patient forget" those ideas that were at the core of their symptoms (Leys, 2000, p. 106).

However, the quest for the patient to forget was not a simple attempt to suppress a memory. It could not be achieved merely by means of a suggestive order to not remember that fixed idea. "The fixed idea seems to be a construction, a synthesis of a great number of images", and, in order to reduce its pathogenic potential, it was "necessary to deconstruct it, to destroy or transform its elements, and then, possibly, the group of elements as a whole would no longer be able to subsist" (Janet, 1894b, p. 128). For this reason, Janet treated "the muscle contractions and olfactory hallucinations" separately, in an attempt to suppress them with "an array of suggestive procedures" (Janet, 1894b, p. 128). However, other elements, such as visual hallucinations, remained "indestructible". Thus, after the deconstruction, Janet sought to modify them instead of suppress them (Janet, 1894b, p. 128). In this way, he was able to dress the naked corpses that appeared in each attack and was even able to transform one of them into a Chinese general (whose name would be "Cho-le-ra") that Justine had seen in an exposition. "It was a complete success" when Justine was able to watch the General stand up and march: "he was no longer horrific" but "hilarious" (Janet, 1894b, p. 128).

In short, after having successfully recovered the memory that was at the origin of the fixed idea, Janet took on the work of deconstructing it in order to later suppress or modify its elements, a process much more complex than simply using suggestion (although, this technique still played a central role in his therapy). Furthermore, this work did not include the process of integrating the traumatic memory into the personality. The memory was transformed (a part of it was forgotten and another remained, albeit altered) and, in this process, the effect it produced (or the affect provoked) on the person was also modified: from horrific to hilarious.

When there was no longer any trace in Justine of the scene of the corpses, the only thing left was the word, which made it possible to "ceaselessly confirm the role of language in obsessions" (Janet, 1894b, p. 131). Although no longer suffering attacks, the word continued to impose itself on her (in her thoughts, in her writing) in the form of an obsessive idea or even as an auditory hallucination (she heard an external voice) or verbal kinaesthetic hallucinations (like those described by Seglas; Janet, 1894b, pp. 131–132). All these phenomena denoted a very clear splitting of the personality. In this sense, Justine affirmed: "it is my head that says the word cholera, it is not me" or "*something* says it in spite of me" (Janet, 1894b, p. 132; italics in original). "To make this last symptom disappear -Janet continued-, we use the same procedures of division and substitution" (Janet, 1894b, p. 132). Using the power of suggestion, he transformed the word *cho-lé-ra* into the name of the Chinese general. In automatic writing, he led Justine to write *choclat, coton, coqueluche, cocoriko*, which resulted in her seeing a *coq* – rooster – every time she thought of words beginning with *co*. These "practical procedures" served to "decompose and *destroy the memories*" (Janet, 1894b, p. 132; italics added), to such an extent that Justine no longer remembered the word that had tormented her or, if she came to recall the term, it seemed to her like a foreign word whose meaning was unknown.

As can be seen, the recovery of the memory that was at the root of the fixed idea, which remained forgotten because it was split from the conscious personality and which was repeated (in an identical and hallucinatory manner) in each attack, was far from being an end in itself; rather, Janet was willing to transform and to destroy that memory. *Recover and transform, remember and forget: the therapy consisted of a complex interplay between the two poles of the memory process.*

Twenty-five years later, in one of his most important works, *Les Medications Psychologiques* (1919a,b,c), Janet continued to appeal to a similar model, although the terms had changed: as part of the therapeutic process, some of the past experiences had to be "eliminated" (Janet, 1919b, p. 290). At the same time, others would be "assimilated" into the personality (Janet, 1919b p. 291). Without this process that implies a simultaneous movement between assimilation and elimination, retrieval and transformation, remembering would be impossible. "The individual who maintains a fixed idea of an event does not necessarily remember it" (Janet 1919b, p. 274). Thus, the therapy consisted of eliminating certain aspects of this past experience in order to assimilate it to the subject's personality in the form of a narrative that avoids repetition.

However, neither Ruth Leys nor other authors who have studied the subject pointed out the fact that this clinical perspective – that gave a central role to how the memory processes traumatic experiences – was focused on the treatment of a few accidental symptoms of a neurosis. These symptoms were caused by a fixed idea whose origin could be found in a past experience. Once again, for a past experience to become a fixed idea, a pre-existing deficit was necessary: "The dissociation of certain functions, the loss of unity, the decrease in the ability to synthesise" (Janet, 1894b, p. 150). This was a factor that Janet considered to be fundamental throughout all of his work, from his first doctoral dissertation theses to his final publications. As he put it, "It is precisely this general characteristic that explains the vulnerability to suggestion and the multiplication of fixed ideas" (Janet, 1894b, p. 150). For Janet, the opposite (the idea that a traumatic event could cause dissociation and a failure to synthesise) was incorrect. In fact, the final 12 pages of his 1894 article were dedicated to describing Justine's hereditary background, where there was a "fundamental psychological lesion" present in "all members of the family", which caused "the superior mental functions—the capacity for synthesis—to decrease and disappear" (Janet, 1894b, p. 163). He proceeded to state clearly that the illness was caused by a "mental degeneration" and not a traumatic event, thus dispelling any doubts as to what he identified as being its true origin (Janet 1894b, p. 163). In this way, the interpretation given by Janet outlined a somewhat opposite *image* to what we could read in Erichsen's text: Justine's symptoms were not so much linked to the accident as to her blood ties, which were the cause of the *weakness* that made her powerless to assimilate certain events. Justine *was not a victim of trauma; she was a degenerate with a weakness in synthesis.*

Nevertheless, Janet was "far from considering these hereditary diseases as incurable" (Janet, 1894b, p. 164). In fact, once the symptom upheld by the fixed idea was cured, the most important part of the therapeutic process began: that of the "education of the spirit", a sort of "exercise" to "increase the ability to synthesise" (Janet, 1894b, pp. 151–152).

In short, if the recovery of the memory or its expression were not enough to cure the hysteria, the processes of deconstruction, elimination or substitution of the remembrance would also be insufficient. The cure would require a "spiritual education" whose objective was to increase the mind's ability to synthesise and overcome the inherited weakness that was the cause of the illness. In this way, Janet inscribed his modern psychological perspective within a historical tradition: the educational and hygienist perspective, fond of French hereditarianism.[32]

Although he agreed with Janet about the fact that the recovery of a memory was not enough to cure the neurosis, Freud took a different path. If the splitting of consciousness (provoked by an inherited weakness) were not the cause but the result of a defence against a conflict, the cure would then necessarily require a modification of the conflicting elements. In his early work "The Neuro-Psychoses of Defence", there is a phrase already suggesting this direction. The phrase outlined a cathartic method that introduced an element that had not been included in the previous description of this technique in his Preliminary Communication:

> The operation of Breuer's cathartic method lies in leading back the excitation in this way from the somatic to the psychical sphere deliberately, and in then forcibly *bringing about a settlement of the contradiction by means of thought-activity* [*Denkarbeit*] and a discharge of the excitation by talking.
>
> (Freud, 1894, p. 50; italics added)

The novelty of these statements lies in the need for a certain amount of *mental work* [*Denkarbeit*] to be carried out on the contradiction. If an idea were repressed due to its incompatible nature, finding it and expressing it would not be enough to bring it to consciousness; in fact, it would also be necessary to transform the relationship between the memory and the ego. Otherwise, nothing would prevent it from reappearing and laying the groundwork for a new act of repression. In other words, locating a repressed memory was not sufficient; it was also necessary to modify the stance the repressive agencies took concerning this fragment of the past, considering that those elements certainly played a part in preventing the return of this fragment of the past to the present. At the same time, although the question of the discharge of affect by means of talking remained valid, it is not possible to find in this reference the importance that was previously given to repeating "as vividly as possible" (Breuer & Freud, 1893, p. 6). For this reason, it does not seem risky to affirm that a difference was beginning to be introduced in the Freudian therapeutic conception between the *repetition* or reliving of the trauma (as occurred in spontaneous hysterical attacks or in those provoked by hypnosis) and the *recalling* of it during the treatment (an issue that, as we have seen, was also underlined by Janet).

These affirmations would be mere speculation were it not for the publication of "Studies on Hysteria" one year later (Breuer & Freud, 1895). In that book, the authors presented a series of cases (one carried out by Breuer, the remaining four by Freud) in which we can observe in greater detail the particularities of their practice and their conceptions. We would like to highlight three main points from this extensive work: first, the debate with the French tradition and, in particular, with Janet, regarding the role played by heredity and trauma in causing the illness; second, the wide array of techniques implemented as well as the transformations undergone by the clinical method; and last, the introduction of the problem of resistance against the act of remembering and narrating, an element that became central to Freud's therapeutic and psychopathological framework and that sheds light on his conception of trauma and memory.

With regard to the issue of heredity, the debate with "the French school of psychiatrists" (Breuer & Freud, 1895, p. 87) was present in the case study of the first treatment directed by Freud: that of Frau Emmy von N. The Viennese doctor sought to demonstrate that some of the patient's symptoms, such as her phobias and apathy, "were for the most part of a traumatic origin" and could not be considered "as stigmata of neurotic degeneracy" (Breuer & Freud, 1895, p. 87).

On the other hand, Freud admitted that "the therapeutic process on the whole was considerable; but it was not a lasting one", for it did not eliminate "the patient's tendency to fall ill in a similar way under the impact of fresh traumas" (Breuer & Freud, 1895, p. 101). In doing so, he also had to recognise that Frau Von N "was undoubtedly a personality with a severe neuropathic heredity" since "there can be no hysteria apart from a disposition of this kind" (Breuer & Freud, 1895, p. 102). However, he insisted that there needed to be an effort to avoid the confusion between a predisposition and degeneracy: "To describe such a woman as a degenerate would be to distort the meaning of the word out of all recognition" (Breuer & Freud, 1895, p. 104). If any doubt remained as to whom he was debating with, in the next paragraph the Viennese doctor concluded that he "can see no sign in Frau von N.'s history of the 'psychical inefficiency' to which Janet attributes the genesis of hysteria" (Breuer & Freud, 1895, p. 104).

This questioning of the idea of heredity was also present in subsequent case studies. In the Elizabeth von R. case study, Freud thought he had found "the features which one meets with so frequently in hysterical people and which there is no excuse for regarding as a consequence of degeneracy: her giftedness, her ambition, her moral sensibility… " (Breuer & Freud, 1895, p. 161). Similarly, the Miss Lucy R. case study was presented

> as a model instance of one particular type of hysteria, namely the form of this illness which can be acquired even by a person of sound heredity, as a result of appropriate experiences (…) In cases of this kind, however, the main emphasis falls upon the nature of the trauma, though taken in conjunction, of course, with the subject's reaction to it.
>
> (Breuer & Freud, 1895, p. 122)

In short, for Freud, trauma can cause hysteria without the presence of heredity. Furthermore, trauma does not act only because of its intrinsic characteristics: the subject's reaction to it is also important. *The notion of trauma is not defined in absolute terms but in relative terms*. "It turns out to be a sine qua non for the acquisition of hysteria that an *incompatibility should develop between* the ego and some idea presented to it (…) The actual traumatic moment, then, is the one at which the incompatibility forces itself upon the ego and at which *the latter decided on the repudiation of the incompatible idea*" (Breuer & Freud, 1895, pp. 122–123; italics added).

Thus, Elizabeth's *image* was explicitly opposed to that of degeneracy. If Justine bore the signs of weakness typical of an injury that affected her entire family, Elizabeth represented the image of a *divided subject*, split between the desire for a man and the commitment she had taken on to care for her father.

Leaving aside his discussion with heredity and addressing the problem of a clinical methodology, any interpretation of the text "Studies on Hysteria" can appreciate that the interventions conducted on the patients were not limited to inciting the catharsis of a traumatic memory or the "expression of (…) ideas" (Janet, 1894b, p. 127).

In the case of Emmy von N., Freud carried out interventions far removed from psychotherapy in the classical sense of the term, such as suggesting she have a "warm bath" or "massage her whole body twice a day" (Breuer & Freud, 1895, p. 50). At the same time, he did not use hypnosis and suggestion as a means of retrieving memories but of erasing them. He took this strategy to such an excessive extent that he admitted, in a footnote, that after she had completed the treatment, he ran into Emmy and heard her complain about being unable to access certain significant moments of her life history (Breuer & Freud, 1895, p. 61, footnote 1).

Towards the end of the case, the Vienesse doctor explicitly recognised that abreaction was not yet the only method used during treatment, but rather an addition that was beginning to gain more and more ground. However, it continued to operate together with conventional suggestive therapy:

> As is the usual practice in hypnotic psychotherapy, I fought against the patient's pathological ideas by means of assurances and prohibitions, and by putting forward opposing ideas of every sort. But I did not content myself with this. I investigated the genesis of the individual symptoms so as to be able to combat the premises on which the pathological ideas were erected.
>
> (Breuer & Freud, 1895, p. 101)

At the beginning of the Lucy R. case study, Freud presented the most important change in his methodology up until this point. Whenever the patients stated they were unable to remember the origin of their symptom, the Vienesse psychoanalyst used the following strategy:

> I placed my hand on the patient's forehead and took her head between my hands and said: 'You will think of it under the pressure of my hand. At the moment at which I relax my pressure you will see something in front of you or something will come into your head. Catch hold of it. It will be what we are looking for.
>
> (Breuer & Freud, 1895, p. 110)

Freud's certainty about the existence of an idea and his insistence that it had to be communicated were coherent with his new hypothesis on the role of conflict in the mechanism that produced symptoms. If the "forgetting is often intentional and desired" given the incompatible nature of the idea (Breuer & Freud, 1895,

p. 111), and if "the hysterical patient's 'not knowing' was in fact a 'not wanting to know'" (Breuer & Freud, 1895, pp. 269–270), then the psychoanalyst believed he had enough arguments to state that "under the pressure of my hand some idea occurred" to the patient. "But (…) she was not always prepared to communicate it to me, and tried to suppress once more what had been conjured up" (Breuer & Freud, 1895, p. 153). The technique sought to relieve the patient of the power to decide what to communicate and what to keep silent. When the conflict came into sight, through suggestion, Freud hoped to counteract the inclination towards an act of repression that, in the present, continued to operate in the form of a *resistance* against remembering. Certain gaps in the patient's narratives, their lack of ideas, were not simply the manifestation of a gap in memory; rather, they were a sign of resistance, that is, of an active process that sought to exclude from memory a part of an idea which was incompatible with respect to what was trying to be remembered.

Furthermore, a patient's illness is not made up of one single incompatible idea. In Freud's opinion, it would be rare to find:

> …one symptom only, which has arisen from one major trauma. We do not usually find a single hysterical symptom, but a number of them, partly independent of one another and partly linked together. We must not expect to meet with a single traumatic memory and a single pathogenic idea at its nucleus; we must be prepared for successions of partial traumas and concatenations of pathogenic trains of thought.
>
> (Breuer & Freud, 1895, pp. 287–288)

Therefore, the "clearing away -of- the pathogenic psychical material" was not carried out all at once but rather "layer by layer", being compared to "the technique of excavating a buried city" (Breuer & Freud, 1895, p. 139).[33] Given this complex linking of memories and symptoms, which "corresponds not only to a zig-zag, twisted line, but rather to a ramifying system of lines and more particularly to a converging one" around one or more nuclei (Breuer & Freud, 1895, p. 290), Freud refused to compare the treatment of a neurosis with an extirpation. The objective, rather, would be to cause

> the resistance to melt (…) thus enabling the circulation to make its way into a region that has hitherto been cut off. (…) If the patient does not relax his resistance against it -a pathogenic memory-, if he tries to repress or mutilate it, then (…) the work is at a stand-still (…) until he has taken it -the memory- up into the breadth of his ego.
>
> (Breuer & Freud, 1895, p. 291)

In summary, the act of retrieving what is forgotten due to its conflictive nature is never a simple task, reduced to a mere "expression" or narration of the trauma experienced, nor is it an unproblematic recovery of a past fragment of the memory. The memory was not forgotten due to a lack of interest; in fact, there was an interest in maintaining its status of being forgotten. Thus, the act of remembering involves an interplay of forces, where the admission of an idea is "dependent on the nature and trend of the ideas already united in the ego" (Breuer & Freud, 1895, p. 269). Remembering involved a double effort: that of recovering the past by means of fragments and that of modifying the organisation of the ideas that make up the ego. If the ego continues to find reasons to resist the admission of an idea because of its incompatible nature, then this idea will not be admitted and will once again be forgotten.

This reasoning may further clarify what Freud was referring to when he wrote that, after conducting the quota of affect from the symptom to the repressed idea, a certain amount of "thought-activity [*Denkarbeit*]", directed at overcoming the contradiction was still necessary (Freud, 1894, p. 48). The act of remembering is made possible only by *an activity* that modifies the *conflictive relationship* with a fragment of the past.

2.5 The Debate's Revival, Twenty Years Later (1913–1914)

In 1913, Janet gave a conference on "Psychoanalysis" at the XVII International Congress of Medicine, held in London (Janet, 1914). By then, the French doctor and philosopher was internationally renowned and considered one of the main figures within the world of academic psychology (Dagfal, 2013, pp. 332–335). In this context, the content of his presentation became a sort of "authorised opinion" on a theory and a movement that were rapidly expanding, but that still did not have the recognition that they would only acquire a few years later.

From this long report, we would like to highlight a few points illustrating what Janet understood about the role of traumatic memories and their clinical treatment around 1913. From Janet's point of view, psychoanalysis "accepts, as a proven fact, that in all cases of neuroses, there exists a traumatic memory (...) which is the cause of all the [pathologic] phenomena, which constitutes the illness as a whole" (Janet, 1914, p. 189). On the other hand, Janet considered that:

> Traumatic memories seemed to play an essential role in a great number of the cases, yet it is indisputable that they may not play any role (...) The memory does not act on its own (...) It is necessary, for the memory to pose a threat, that it concurs with a particular mental state (...): the narrowing of the field of consciousness, the weakness in the ability to synthesise, the lowering of psychological tension.
>
> (Janet, 1914, pp. 179–180, italics in original)

It is true that, in this conference, Janet came to admit that "in certain cases – but only in a *certain* few – the depression may have initiated at the same time as the traumatic memory and as result of the same event" (Janet, 1914, p. 180; italics in original). In this sense, he seemed to recognise something that he himself did not admit in 1894: the possibility that trauma could cause psychological weakness.

However, for him, this possibility was more an exception than a rule. In many other cases, "there were no traumatic memories" and it would therefore be necessary to "seek the origin of the depression in the hereditary constitution" (Janet, 1914, p. 181). In contrast, psychoanalysis supposedly maintained that all neurotic symptoms find their cause in the memory of a trauma, for which this doctrine would attribute universal status to that which is only particular.

As we will see in the following two chapters, around 1913, after abandoning his "Seduction Theory", Freud no longer believed that all neuroses had a traumatic origin. However, we are not interested in criticising Janet's inaccuracies. We are trying to analyse the correspondence of his positions with the historiographical accounts we mentioned at the beginning (Van der Hart & Horst, 1989; Van der Kolk & Van der Hart, 1995). We argue that the French philosopher's own ideas, as well as the ones he had about psychoanalysis, went in the opposite direction of the hypothesis of those who have tried to present him as a predecessor of contemporary neurological developments on trauma. In fact, according to Janet, his theory was not centred on trauma, while psychoanalysis was, which was something he strongly criticised.

Furthermore, Janet stated that psychoanalysis implemented only two types of treatments. The first one was the recommendation to engage in "regular and normal intercourse" (Janet, 1914, p. 225), a prescription proposed by Freud towards the end of the nineteenth century as a treatment for neurasthenias and psychoneurosis (Freud, 1895a,b), but that he had already questioned well before 1913 (Freud, 1910). The second type of treatment that, according to Janet, psychoanalysts carried out

> consisted of (…) generalising an application of a type of examination that I myself had indicated in my early studies. I demonstrated that it could be convenient, in certain cases of hysteria, to search for the traumatic memory, which appeared to have been forgotten (…) and guide the subject towards clearly expressing that memory.
>
> (Janet, 1914, p. 225)

This is the same argument put forth almost 20 years earlier. Janet suggested that Freud had merely generalised a part of a treatment that he himself had already proposed. In his opinion, it continued to be true that the expression of a forgotten memory was a "mere preamble (…) Right after, it was necessary to work towards the dissociation of the traumatic memory" (Janet, 1914, p. 225). For him, the "elimination" continued to be "the most difficult part of this type of treatments, for which the search for the subconscious memory was only an introduction" (Janet, 1914, p. 225). Probably in response to the return of this age-old critique, in 1914, Freud published a fundamental text: "Remembering, Repeating and Working Through" (Freud, 1914). "It seems to me not unnecessary to keep on reminding students of the far-reaching changes which psycho-analytic technique has undergone since its first beginnings" (Freud, 1914, p. 147). Whether he was thinking about future therapists or his famous French colleague, Freud presented an overview of the various modifications his practice had undergone with the passing of the years. If, "in its first phase — that of Breuer's catharsis", the technique had been centred on, "remembering and abreacting", the renouncement of hypnosis as a method (declared already in "Studies on Hysteria" in 1895) had given the need for "resistance (…) to be circumvented" a central role (Freud, 1914, p. 147). When, around 1900, the concentration method was replaced by free association, the goal was still the same: "Descriptively speaking, it is to fill in gaps in memory; dynamically speaking, it is to overcome resistances due to repression" (Freud, 1914, p. 148).

In this brief description, the struggle against resistance had already revealed the need for *something other* than the mere expression of a memory in order to complete a treatment. It was followed up by a series of issues that made the nature of memory, and the operations carried out during an analysis even more complex. First, Freud referred to the characteristics of forgetting. Usually, forgetting impressions, scenes or experiences does not indicate a void in memory, but rather, given the conflictive nature of these, it "nearly always reduces itself to shutting them off" (Freud, 1914, p. 148). Counterbalancing the censored scenes, the "screen memories" would retain "all of what is essential from childhood", albeit in a disfigured way (Freud, 1914, p. 148). Finally, there were certain very early childhood experiences from which no memory could be recovered, the reason for which they would always represent a hole regarding recollection. They were those experiences that "were not understood at the time but which were subsequently understood and interpreted" (Freud, 1914, p. 149). However, and above all, they were those which we can only take notice of through dreams or through "the fabric of the neurosis", whose characteristics make one "obliged to believe in them" (Freud, 1914, p. 149). In other words, a complete memory of these scenes would never be obtained; the occurrence of these could only be inferred through a process of construction that makes use of pieces that seem to imply the existence of these scenes. This idea was further developed in the case study known as "The 'Wolf Man'" (Freud, 1918) and in the article entitled "Constructions in Analysis" (Freud, 1937). But in some way, it was already present in "The Psychotherapy of Hysteria" which was a part of "Studies on Hysteria". In that article, Freud stated that

> The whole spatially-extended mass of psychogenic material is in this way drawn through a narrow cleft and thus arrives in consciousness *cut up*, as it were, *into pieces or strips*. It is the psychotherapist's business to *put these together* once more into the organization *which he presumes* to have existed. Anyone who has a craving for further similes may think at this point of a Chinese *puzzle*.
>
> (Breuer & Freud, 1895, p. 291; italics added)

In summary, memory would include three types of complex processes: processes of forgetting, which were a form of shutting off experiences in response to a conflict between opposing forces; screen memories that simultaneously veiled and unveiled the past; and disconnected pieces of scenes that produced effects even if they could never be remembered, but only conjectured or constructed.

However, the point we are interested in highlighting can be found in Freud's affirmation that

> the patient does not *remember* anything of what he has forgotten and repressed, but *acts* it out. He reproduces it not as a memory but as an action; he *repeats* it, without, of course, knowing that he is repeating it.
>
> (Freud, 1914, pp. 151–152; italics in original)

In the times of the cathartic method, the repetition or re-experience of traumas was promoted by the treatment. In 1914, Freud underlined "the part played by resistance" in the

> compulsion to repeat, which now replaces the impulsion to remember, not only in his personal attitude to his doctor -even though the relationship between repetition and transference was here central- but also in every other activity and relationship which may occupy his life at the time.
>
> (Freud, 1914, p. 151)

Even though "remembering in the old manner – reproduction in the psychical field – and not through action – is the aim" of the treatment (Freud, 1914, p. 153), Freud considered it necessary to grant this compulsion to repeat

> the right to assert itself in a definite field. We admit it into the transference as a playground in which it is allowed to expand (…) and in which it is expected to display to us everything in the way of pathogenic instincts that is hidden in the patient's mind.
>
> (Freud, 1914, p. 154)

Only in this way would it be possible to have news of certain repressed pieces of the past. Thus, repetition was not merely a resistance to remembering; it was, at the same time, a pathological, symptomatic way to remember. Likewise, remembering would imply overcoming the resistance that prevented the recovery of the past as such, re-living the past and thus making it present. Finally, psychoanalytic therapy did not simply attempt to encourage the patients to express the past, but also to locate the resistance that made it impossible for them to remember it. In fact:

> Giving the resistance a name could not result in its immediate cessation. One must allow the patient time to (…) work through it [durcharbeiten] (…) This working-through of the resistances may in practice turn out to be an arduous task (…) Nevertheless it is a part of the work which effects the greatest changes in the patient and which distinguishes analytic treatment from any kind of treatment by suggestion.
>
> (Freud, 1914, pp. 155–156)

In other words, therapy was not limited to merely recovering a memory or signalling the resistance; it had to lead to something else: a *work* on the resistances that, in the present, were blocking the acceptance of a fragment of the past.

2.6 Final Comments

Throughout this chapter, we attempted to show that it was Freud – and not Janet – who gave more importance to the issue of trauma, not only in the construction of hypotheses about the causal mechanism of neurotic symptoms but also in the development of a therapeutic method to cure them.

On a theoretical level, both authors conceived the existence of elements split off from consciousness, which formed a system that functioned independently of the ego (a subconscious second personality for Janet, an unconscious system for Freud). They also agreed, on a clinical level, that it was not enough to recover those isolated and forgotten elements to cure the neurosis. Their differences were more subtle and needed to be specified against the backdrop of what those authors had in common.

Even though for Janet and Freud the splitting of consciousness was a secondary phenomenon, the French doctor thought that this splitting was the result of a hereditary weakness in synthesis, while his Viennese colleague proposed an accidental cause: it was the effect of a "traumatic" situation, during which an incompatible idea emerged, which the patient tried to forget.

In other words, for none of the two, the traumatic nature of an idea depended, in any case, on its isolation from consciousness or on its intrinsic value. For Janet, an idea could become pathogenic if and only if it affected an especially predisposed person, with repetitive difficulties to integrate new elements into the ego. This weakness in synthesis preceded the splitting, which made the traumatic factors less relevant. On the other hand, for Freud, an idea became pathogenic because it entered into a relationship of incompatibility with the group of ideas making up the ego. Thus, it was the ego that provoked the repression (and, therefore, the isolation) of the "traumatic" idea. The conflict (and the response given to it by the subject) preceded the splitting, which made the hereditary factors less relevant as a causal agent.

We have shown that these different theoretical positions were correlated to divergences in their therapeutic orientations with regard to trauma. Both authors agreed that it was not enough to recover the memory of a trauma to overcome it. Janet considered that it was also necessary to deconstruct the past idea in fragments, to suppress some of them and to transform some others. However, he thought that the most important task was to strengthen the personality, diminishing its hereditary weakness in synthesis. On the other hand, Freud put the accent on the resistances to remembering. If an idea became traumatic because it was incompatible with the ego, then it was necessary to modify that contradictory relationship, that is to say, to change the subject's response to that idea. In other words, during the treatment, Janet insisted on modifying the past (the old memory and the hereditary predisposition), whereas Freud aimed to modify the present (the current resistance to a fragment of the past).

Notes

1 A preliminary and shorter version of this chapter was published in 2020: Luis César Sanfelippo and Alejandro Antonio Dagfal (2020) The Debate Between Janet and Freud Revisited: Trauma and Memory (1892–1895/1913–1914). *The Psychoanalytic Quarterly*, 89:1, 119–141, DOI: 10.1080/00332828.2020.1688549.

2 The best biographical work on the life of Pierre Janet continues to be the fourth chapter of *The Discovery of the Unconscious: The History and Evolution of Dynamic Psychiatry* by Henri Ellenberger (1970, pp. 378–471).

3 It was a philosophical thesis for a doctorate in letters. In 1893, he defended his medical doctoral thesis entitled *Contribution à l'etude des accidents mentaux chez les hystériques.*

4 "Finally, human activity sometimes presents itself in abnormal forms, incoherent and convulsive movements, unconscious acts ignored by the very person who performs them, impulsive desires contrary to the will and which the subject cannot resist" (Janet, 1889, p. 4).

5 As a sign of evolutionary thinking typical of that time, Janet maintains that: "The individuals whose field of consciousness is abnormally restricted seem to me to form two groups: they are sick or children" (Janet, 1889, p. 196).

6 Partial automatisms imply the presence of automatic phenomena without the self and will being completely abolished.

7 There would be "suggestible" individuals since not all people would be so: only those conditioned by a "narrowing of the field of consciousness" (Janet, 1889, pp. 139 and 190). On this point, he showed his closeness to the Salpêtrière school for which suggestibility was a sign of illness.

8 Unlike Janet's life, there are many good biographies on Freud's (Jones, 1953–57; Roudinesco, 2014).

9 The orientation of this laboratory was quite far from French experimental physiology. As Assoun has emphasised, the procedures carried out there consisted, above all, of the anatomical study of body tissues and in the deduction of their functions based on their location (Assoun, 1981).

10 His fascination can be observed in passages like the following: "it will be understood how it is that the writer of this report, like every other foreigner in a similar position, left the Salpêtrière as Charcot's unqualified admirer" (Freud, 1886a, p. 10).

11 We can mention another sentence that points in the same direction: "It may be said that hysteria is as ignorant of the science of the structure of the nervous system as we ourselves before we have learnt it" (Freud, 1888a, p. 49). This same idea was once again taken up by Freud a few years later, in a text published in French on hysterical paralysis (Freud, 1893a).

12 For example, further above, we saw that Janet placed emphasis on the loss of the ability for synthesis and the consequent disintegration of the personality, and not on the distribution of nervous excitations.

13 Breuer's method was presented by Freud in this article and had not been mentioned in any of the more technical texts devoted to hypnosis and suggestion. Only in 1893 Freud came to publicly admit his adherence to this method that he, however, knew about long before. As Mauro Vallejo pointed out to us, the decade following Freud's visit to the Salpêtrière and the publication of "Studies on Hysteria" is full of hesitations and trials with different therapeutic techniques.

14 In the text "The Unconscious" from 1915, Freud defined the economic point of view as that which "endeavours to follow out the vicissitudes of amounts of excitation and to arrive at least at some relative estimate of their magnitude" (Freud, 1915a, p. 181). To further explore the conceptual roots of said point of view, see Asoun's book, *Introduction à la métapsychologie freudienne* (Assoun, 1981, pp. 143–183). For this author,

the role that Freud attributed to the quantitative dimension inscribed his endeavour in the epistemic problem of many nineteenth-century psychologies: the attempt to overcome Kant's refusal to admit psychology within the field of science because it could not be supported by mathematics. By taking quantities into consideration, which Freud recognised were not measurable but which he aspired to, at least, "arrive (…) at some relative estimate of their magnitude", he linked psychoanalytic thought with the energetic models in force at the time, within the field of psychology (Fechner) and outside of it (Mayer, Helmholtz, Ostwald).

15 They played the part of a triggering factor and generator of the illnesses' symptoms, not as the first cause of the illness and cause of its disposition, since this role was entirely reserved for heredity.

16 This statement was made by the French philosopher in the first of the three lectures that he gave at the Salpêtrière in 1892. His presentation was focused on hysterical anaesthesia and will be worked on in depth in the following section.

17 There is also a lecture given by Freud contemporaneously with the publication of the article, which had the same title: "On the Psychical Mechanism of Hysterical Phenomena" (Freud, 1893b). In it, he presented at a meeting of the Vienna Medical Club the main ideas constructed together with Breuer, almost in the same terms as in the jointly written article.

18 After this quote, which closed the first section of the article, the authors introduced a footnote in which they recognised that it was not possible to distinguish which part of their hypotheses were new and which part could already be found in other authors such as Möebius (1888) o Strümpell (1892). These authors had already suggested that the bodily disturbances typical of hysteria were caused by ideas. Janet pointed this out in a paper that very well described hysteria's state of the art halfway through 1893 (Janet, 1893a,b).

19 Here is an example of associative thinking that allows for the discharge of affects: "After an accident, for instance, the memory of the danger and the (mitigated) repetition of the fright becomes associated with the memory of what happened afterwards – rescue and the consciousness of present safety" (Breuer & Freud, 1893, p. 9).

20 "On the Theory of Hysterical Attacks" is the third of the three manuscripts published under "Sketches for the 'Preliminary Communication' of 1893". In this draft, Freud affirmed that "any impression which the nervous system has difficulty in disposing of by means of associative thinking or of motor reaction becomes a psychical trauma" (Freud, 1892, p. 154). In this context, "disposing of" was equivalent to discharging, as suggested by the statement that the psychical experiences repeated in a hysterical attack were "impressions which have failed to find adequate discharge" (Freud, 1892, p. 154). The difficulties in disposing-of/discharging come from the situation's characteristics and the response (or lack of response) given to it.

21 Much of the conceptual schema presented in the "Preliminary Communication" was based on an assumption not made explicit in the said text, although it was in the draft on hysterical attacks. We are referring to the "principle of constancy", which was defined there for the first time in the following terms: "The nervous system endeavours to keep constant something in its functional relations that we may describe as the 'sum of excitation'. It puts this precondition of health into effect by disposing associatively of every sensible accretion of excitation or by discharging it by an appropriate motor reaction" (Freud, 1892, pp. 153–154). This principle, which linked Freud's thought with energy models and reflex models of the nervous system in force at the end of the nineteenth century, allows us to observe the importance given by the author to the economic point of view in considerations of the functioning of the nervous system and the psychical apparatus. On this point, we disagree with Levin, who, by attempting to move Freud away from neurophysiological thought and towards psychology, maintained that the constancy theorem was derived solely from clinical observations and the tendency to

quantify present in Herbart's thinking, which dispensed with physiology (Levin, 1985, p. 108). The fact that Herbart's ideas made it possible to reconcile the idea of a conflict between ideas with quantification in no way annulled the connection of the principle of constancy with reflex physiology and energy models. As we have already seen, the idea of a shock from an emotion that would deregulate nervous functioning (Page) shares the same terrain of ideas in which said principle is rooted.

22 In turn, in 1893, Janet defended his doctoral thesis in medicine, which was directed by Charcot, and entitled "*Contribution à l'étude des accidents mentaux chez les hystériques*" (Janet, 1893d). In 1894, this thesis was published as "*L'État mental des hystériques. Les accidents mentaux*" (Janet, 1894a). Only in the second edition of *L'État mental des hystériques* were the works dedicated to accidents and stigmata brought together. This editorial precision has already been pointed out by Serge Nicolas (in https://sites.google. com/site/pierrejanet18591947/home/oeuvres) and by Alejandro Dagfal (2013).

23 Anaesthesias were considered "diseases of the personality". We also have disorders of memory and will, which were addressed in the following lectures. It is not by chance that we again come across a system that reminds us of the three works by Théodule Ribot on diseases of memory, will and personality. Outside of the *Archives de Neurologie*, Janet published much of his scientific papers in Ribot's journal, the *Revue philosophique de la France et de l'étranger*. Ribot's works and teaching at the *Collège de France* were fundamental milestones in the conformation of an experimental psychological discipline in France. In 1901, Janet replaced him in the "Chair of Experimental and Comparative Psychology" at the *Collège de France*.

24 The idea of conflict between psychical and temporal agencies was not explicitly raised by Janet but by Freud.

25 Freud did not yet use the term unconscious to refer to the psychical group opposed to consciousness.

26 In parallel, Freud was developing a hypothesis about the mechanism of neurasthenic symptoms and what he came to one year later call "anxiety neurosis" (Freud, 1895a,b). In this field, sexuality did not refer to certain incompatible ideas. Instead, it was understood from an economic point of view and denoted a sum that the psyche could not adequately process.

27 Sulloway makes a similar assessment by considering that "certain (…) features of the Breuer-Freud theory (…) have manifest historical roots in the psychological writings of Johann Friedrich Herbart" (Sulloway, 1979, p. 67).

28 As in Janet's texts, neurotic forgetting would not imply a lack of registration of the psychical fact but rather an inability to connect it with consciousness.

29 Acts of will that are not sustained in later texts.

30 As Dagfal stated, "lacking a unified therapeutic model, Janet resorted, by trial and error, to a whole series of techniques and procedures" (2013, p. 331).

31 As we will see, Freud reached the same conclusion, although his proposals differed.

32 Unlike British hereditary conceptions, which were much more deterministic, in France, both heredity and hygiene were considered important. To address this issue in depth, we again recommend Mauro Vallejo's doctoral thesis (2011).

33 This archaeological metaphor used by Freud to account for psychoanalytic practice and the structure of memories that were at the base of a neurosis, remained in force in his work until the end of his days. Thus, for example, in the paper "Constructions in Analysis" he stated: "just as the archaeologist builds up the walls of the building from the foundations that have remained standing, determines the number and position of the columns from depressions in the floor and reconstructs the mural decorations and paintings from the remains found in the débris, so does the analyst proceed when he draws his inferences from the fragments of memories, from the associations and from the behaviour of the subject of the analysis" (Freud, 1937a, p. 259).

References

Assoun, P.-L. (1981). *Introducción a la epistemología freudiana.* México: Siglo XXI, 1987.

Breuer, J. & Freud, S. ([1893] 1955). On the physical mechanism of hysterical phenomena: Preliminary communication. In Freud, S. (Ed.), *The Standard Edition of the Complete Psychological Works of Sigmund Freud Vol. II: Studies on Hysteria* (pp. 3–47). London: The Hogarth Press and the Institute of Psycho-Analysis.

Breuer, J. & Freud, S. ([1895] 1955). Studies on hysteria, 1893–1895. In Freud, S. (Ed.), *The Standard Edition of the Complete Psychological Works of Sigmund Freud, Vol. II: Studies on Hysteria* (pp. 1–335). London: The Hogarth Press and the Institute of Psycho-Analysis.

Caruth, C. (Ed.). (1995). *Trauma: Explorations in Memory.* Baltimore, MD: The Johns Hopkins University Press.

Charcot, J.-M. (1889). *Clinical Lectures on Diseases of the Nervous System,* Volume III. London and New York: Routledge (2014)

Dagfal, A. (2013). 1913–2013: A un siglo de "El psico-análisis' según Janet. *Estudos e Pesquisas em Psicología, 13* (1), 320–376.

Ellenberger, H. (1970). *The Discovery of the Unconscious: The History and Evolution of Dynamic Psychiatry.* New York: Basic Books.

Freud, S. ([1886a] 1966). Report on my studies in Paris and Berlin. In Freud, S. (Ed.), *The Standard Edition of the Complete Psychological Works of Sigmund Freud, Vol. I: Pre-Psycho-Analytic Publications and Unpublished Drafts* (pp. 5–15). London: The Hogarth Press and the Institute of Psycho- Analysis.

Freud, S. ([1886b] 1966). Observation of a severe case of hemi- anaesthesia in a hysterical male. In Freud, S. (Ed.), *The Standard Edition of the Complete Psychological Works of Sigmund Freud, Vol. I: Pre-Psycho-Analytic Publications and Unpublished Drafts* (pp. 23–31). London: The Hogarth Press and the Institute of Psycho- Analysis.

Freud, S. ([1887] 1966). Two short reviews. In Freud, S. (Ed.), *The Standard Edition of the Complete Psychological Works of Sigmund Freud, Vol. I: Pre-Psycho-Analytic Publications and Unpublished Drafts* (pp. 34–36). London: The Hogarth Press and the Institute of Psycho- Analysis.

Freud, S. ([1888a] 1966). Hysteria. In Freud, S. (Ed.), *The Standard Edition of the Complete Psychological Works of Sigmund Freud, Vol. I: Pre-Psycho-Analytic Publications and Unpublished Drafts* (pp. 38–59). London: The Hogarth Press and the Institute of Psycho- Analysis.

Freud, S. ([1888b] (1966)). Preface to the translation of Bernheim's suggestion. In Freud, S. (Ed.), *The Standard Edition of the Complete Psychological Works of Sigmund Freud, Vol. I: Pre-Psycho-Analytic Publications and Unpublished Drafts* (pp. 75–87). London: The Hogarth Press and the Institute of Psycho-Analysis.

Freud, S. ([1892] 1966). Sketches for the 'Preliminary communication' of 1893. In Freud, S. (Ed.), *The Standard Edition of the Complete Psychological Works of Sigmund Freud Vol. I: Pre-Psycho-Analytic Publications and Unpublished Drafts* (pp. 147–156). London: The Hogarth Press and the Institute of Psycho-Analysis.

Freud, S. ([1892–1893] 1966). A case of successful treatment by hypnotism. In Freud, S. (Ed.), *The Standard Edition of the Complete Psychological Works of Sigmund Freud Vol. I: Pre-Psycho-Analytic Publications and Unpublished Drafts* (pp. 115–130). London: The Hogarth Press and the Institute of Psycho-Analysis.

Freud, S. ([1892–1894] 1966). Preface and footnotes to Charcot's Tuesday lectures. In Freud, S. (Ed.), *The Standard Edition of the Complete Psychological Works of Sigmund*

Freud Vol. I: Pre-Psycho-Analytic Publications and Unpublished Drafts (pp. 130–143). London: The Hogarth Press and the Institute of Psycho- Analysis.
Freud, S. ([1893a] 1966). Some points for a comparative study of organic and hysterical motor paralyses. In Freud, S. (Ed.), *The Standard Edition of the Complete Psychological Works of Sigmund Freud, Vol. I: Pre-Psycho-Analytic Publications and Unpublished Drafts* (pp. 160–172). London: The Hogarth Press and the Institute of Psycho-Analysis.
Freud, S. ([1893b] 1962). On the psychical mechanism of hysterical phenomena: A lecture. In Freud, S. (Ed.), *The Standard Edition of the Complete Psychological Works of Sigmund Freud Vol. III: Early Psycho-Analytic Publications.* (pp. 25–39). London: The Hogarth Press and the Institute of Psycho-Analysis.
Freud, S. ([1894] 1962). The neuro-psychoses of defence. In Freud, S. (Ed.), *The Standard Edition of the Complete Psychological Works of Sigmund Freud Vol. III: Early Psycho-Analytic Publications* (pp. 41–68). London: The Hogarth Press and the Institute of Psycho-Analysis.
Freud, S. ([1895a] 1962). On the grounds for detaching a particular syndrome from neurasthenia under the description 'anxiety neurosis'. In Freud, S. (Ed.), *The Standard Edition of the Complete Psychological Works of Sigmund Freud Vol. III: Early Psycho-Analytic Publications* (pp. 85–117). London: The Hogarth Press and the Institute of Psycho-Analysis.
Freud, S. ([1895b] 1962). A reply to criticisms of my paper on anxiety neurosis. In Freud, S. (Ed.), *The Standard Edition of the Complete Psychological Works of Sigmund Freud Vol. III: Early Psycho-Analytic Publications* (pp. 119–139). London: The Hogarth Press and the Institute of Psycho-Analysis.
Freud, S. ([1896] 1962). Further remarks on the neuro- psychoses of defence. In Freud, S. (Ed.), *The Standard Edition of the Complete Psychological Works of Sigmund Freud Vol. III: Early Psycho-Analytic Publications* (pp. 157–185). London: The Hogarth Press and the Institute of Psycho-Analysis.
Freud, S. ([1910] 1957). Wild' psycho-analysis. In Freud, S. (Ed.), T*he Standard Edition of the Complete Psychological Works of Sigmund Freud Vol. XI: Five Lectures on Psycho-Analysis Leonardo da Vinci and Other Works* (pp. 219–227). London: The Hogarth Press and the Institute of Psycho-Analysis.
Freud, S. ([1914] 1958). Remembering, reapeating and working through (Further recomendations on the technique of psycho-analysis II). In Freud, S. (Ed.), *The Standard Edition of the Complete Psychological Works of Sigmund Freud Vol. XII: The Case of Schreber Papers on Technique and Other Works* (pp. 145–156). London: The Hogarth Press and the Institute of Psycho-Analysis.
Freud, S. ([1915a] 1957). The unconscious. In Freud, S. (1957) (Ed.), *The Standard Edition of the Complete Psychological Works of Sigmund Freud Vol. XIV: On the History of the Psycho- Analytic Movement, Papers on Metapsychology and Other Works* (pp. 159–215). London: The Hogarth Press and the Institute of Psycho-Analysis.
Freud, S. ([1918] 1955). From the history of an infantile neurosis. In Freud, S. (Ed.), *The Standard Edition of the Complete Psychological Works of Sigmund Freud Vol. XVII: An Infantile Neurosis and Other Works* (pp. 1–123). London: The Hogarth Press and the Institute of Psycho-Analysis.
Freud, S. ([1925] 1959). An autobiographical study. In Freud, S. (Ed.), *The Standard Edition of the Complete Psychological Works of Sigmund Freud Vol. XX: An Autobiographical Study. Inhibitions, Symptoms and Anxiety. The Question of Lay Analysis and Other Works* (pp. 1–70). London: The Hogarth Press and the Institute of Psycho-Analysis.

Freud, S. ([1937a] 1964). Constructions in analysis. In Freud, S. (Ed.), *The Standard Edition of the Complete Psychological Works of Sigmund Freud Vol. XXIII: Moses and Monotheism, an Outline of Psycho- Analysis and Other Works* (pp. 255–270). London: The Hogarth Press and the Institute of Psycho-Analysis.

Gauchet, M. (1994). *El inconciente cerebral.* Buenos Aires: Nueva Visión.

Gauchet, M & Swain, G. (2000). *El verdadero Charcot.* Buenos Aires: Nueva Visión.

Hacking, J. (1995). *Rewriting the Soul: Multiple Personality and the Sciences of Memory.* Princeton, NJ: Princeton University Press.

Hartog, F. (2003). *Régimes d'Historicité. Présentisme et expériences du temps.* Paris: Seuil.

Janet, P. (1889). *L'automatisme psychologique: Essai de psychologie expérimentale sur les formes inférieures de l'activité humaine.* París: Alcan.

Janet, P. (1892a). L' anesthésie hystérique. Conférence faite a la Salpêtrière le vendredi 11 mars 1892. *Archives de Neurologie, XXIII* (67), 323–352. Janet, P. (1892b). L' amnesia hystérique. 2' Conférence faite a la Salpêtrière le vendredi 17 mars 1892. *Archives de Neurologie, XXIV* (70), 29–55. Janet, P. (1892c). La suggestion chez les hystériques. 3' Conférence faite a la Salpêtrière le 1er Avril 1892. *Archives de Neurologie, XXIV* (70), 448–470. Janet, P. (1893a). Quelques définitions récentes de l' hysterie. *Archives de Neurologie, XXV* (76), 417–438.

Janet, P. (1893b). Quelques définitions récentes de l' hysterie (2' parte). *Archives de Neurologie, XXVI* (77), 1–29. Janet, P. (1893c). *Etat mental des hystériques: Les stigmates mentaux.* París: Rueff.

Janet, P. (1893d). *Contribution à l'étude des accidents mentaux chez les hystériques.* Doctoral thesis in medicine.

Janet, P. (1894a). *L'État mental des hystériques. Les accidents mentaux.* París: Rueff.

Janet, P. (1894b). Histoire d'une idée fixe. *Revue Philosophique de la France et de l'Etranger, 37*, 121–168.

Janet, P. (1914). El psico-análisis. *Archivos de Ciencias de la Educación, 1*, 175–229. La Plata.

Janet, P. (1919a). *Les Médications Psychologiques. Études historiques, psychologiques et cliniques sur les méthodes de la psychoterapie. Vol 1. L'action morale.* Paris: Alcan.

Janet, P. (1919b). *Les Médications Psychologiques. Études historiques, psychologiques et cliniques sur les méthodes de la psychoterapie. Vol 2. Les économies psychologiques.* Paris: Alcan.

Janet, P. (1919c). *Les Médications Psychologiques. Études historiques, psychologiques et cliniques sur les méthodes de la psychoterapie. Vol 3: Les acquisitions psychologiques.* Paris: Alcan.

Jones, E. (1953–57). *The Life and Work of Sigmund Freud: Volume I, II and III.* New York: Basic Books.

Koselleck, R. (1993). *Futuro pasado. Para una semántica de los tiempos históricos.* Barcelona: Paidós.

Levin, K. (1985). *Freud y su primera psicología de las neurosis.* México, DF: F.C.E.

Leys, R. (2000). *Trauma. A Genealogy.* Chicago, IL: The University of Chicago Press.

Roudinesco, E. (2014). *Sigmund Freud en son temps et dans le notre.* Paris: Seuil.

Sanfelippo, L. & Dagfal, A. (2020). The debate between Janet and Freud revisited: Trauma and memory (1892–1895/1913–1914). *The Psychoanalytic Quarterly, 89* (1), 119–141, DOI: 10.1080/00332828.2020.1688549

Sulloway, F. (1979). *Freud Biologist of the Mind. Beyond the Psychoanalytic Legend.* New York: Basic Books.

Vallejo, M. (2011). *Teorías hereditarias del siglo XIX y el problema de la transmisión intergeneracional. Psicoanálisis y Biopolítica.* Doctoral thesis, UNLP.

Van der Hart, O. & Horst, R. (1989). The dissociation theory of Pierre Janet. *The Journal of Traumatic Stress, 2* (4), 397–412.

Van der Kolk, B. & Van der Hart, O. (1995). The intrusive past: The flexibility of memory and the engraving of trauma. In Caruth, C. (Ed.), *Trauma: Explorations in Memory* (pp.158–182). Baltimore, MD: The Johns Hopkins University Press.

Chapter 3

Sexual Cause and Traumatic Testimonies

The Versions of the Neurotica and Its Abandonment (1896–1933)

In the previous chapter, dedicated to the intersection between trauma and memory, the debate on the aetiology of the neuroses appeared, although in a marginal way. While the French tradition of psychopathology still maintained that hereditary factors constituted the ultimate cause of neurotic illness, Sigmund Freud seemed increasingly determined to defend the acquired nature of these pathologies and to replace the importance given to heredity with the causal power of certain accidental factors.

Nevertheless, Freud found it difficult to justify his aetiological hypotheses. As we have seen, by presenting his theory of defence hysteria, he was disputing with Janet about the nature of the splitting of consciousness. For the Viennese doctor, it was not the immediate effect of an inherited weakness but the consequence of the attempt to forget an incompatible idea. However, he immediately recognised that he was unaware of the reasons why some people remained healthy in the face of the same conflictual circumstances that in his patients led to defence and illness. He then introduced a sentence that clearly showed the problem he was facing and the insufficiency of the answers he had given up until that point:

> The ability to bring about one of these states [hysteria, obsession or hallucinatory psychosis] – which are all of them bound up with a splitting of consciousness – by means of an effort of will of this sort [to forget the incompatible idea].is to be regarded as the manifestation of a pathological disposition, although such a disposition is not necessarily identical with individual or hereditary 'degeneracy'.
>
> (Freud, 1894, p. 48)

What could be, in 1894, a disposition that was not hereditary? If a new hypothesis were not to appear, any nineteenth-century doctor would notice the insufficiency of the Freudian approach and would continue clinging to the certainties that the theory of degeneracy granted in regard to understanding the cause of nervous illnesses.

In 1896, Freud published a series of articles in which he believed he had found the answer to the pending question:

DOI: 10.4324/9781003380016-4

> In my first paper on the neuroses of defence there was no explanation of how the efforts of the subject, who had hitherto been healthy, to forget a traumatic experience of this sort could have the result of actually effecting the intended repression and thus opening the door to the defence neurosis. It could not lie in the nature of the experiences, since other people remained healthy in spite of being exposed to the same precipitating causes. Hysteria, therefore, could not be fully explained from the effect of the trauma: it had to be acknowledged that the susceptibility to a hysterical reaction had already existed before the trauma. The place of this indefinite hysterical disposition can now be taken, wholly or in part, by the posthumous operation of a sexual trauma in childhood. 'Repression' of the memory of a distressing sexual experience which occurs in maturer years is only possible for those in whom that experience can activate the memory-trace of a trauma in childhood.
>
> (Freud, 1896b, p. 166)

This passage shows Freud's attempt to erect an infantile sexual trauma in the place that heredity once occupied. Neuroses would only be developed in adulthood by those people who, during childhood, went through an experience of sexual abuse. This experience became traumatic if its memory was awakened after puberty. In this way, the neuroses came to be considered illnesses of traumatic origin. However, the enthusiasm for these revolutionary hypotheses was short-lived. Only one year and a half after presenting his theory to the public, the Viennese psychoanalyst confessed to his friend Fliess that he no longer believed in his *Neurotica* (Masson, 1985, p. 264).[1]

Since the beginning of the twentieth century, Freud presented different versions of what happened at that early moment in his thought. For many decades, the reconstructions put forward by the creator of psychoanalysis constituted the only available historical material regarding that period of his work. They contributed to consolidating a canonical version of the reasons for the abandonment of his theory. His *Neurotica* would have been disregarded when Freud adverted that his patient's testimonies of childhood traumas did not refer to events that actually occurred but to phantasies.

However, the readings on this period of the Freudian works underwent transformations at three different moments during the second half of the twentieth century. First, in 1951, the first version, partial and reduced, of the letters that Freud had sent to Fliess was published. The material selected for its edition highlighted the journey from general neurological concerns to the clinic of the neuroses and the implementation of the psychoanalytic method. It also showed the emergence of the first hypotheses about the role of the Oedipus Complex, infantile sexuality and phantasies regarding the neuroses. Furthermore, in the introduction to that fragmented epistolary compilation, Ernst Kris gave a name to the hypotheses put forward by Freud in 1896, which have since come to be known as the "Seduction Theory" (Triplett, 2004).

Freud's versions of the period seemed to be reinforced by the 1951 edition of the letters and by the readings promoted by some of the leading figures of the International Psychoanalytic Association: Anna Freud, Ernest Jones and Ernst Kris. Everything seemed to indicate that the episodes of seduction no longer aroused much interest: they would simply be an initial error prior to the great oedipal discovery, thus forcing the scenes recounted by Freud's patients to be considered phantasies.

However, in 1984, the publication of Jeffery Masson's best-seller, *The Assault on Truth. Freud's Suppression of the Seduction Theory* (Masson, 1984), introduced an alternative explanation. Masson was not an outsider to the psychoanalytic movement; rather, he was the guardian of the Freud Archives and, therefore, had access to a large amount of unpublished material inaccessible to the general public. In fact, it was he who, just one year later, led the publication of the complete version of Freud's correspondence with Fliess (Masson, 1985). In this context, his rejection of the official version and his hypothesis that the Seduction Theory had been abandoned due to Freud's cowardice in admitting the existence of child abuse could not go unnoticed. According to his interpretation, Freud did not give up his initial hypothesis because he discovered that the stories he was listening to were phantasies, but because of the fear of the disapproval of his medical colleagues, within a Victorian society that could not see with good eyes to whoever denounced what supposedly happened in the bedrooms of bourgeois families. This version reopened a debate that seemed closed off: do narrations, especially those that refer to a distant past on the scale of a lifetime, refer to events that actually occurred or to phantasised scenes that never took place? Do they correspond to *reality,* or to *phantasy*? Moreover, due to a common shift (which tends to view truth as the correspondence between statements and entities), are they *true* or are they *false*?

Finally, new discussions about the Seduction Theory appeared towards the end of the twentieth century and the beginning of the following century. These arose from a series of (fundamentally Anglo-Saxon) historical investigations that questioned not only the realness of the scenes of abuse but also the very existence of the narratives of seduction allegedly heard by Freud. These works are based on careful readings of certain passages of the papers published in 1896, which were not usually highlighted in the official version of psychoanalytic history or Masson's criticism. If we were to pay attention only to what the founder of psychoanalysis stated in later accounts when he affirmed that "almost all my women patients told me that they had been seduced by their father" (Freud, 1933, p. 120), we might be convinced that these patients spontaneously recounted traumatic childhood scenes. However, the original texts challenge this assumption, as can be seen in the following passages:

> But the fact is that these patients never repeat these stories spontaneously, nor do they ever in the course of a treatment suddenly present the physician with the complete recollection of a scene of this kind. One only succeeds in awakening the psychical trace of a precocious sexual event under the most energetic pressure

> of the analytic procedure, and against an enormous resistance. Moreover, the memory must be extracted from them piece by piece.
>
> (Freud, 1896a, p. 153)

> Before they come for analysis the patients know nothing about these scenes (…) Only the strongest compulsion of the treatment can induce them to embark on a reproduction of them. While they are recalling these infantile experiences to consciousness, they suffer under the most violent sensations, of which they are ashamed and which they try to conceal; and even after they have gone through them once more in such a convincing manner, they still attempt to withhold belief from them, by emphasizing the fact that, unlike what happens in the case of other forgotten material, they have no feeling of remembering the scenes.
>
> (Freud, 1896c, p. 204)

By taking fragments like the ones presented here, several authors rushed to conclusions that can be grouped into two general orientations. On the one hand, they considered that the stories never existed and that Freud derived them from interpretations or reconstructions (Esterson, 2001; Schimek, 1987). Or even that they were inventions made by someone who lied, who lacked integrity (Israel & Schatzman, 1993), who was dishonest (Esterson, 1993), and who had never brought forward evidence of the alleged seduction (Triplett, 2004). On the other hand, they considered it probable that the patients had come to recount the scenes, but that they would have done so due to the suggestive nature of the procedure used by Freud. According to this hypothesis, Freud's procedure led to them "*reproducing* all the scenes that he expected of them" (Borch-Jacobsen, 1996, p. 38; italics in original). In both orientations, the Freudian statements would be *false* because they did not refer to *real* events.

However, we consider that at least three issues have not been analysed in depth by any of these historical versions of the Seduction Theory. First, none of them deeply address what Freud was trying to solve with his hypothesis about the existence of childhood sexual traumas. Whether he made the mistake of interpreting the stories as real events when they were phantasies, whether he did not dare to affirm that they were events that actually took place, whether he constructed specific stories that he never actually heard or produced them by suggestion, we consider it necessary to establish why Freud needed those scenes. In other words, what were the reasons for his enthusiasm when he believed to have discerned them? How did they tie in with his immediately preceding writings? With whom was he arguing, and about what issues? Few authors can take distance from the debates biased by a supposed exclusionary disjunction between reality (truth) and phantasy (falsehood) and investigate the reasons for the importance given by Freud to these hypotheses of 1896. Codell Carter was the first to point out the relationship between these hypotheses and germ theory, the latter having revolutionised European medical thought of the time (Carter, 1980). If the tradition of pathological anatomy had made it possible to better clinically distinguish the different illnesses by anchoring their symptoms to an injured material substrate, and if experimental physiology made it possible to illuminate the functions and better explain the mechanisms behind the pathological phenomena, Pasteur and Koch's innovations had succeeded in imposing the ideal of a strictly causal understanding of pathology. Illnesses had to be distinguished not only by their symptomatic presentation and by their pathogenic mechanism but also by the *specific* cause that gave rise to them. Each cause (for infectious diseases, each germ) could produce only one type of illness; conversely, each illness would have only one noxa. According to Carter, the Seduction Theory constituted an ambitious attempt to transplant this revolutionary aetiological perspective to the field of the neuroses. Many years later, several works by Mauro Vallejo (2011, 2012), Sanfelippo and Vallejo (2013a) attempted to broaden Carter's viewpoint. This was done by relating the Seduction Theory not only with the new infectious theories but also with the medical sphere bound to neuropathology and with Freud's growing interest in aetiology in his early texts on the neuroses. In this chapter, we set out to deepen these previous developments.

First, we will try to demonstrate that Freud's "*Neurotica*" was important for him because he expected it to be a great discovery in the field of aetiology. Furthermore, he believed his theory could function as the missing piece of a puzzle he was obsessed with throughout those years: the "Project for a Scientific Psychology" (1895d). If the temporality he outlined regarding childhood sexual trauma were correct, then it would be possible to explain the problem of repression or pathological defence, which was one of the main unresolved issues of the Project.

Second, we will attempt to explain the conception of trauma that emerges from the texts of 1896. In them, the founder of psychoanalysis established a complex link between lived events, memory-traces, memories, ideas and sums of affects. According to this conceptual configuration, childhood experiences of abuse were not traumatic due to their mere occurrence but because, after puberty, their memory-traces were linked to an idea that aroused them. To explain this process, Freud introduced the *nachträglich* temporality. This hypothesis prevents conceiving the relationship between experiences and symptoms in terms of linear causality. In this sense, we will try to explain that the power of determination granted to events that actually occurred already had nuances even before the doubts regarding the veracity of the testimonies and the problems around phantasies were introduced.

The third issue we propose to develop in this chapter refers precisely to the opposition between reality and phantasy. Is it true that Freud first privileged reality and then denied its importance after discovering phantasies? Does the relationship between the two terms of the debate consist of an exclusive disjunction? Undoubtedly, in Freud's writings, some references seem to establish a clear opposition between experiences and phantasies. However, many other references make it necessary to question this idea, which is quite widespread both among detractors of psychoanalysis (who, as we saw in the previous chapter, consider that Freud privileged a supposed internal world to the detriment of lived contingencies) and among certain psychoanalysts (who repeat the canonical version that states that Freud abandoned his *Neurotica* after discovering phantasies). As we shall see, in many texts, Freud did not establish a disjunction but a *conjunction* between phantasy and reality.

In short, in this chapter, we seek to address the three issues neglected by the different versions of the *Neurotica's* abandonment, in order to account for the transformations of the Freudian notion of *trauma* in regards to the problems of aetiology, *nachträglich* temporality and the relationship between reality and phantasy. At the end of this development, we will find ourselves on the verge of the final significant issues linked to trauma in the Freudian work: on the one hand, economic disturbances and the limits of representation (regarding the War Neuroses); on the other hand, collective traumas and their intergenerational transmission.

3.1 "Neurotica": A General Theory of the Neuroses Centred on Aetiology

3.1.1 A Mechanism That Does Not Define Aetiology: A Non-Causal Therapy

In the preceding chapter, we developed some features of Freud's work prior to 1896 that allowed us to see his relationship with the French neuropathological and hereditary tradition. In general terms, it could be affirmed that, immediately after his stay at *La Salpêtrière*, Freud seemed to be very close to this tradition, mainly due to his attempt to delimitate the neuroses based on symptoms and the search for the underlying pathological mechanism. However, he gradually began to distance himself from the Charcotian legacy (as we pointed out, starting in 1894, with his first controversies with Janet).

The basis for the distancing revolved around the issues of heredity and aetiology. In 1888, Freud still fully adhered to the teachings of Charcot when he stated that hysteria must be regarded as a *status* whose aetiology "is to be looked for entirely in heredity" (Freud, 1888a, p. 50). A few years later, he published "A Case of Successful Treatment by Hypnotism" (Freud, 1892–1893), demonstrating the efficacy obtained by using suggestion to treat symptoms. However, he also recognised the limits of the therapy. Through the use of hypnotic suggestion he was able to help his patient overcome the inhibition that impeded her from breastfeeding her second child, but he could not prevent the same symptom from reappearing following the birth of her third child. As the Vienesse doctor did not theorise about the issue of the ultimate cause of the neuroses, his treatment remained limited to the symptoms, but he could do nothing regarding the patient's disposition to fall ill.

The paper written alongside Breuer in 1893 illustrates this problem. The authors insisted that the causes of neurotic phenomena were accidental, that is, traumatic. However, it is necessary to read the text carefully to elucidate what exactly a trauma could *cause* in a case of hysteria. We can observe the authors' intention that certain symptoms, once considered signs of a pathological inheritance, be conceived as the direct consequence of trauma.

> External events determine the pathology of hysteria to an extent far greater than is known and recognized. (...) *Our experiences have shown us, however, that the most various* ***symptoms****, which are ostensibly spontaneous and, as one might say, idiopathic products of hysteria, are just (...) strictly related to the precipitating trauma.*
>
> (Breuer & Freud, 1893, p. 4; italics in original; bold added)

However, we consider it necessary to emphasise that in these references, the traumatic event was interpreted as being the cause of the *symptoms*, of the hysterical *phenomena*, but *not of hysteria itself*. An event can provoke symptoms only in those cases where predisposition for the illness existed. It is necessary to distinguish the *phenomenon* (the symptoms and the splitting-off) from the *illness itself* (hysteria) to understand the conclusion of the two versions of *On the Psychical Mechanism of Hysterical Phenomena*:

> Thus *we cure – not hysteria but some of its individual symptoms* – by causing an unaccomplished reaction to be completed (...) *Hysteria, like the neuroses, has its deeper causes*; and it is those deeper causes that set limits (...) to the success of our treatment.
>
> (Freud, 1893, p. 39; italics added)

> It is of course true that *we do not cure hysteria in so far as it is a matter of disposition.* (...) we cannot conceal from ourselves that this has brought us nearer to an understanding only of the mechanism of hysterical symptoms and *not* of the *internal causes of hysteria.*
>
> (Breuer & Freud, 1893, p. 17; italics added)

As we have seen in the previous chapter, by 1894, the signs that indicated his change of attitude regarding heredity and aetiology increased significantly. The subtitle of his article "The Neuro-Psychoses of Defence" is quite eloquent of the direction that Freudian thought was taking: "An Attempt at a Psychological Theory of *Acquired* Hysteria, of Many Phobias and Obsessions and of Certain Hallucinatory Psychoses" (Freud, 1894, p. 41; italics added). In that article, Freud defended the existence of acquired neuroses, and he explicitly criticised Janet for assuming an innate weakness in cases of hysteria. From his perspective, the splitting of consciousness was a phenomenon secondary to the appearance of a psychical conflict. However, as we have stated at the beginning of this chapter, a margin of disposition remained in force, since he could not explain why some people remained healthy after facing the same incompatible situations that made others fall ill (Freud, 1894, p. 48). A disposition should therefore exist in those who became ill. Moreover, for it to be plausible that this disposition was not equivalent to heredity, it would be necessary to construct an aetiological theory that would take its place.

He was unable to construct an alternative theory throughout the following year. For this very reason, he made statements such as the following: "At any rate, 'similar heredity' is often enough found in obsessional cases, as in hysteria" (Freud, 1895a, p. 79). Or he continued to admit the same type of limits to his therapeutic practice: "-the cathartic method- cannot affect the underlying causes of hysteria: thus it cannot prevent fresh symptoms from taking the place of the ones which had been got rid of" (Breuer & Freud, 1895, p. 261).

However, in the chapter from *Studies on Hysteria* entitled "The Psychotherapy of Hysteria" (Breuer & Freud, 1895, pp. 253–312) the framework of what would be completed in 1896 appeared for the first time. Here, Freud began to conceive the possibility that each differential clinical picture of the neuroses (hysteria, obsessional neurosis, neurasthenia, anxiety neurosis) corresponded to a specific aetiology:

> In the first place I was obliged to recognize that, in so far as one can speak of determining causes which lead to the *acquisition* of neuroses, their aetiology is to be looked for in *sexual* factors. There followed the discovery that different sexual factors, in the most general sense, produce different pictures of neurotic disorders. And it then became possible, in the degree to which this relation was confirmed, to venture on using aetiology for the purpose of characterizing the neuroses and of making a sharp distinction between the clinical pictures of the various neuroses. Where the aetiological characteristics coincided regularly with the clinical ones, this was of course justified.
>
> (Breuer & Freud, 1895, p. 257; italics in original)

There are several points to underline in the preceding paragraph. First, the conditional and cautious tone that reigns throughout it, which contrasts enormously with the texts that made up his *Neurotica*. Only in 1896 would Freud believe in having obtained the certainties that one year prior were still set to be "confirmed".

Second, we want to underline the role of *sexual* factors in the aetiology of the neuroses. Until now, sexuality, once an obligatory reference in regard to hysteria (due to the role given to the uterus since ancient times; or to the ovary since the middle of the nineteenth century), was not common in Freudian publications. We have seen that in the article "Hysteria", he referred to functional sexual factors but reduced their influence to the role of an *agent provocateur* of an illness conceived hereditarily (Freud, 1888a). Furthermore, this reference appeared in the context of a general criticism towards the importance given in the past to sexuality regarding said illness.

This marginal role given to sexuality was not modified in the publications of 1893. Only on a few occasions did Breuer and Freud allude to this topic in the writings of that year. They did so, first, when giving examples of situations that impeded the reactions that would allow for the discharge of affect. Second, when referring to situations that could produce a splitting of consciousness without a previous disposition. The "sexual affect" is brought forward as an example of the "laborious suppression", which led to dissociation (Breuer & Freud, 1893, p. 38). As can be seen, sexuality was just one example among others.

Sexuality indeed acquired a much more prominent place in "The Neuro-Psychoses of Defence" (Freud, 1894). As we have underlined, Freud maintained that, in the case of hysterical women, the incompatible ideas which generated the conflict with the ego and aroused the defence, "arise chiefly on the soil of sexual experience and sensation" (Freud, 1894, p. 47). He also affirmed that "in all the cases" of obsessional neurosis he had analysed, "it was the subject's sexual life that had given rise to a distressing affect" and that led to repression (Freud, 1894, p. 52). However, it could not be ruled out that "this affect should sometimes arise in other fields" (Freud, 1894, p. 52). Thus, sexuality was not yet considered the ultimate cause of *all* cases of neurosis; this shift took place in 1896. Precisely, the cited paragraph from "The Psychotherapy of Hysteria" shows an intermediate moment, because even though Freud considered sexuality to be a fundamental element of the aetiology of the neuroses, he limited the reach of his statements to the cases in which he considered the causes were acquired.

We would like to highlight a third point from the paragraph of 1895. Freud stated there that "different sexual factors (…) produce different pictures of neurotic disorders" (Breuer & Freud, 1895, p. 257). This quote is the first reference of Freud's attempt to apply an aetiological *model* that, thanks to the works of Pasteur and Koch, was beginning to prevail throughout general medicine. Obviously, we are not claiming that Freud assumed that a germ could cause neuroses. What he took from this model is the skeleton, the formal relations, and not its content. Thanks to this he was able to conceive that a single causal factor could correspond to each neurosis. However, this idea was first applied to the "actual" neuroses before it could be applied to the neuro-psychoses of defence.

3.1.2 Aetiology in the "Actual" Neuroses

The first Freudian references to a sexual aetiology of the neuroses correspond to *neurasthenia* and *anxiety neurosis*, as well as the first attempts to discuss the role that was usually given in the field to heredity.

Between 1892 and 1894, Freud produced and published the German translation of the *Lecons du mardi de la Salpêtrière*, which Charcot gave between 1887 and 1888. He added a series of controversial footnotes in these writings that questioned some of his teacher's statements. Also, in these footnotes, he presented a double thesis for the first time: the ('actual') neuroses had a sexual origin, and a different sexual factor caused each clinical picture. Below we include some quotes that exemplify what was stated:

> All these -Charcot's- aetiological discussions on questions of neurasthenia are incomplete so long as no consideration is given to sexual noxae, which,

> in my experience, constitute the most important and only indispensable aetiological factor.
>
> (Freud, 1892–1894, p. 142)

> The more frequent cause of agoraphobia as well as of most other phobias lies not in heredity but in abnormalities of sexual life.
>
> (Freud, 1892–1894, p. 139)

In his translation, it is probable that the most significant attack on Charcot's hereditary theses did not occur in the field of the "actual" neuroses nor the domain of the neuro-psychoses. In the eighth footnote of the original German edition (which is not included in the standard edition of the Complete Psychological Works), the Viennese doctor discussed the aetiology of Tabes. There he stated that, at first, he agreed with his teacher that heredity was the cause of this illness and that syphilis would merely be an *agent provocateur*. But later, after discovering the theories of Fournier and Erb, he turned against the opinion of the great French clinician: syphilis was the true cause of the illness (Charcot, 1894, n.8).

The opinions Freud expressed in the translation's footnotes provoked anger in the Salpêtrière doctor. In a letter dated June 30, 1892, which has been studied in depth by Tony Gelfand, Charcot communicated to the Vienesse doctor his impression regarding the editorial task carried out by the latter and, above all, criticised the content of certain footnotes (Gelfand, 1989). The controversy did not revolve around the role attributed to sexuality but rather around the questioning of heredity as the cause of the neuroses. One of the points the old master questioned the most was the adherence of his former disciple to the theory that established syphilis as the specific cause of nervous diseases such as Tabes and general paralysis. Charcot continued to think that syphilis (and, as Gelfand puts it, also microbes and, by analogy, the sexual factors that Freud refers to with regard to neurasthenia and phobias – Gelfand, 1989, p. 302) were *external* elements that could only function as *agents provocateurs*. Thus, the *internal* cause of the illness was a hereditary disposition. With these arguments, Charcot once again reaffirmed the same belief in hereditary doctrines and the same resistance to admitting the veracity of Pasteur's, Koch's or Fournier-Erb's theories.

As can be seen, for Charcot, the main point of the Freudian "rebellion" was found in the aetiological discussion and not in the problem of sexuality. Would the same be true for his disciple? Is it not true that the "reaction of distaste and repudiation" (Freud, 1914a, p. 12) that Freud received in those years was due to his theses on sexuality?[2] It is true that, in 1914, when Freud wrote "On the History of the Psycho-Analytic Movement" (Freud, 1914a), sexuality was the subject of debate. Freud, who had become the teacher and head of the movement, reproached Jung for his tendency to relativise the importance of sexuality in psychoanalysis. But, during the first five years of the 1890s, was sexuality the main driver of the controversy that Freud intended to establish in the field of the clinic of the neuroses? Or, as Charcot read in the footnotes of the translation, was Freud beginning to be interested in discussing the "more-than-thousand-year-old problem" (Masson, 1985, p. 184, letter of 26/04/1896) of aetiology?[3]

Before fully addressing these questions, we must return to Freud's writings on the "actual" neuroses. In "Draft A", sent to Fliess at the end of 1892 (Masson, 1985, pp. 37–38), Freud put forward the following theses:

1 No neurasthenia or analogous neurosis exists without a disturbance of the sexual function.
2 This either has an immediate causal effect or acts as a predisposition to other factors, but always in such a way that without it the other factors cannot bring about neurasthenia (Masson, 1985, p. 38).

The passage is interesting because of its universal character: all cases of neurasthenia and analogous neurosis would suppose a sexual alteration that served as the cause. But, it is also important because it was the first time that a sexual element was erected not only as the cause of the symptoms but also as the cause of the *disposition* to the illness. If a sexual disturbance could have a predisposing effect, then it could be given the formal role traditionally given to heredity: that of being the *zero point* of the illness. In other words, it is not the starting point of clinically observable phenomena but, rather, the point that becomes necessary to assume at the origin, the condition of possibility for the development of all other pathological phenomena; the true beginning of the series. Nevertheless, in this text, there were still no references to an aetiological model that relates each clinical picture to a specific cause.

"Draft B" was written on February 8, 1893, and was entitled "The Etiology of the Neuroses" (Masson, 1985, pp. 39–44). Despite the breadth of the title, only two clinical pictures were studied in this draft: neurasthenia and anxiety neurosis. It so happens that in those years Freud used to reserve the term *neurosis* for what he later called "*actual*" *neuroses*. The draft began by considering that "neurasthenia is a *frequent* consequence of an abnormal sexual life" (Masson, 1985, p. 39; italics added). However, he immediately extended his claim and made explicit that the assertion he wished to confirm "is that neurasthenia actually can *only* be a sexual neurosis" (Masson, 1985, p. 39; italics in original). In other words, he aimed to demonstrate that neurasthenia was *always* (and not just frequently) a consequence of sexual disturbances.

However, Freud recognised that he could not distinguish if "what appears to be hereditary neurasthenia" was in fact a product of hereditary disposition, of toxic influences, or of "early sexual exhaustion" (Masson, 1985, p. 40). It is worth clarifying that, in this context, "early sexual exhaustion" did not refer to episodes of seduction but, rather, to practices considered harmful, such as masturbation. This, however, did not prevent him from affirming that "sexual exhaustion can by itself alone provoke neurasthenia" (that is, without the influence of heredity) and that "if it fails to achieve this by itself, it (…) predisposes the nervous system" (Masson, 1985, p. 40).

The same reasoning was applied to anxiety neurosis. After raising the following questions:

> "(1) to what extent this condition emerges in hereditary cases, *without* any sexual noxa, (2) whether it is released in hereditary cases by any chance sexual noxa, (3) whether it supervenes as an intensification in common neurasthenia", he affirmed that "there is no question but that it is acquired (…) through coitus interruptus."
>
> (Masson, 1985, p. 43; italics in original)

As can be observed, despite the oscillations and the impossibility of totally ruling out the role of heredity, Freud tended to emphasise more and more the causal role that certain sexual elements had in the production of neuroses. However, he still had not established a one-to-one correspondence between the aetiological factor and the clinical form, since, for example, coitus interruptus could be considered a possible cause of both conditions.

During 1893 and 1894, Freud did not publish any articles on these types of neuroses, although he did make important publications on the neuro-psychoses of defence and even on strictly neurological problems (such as the text, unpublished in English, on infantile paralysis entitled *Zur Kenntnis der cerebralen Dinlegien des Kindesalters*). However, references to neurasthenia and anxiety neurosis were common in the correspondence with Fliess. Near the end of 1893, Freud took a further step towards the conception of a mechanism and an aetiology for anxiety:

> Altogether I have hit upon the idea to tie anxiety not to a psychic but rather to a *physical* consequence of sexual abuse. I was led to this by a wonderfully pure case of anxiety neurosis following coitus interruptus in a totally placid and *totally frigid* woman.
>
> (Masson, 1985, p. 61, letter of 27/11/93; italics in original)

Anxiety, therefore, was not rooted in psychical sensations but rather in the accumulation of somatic tension due to coitus interruptus.

This conclusion was reaffirmed and amplified in Draft E, entitled "How Anxiety Originates", which was supposedly written in June of 1894 (Masson, 1985, pp. 78–83). Many of the ideas that would one year later be expressed in the first publication on the subject were found in it. The different situations of people in which anxiety arose ("virginal" people, abstinent people, those who practise coitus interruptus, etc.) were unified, because in them "an accumulation of physical sexual tension" was present (Masson, 1985, p. 79). When the tension grew past a certain threshold, it was deployed psychically, that is, it entered "into relation with certain groups of ideas, which then set about producing the specific remedies", which in the case of sexual tension would be coitus (Masson, 1985, p. 80). If something (such as the situations previously mentioned) were to interrupt this process that was considered normal, then "the psychic linkage offered to it remains insufficient" since it would not lead to the discharge of the excitation through coitus, and "accordingly, the physical tension, not being psychically bound, is transformed into – anxiety" (Masson, 1985, pp. 80–81).

In summary, while he was publicly presenting the psychical mechanism that produced the neuro-psychoses of defence, Freud was also beginning to conceive a physiological mechanism to account for anxiety neuroses. This double movement allowed him to begin developing a nosography in which the clinical pictures were differentiated not only by the syndromes that characterised them but also by the mechanisms that produced these symptoms. In addition, around the same time, he was drafting for the first time an overview of the aetiology of all the neuroses that made up said nosography. In a letter to Fliess from May 1894, he highlighted the aetiological value of sexual factors. However, he continued to maintain the possibility of heredity being decisive in some cases, as can be observed in the following quote:

> In every case in which neuroses are acquired, it happens as a result of sexual disturbances, but there are people in whom heredity causes a disturbance of their sexual affects and who develop the corresponding forms of hereditary neurosis.
> (Masson, 1985, p. 74, letter of 21/05/94)

On January 15 1895, the article "On the Grounds for Detaching a Particular Syndrome from Neurasthenia Under the Description 'Anxiety Neurosis'" (Freud, 1895b) was published. The reasons that justified the distinction between these two syndromes were found in their symptomatologies, mechanisms and aetiologies (Freud, 1895b, p. 91). Above all, we wish to dwell upon the issues that concern these last two points.

Regarding aetiology, Freud continued to admit the possibility that in some cases "there is seldom any difficulty in establishing evidence of a grave hereditary taint" (Freud, 1895b, p. 99). However, his whole analysis was focused on neuroses acquired from "a set of noxae and influences from sexual life" (Freud, 1895b, p. 99). For neurasthenia, the pathognomonic aetiological condition would be masturbation (Freud, 1895b, pp. 102–109). Anxiety neurosis would instead be caused by abstinence, coitus interruptus or other sexually equivalent conditions (Freud, 1895b, pp. 102–106). This was the first text in which Freud assigned a *specific* aetiology to each one of these clinical pictures.

Regarding the mechanism, although in both syndromes it is explained in relation to somatic sexual excitation, it was also possible to establish a difference between them. Neurasthenia would develop due to an *inadequate unloading* of the sexual excitation. Anxiety neurosis would be produced by an *excess of somatic excitation* which, by not being able to be worked over psychically, "is expended subcortically" in the form of anxiety (Freud, 1895b, p. 109).

To finish with the analysis of this text, we wish to identify the Freudian category of *mixed neuroses*. From his perspective, the presence of anxiety in other neuroses should not annul the specificity of each clinical picture, since it would in fact be due to an "*intermixture of several specific aetiologies*" (Freud, 1895b, p. 113).

As we stated in the introduction of this chapter, on the horizon of this Freudian operation regarding the aetiological problem of the neuroses, was his yearning to adapt these always uncertain illnesses to a model in "vogue in German medicine (…) Many diseases that had previously been defined only by their symptoms could now be defined by the microbes that caused them" (Hacking, 1995, p. 193). Each one of the various and specific sexual noxae that cause each neurosis were considered *analogous* to each one of the different microorganisms that cause different infectious diseases.

The second text on the "actual" neuroses was written in response to criticisms made by Leopold Löwenfeld (Freud, 1895c). In this text, Freud described for the first time the complete and complex aetiological schematic picture that he later repeated in the writings of his *Neurotica*. A specific clinical picture was considered the effect of the following combination of aetiological conditions:

> The factors which may be described as *preconditions* are those in whose absence the effect would never come about, but which are incapable of producing the effect by themselves alone (…)
>
> The *specific cause* is the one which is never missing in any case in which the effect takes place, and which moreover suffices, if present in the required quantity or intensity, to achieve the effect, provided only that the preconditions are also fulfilled.
>
> As *concurrent causes* we may regard such factors as are not necessarily present every time, nor able (…) to produce the effect by themselves alone, but which operate alongside of the preconditions and the specific cause in satisfying the aetiological equation.
>
> (Freud, 1895c, p. 136; italics in original)

When exemplifying this aetiological schematic picture, Freud made clear his intention to make it comparable with the microbial theories of Pasteur and Koch, which were gaining more and more ground at the end of the nineteenth century:

> *Effect:* Phthisis pulmonum.
>
> *Precondition:* Disposition, for the most part laid down through heredity, by the organic constitution.
>
> *Specific Cause:* Bacillus Kochii.
>
> *Auxiliary Causes:* Anything that diminishes the powers – emotions as well as suppurations or colds.
>
> The schematic picture for the aetiology of anxiety neurosis **seems to me to be on the same lines**:
>
> *Precondition*: Heredity.
>
> *Specific Cause:* A sexual factor, in the sense of a deflection of sexual tension away from the psychical field.
>
> *Auxiliary Causes:* Any stock noxae – emotion, fright and also physical exhaustion through illness or over-exertion.
>
> (Freud, 1895c, p. 137; italics in original; bold added)

Apart from the explicit comparison, it should be noted that heredity has not disappeared. It could be thought that it would keep its long-standing status of being a necessary condition, a zero point needed for the rest of the aetiological factors to be included in the illness' causation. This is true, Freud did not entirely exclude this possibility, but he greatly relativised it:

> Whether a special personal constitution (*which need not be produced by heredity*) is absolutely necessary for the production of an anxiety neurosis, or whether any normal person can be made to have an anxiety neurosis by some given quantitative increase of the specific factor – this I am not able to decide with certainty; but I incline strongly to the latter view.
>
> (Freud, 1895c, p. 137; italics added)

We find in this sentence the same acknowledgement of a margin of uncertainty found in earlier texts. However, here the scales are noticeably tipped to one side. The disposition is not necessarily hereditary, and if the specific factor is strong, anyone could develop the illness. In case there was any doubt, in the sentence following the one previously quoted, Freud affirmed that "Hereditary disposition is the most important precondition for anxiety neurosis; but it is not an *indispensable* one, since it is absent in a class of borderline cases" (Freud, 1895c, p. 137; italics in original). Instead, the *specific* sexual factor was the only one found in *all* cases, and it was the condition that differentiated one clinical picture from another. It was the zero point from which all the other factors found their place and function in the causation of the ills.

Additionally, unlike heredity, this specific cause granted therapy more importance. Freud began to believe in the possibility that, once the aetiological factor was eliminated, the illness's effects would cease. In this way, for the first time, the Viennese physician was approaching the hope of constructing a therapeutic approach based on causality that was not restricted to the elimination of symptoms.

However, this entire schema was unbalanced for two reasons. First, because it could not yet be applied to the neuro-psychoses of defence. It was only in October 1895, in a private letter from Fliess, that the first explicit mention of the sexual factors that differentiated the cause of each neuro-psychosis of defence appeared (Masson, 1985, pp. 150–151, letter of 8/10/1895).

Second, this schema was also unbalanced because neurasthenia and anxiety neurosis were clinical pictures that could present psychical symptoms, despite which they were explained in physiological terms. The same did not happen with hysteria and obsessional neurosis. The explanation was "limited" to being psychological. In a context where the physiological approach to disease had great prestige, this would appear to be a glitch.

Perhaps due to this reason, he attempted to "explain defense, (...) to explain something from the very core of nature!" (Masson, 1985, p. 136, letter of 16/8/1895). This sentence sums up the first purpose of his "Project for a Scientific Psychology" (Freud, 1895d): to find for the neuro-psychoses of defence the physiological explanation that he had already found for the other two neuroses. Therefore, this Project was an attempt to find the *aetiological* reasons for defence: why do some people fall under the effects of repression and neuroses, and others, when faced with the same circumstances, do not?

Freud's hopes to construct a complete nosography which followed the model of infectious diseases and included aetiology merged with his dream of finding an explanation for the pathological processes, consistent with physiological medicine. Both yearnings required a hypothesis that would account for the specific causes of the neuro-psychoses of defence. His *Neurotica* would be the missing piece of this puzzle.

However, before diving into this, we will analyse Freud's physiological obsession in the Project.

3.1.3 The Project for a Scientific Psychology

"Psychology"[4] was, without a doubt, passionately written. Freud felt plagued by it (Masson, 1985, p. 123, letter of 28/03/1895); it regularly consumed him until he was overworked (Masson, 1985, p. 127, letter of 27/04/1895). He devoted "every free minute" to it for weeks and spent "the hours of the night from eleven to two with such fantasizing, interpreting and guessing" (Masson, 1985, p. 129, letter of 25/05/1895). He also, at times, attempted to persuade himself that the "cross to bear" that he had taken up was no longer of his interest (Masson, 1985, pp. 135–136, letter of 16/08/1895). Finally, on October 8, 1895, he finished outlining and sent his friend the only surviving manuscript. That was the same day that the first reference to his *Neurotica* appeared. Moreover, he kept expanding and modifying his speculative physiology in numerous later letters.

Our purpose is not to explain the theses from the Project but, instead, to limit ourselves to the points connected to the *Neurotica*. Freud began his manuscript by proposing the existence of neurons in the nervous system and of a quantity (Q) that circulates through them. To this, he added the hypothesis that the system tends towards the discharge of Q, or at least to keep the amount as low and constant as possible.[5] Following on from this simple beginning, Freud classified the neurones into three groups: *phi* (in charge of receiving the quantity from the external world), *psi* (they receive the quantity exclusively from the internal world and are modified by it, the reason for which they were linked to the function of memory), and *omega* (which give rise to the perception of conscious qualities). The passages of quantity through the psi neurons leave *traces*, in the form of facilitations, increasing the probability of Q following the same path the next time.

In Part II of the *Project*, entitled "Psychopathology" (Freud, 1895d, pp. 347–359), Freud took it upon himself to explain in physiological terms the problem of pathological defence, which had, up until then, only been explained in psychological terms. From his perspective, "clinical experience" taught that: "First, repression is brought to bear invariably on ideas which evoke a distressing affect (unpleasure) in the *ego*, secondly on idea(s) from sexual life" (Freud, 1895d, p. 350; italics in original). But why would *only* sexual ideas evoke unpleasure in the ego and put repression into operation? Could it be because of their intensity? Freud flatly ruled out this possibility:

> It is quite impossible to suppose that distressing sexual affects so greatly exceed all other unpleasurable affects in intensity. It must be another characteristic of sexual ideas that can explain how it is that sexual ideas are alone subjected to repression.
>
> (Freud, 1895d, p. 352)

Being interested in demonstrating this particularity of sexuality, which would make it the only area capable of provoking pathological defence, Freud embarked on the exposition of a clinical case. The symptom of his patient, Emma, consisted in being subject to "a compulsion of not being able to go into shops alone" (Freud, 1895d, p. 353). Linked to this symptom was the memory of an event that took place shortly after puberty, when two shop assistants had laughed at her due to her clothes. Following that first scene, a second memory emerged, from a time prior to puberty and not remembered by her until then. She recalled a shopkeeper having grabbed at her genitals through her clothes. Scene I "unconsciously" aroused the memory of the earlier one (Scene II) (Freud, 1895d, p. 354). This memory did not, however, cause the sexual idea to enter consciousness, but rather, it "aroused what it was certainly not able to at the time, a *sexual release*, which was transformed into anxiety (Freud, 1895d, p. 354; italics in original). When it comes to *sexual* experiences that took place in *childhood*, these would be the only cases "of a memory arousing an affect which it did not arouse as an experience, because in the meantime the change (brought about) in puberty had made possible *a different understanding of what was remembered*" (Freud, 1895d, p. 356; italics added). If a current situation in adult life were to arouse the memory of a sexual scene from childhood, greater unpleasure would be produced (a greater release of Q in the nervous system) than that produced in the original experience. This is explained by the fact that the person's condition changed (thanks to the level of sexual development that had been absent in childhood), allowing them to *resignify* the memory. Previously insignificant, the latter "has only become a trauma by *deferred action*" (Freud, 1895d, p. 356). In the following section, we will analyse in greater detail this deferred temporality, which was outlined by Freud in the Project and is central to his *Neurotica*. However, before that, we wish to continue exploring the reasons for repression.

So far Freud had explained a characteristic of childhood sexual experiences: the memory of them in adulthood generates an unpleasant reaction that had not been present at the time of their occurrence. However, why would this (and not a non-sexual experience) lead to repression, even when its non-sexual counterpart is capable of releasing unpleasure when it occurs? Having reached this point, Freud embarked on a complex explanation of the differences between normal and pathological defence:

> If the trauma (experience of pain) occurs (…) at the time when there is already an ego, there is to begin with a release of unpleasure, but simultaneously the ego

> is at work too, creating side-cathexes. If the cathexis of the memory is repeated, the unpleasure is repeated too, but the ego-facilitations are there already as well; experience shows that the release (of unpleasure) is less the second time, until, after further repetition, it shrivels up to the intensity of a signal acceptable to the ego. It is therefore only a question of the ego's inhibition not being absent at the *first* release of unpleasure, of the process not occurring as a posthumous primary affective experience; and this (condition) is precisely fulfilled if (...) the memory is what first brings about the release of unpleasure.
>
> (Freud, 1895d, p. 359)

Any situation capable of producing unpleasure would push the ego to create side-cathexes, allowing the excitation to be discharged. This process would produce connections (facilitated "pathways of passage" – Freud, 1895d, p. 358) between the memory of the experience (and its unpleasure) and the side-cathexes (which alleviated the unpleasure). These connections work so that in every successive recollection of the memory, the arousal of unpleasure would become increasingly inhibited. This normal defensive process would not be possible in cases where the unpleasure was only released posthumously due to the recall of the memory and not during the experience. When "what has appeared is no perception but a *memory*, which unexpectedly releases unpleasure, and the ego only discovers this too late", the ego will not be able to produce the inhibitory side-cathexes that characterise normal defence: the path towards repression is opened (Freud, 1895d, p. 358).

This explanation is probably insufficient. In the letter with which he sends the notebooks containing the manuscripts of "Psychology" to Fliess, Freud confessed to his friend that "it does not yet, perhaps never will, hang together. What does not yet hang together is not the mechanism (...) but the elucidation of repression, the clinical knowledge of which has in other respects greatly progressed" (Masson, 1985, p. 141). The physiological hypothesis explaining the reasons for repression did not seem to satisfy the psychoanalyst. However, his expected means of answering the fundamental aetiological question ('why do some fall ill while others do not?') immediately shifted from neurological speculations to his patients' narratives. In order to dethrone heredity, Freud needed to find in these narratives certain elements that would simultaneously explain the defence ('why do they repress and fall ill?') and the choice of neurosis ('why do they develop hysteria or obsessional neurosis?'). In the same epistle where he announced to his friend that he had sent him the "Project", the founder of psychoanalysis also announced the first version of his new hope:

> Just think: among other things I am on the scent of the following strict precondition for hysteria, namely, that a primary sexual experience (before puberty), accompanied by revulsion and fright, must have taken place; for obsessional neurosis, that it must have happened, accompanied by pleasure.
>
> (Masson, 1985, p. 141)

Sigmund Freud would later call this new hope his *Neurotica*.

It did not take long for the conjectures that he had been on the scent of towards the end of his "Project" to reach public exposure. On the 14th, 21st and 28th of the same month of October 1895, Freud gave a lecture entitled "On Hysteria", in which he laid down a good part of the foundations on which his Seduction Theory would stand. This conference has reached us in the form of two extensive summaries, written anonymously and only partially translated into Spanish by Mauro Vallejo (Sanfelippo & Vallejo, 2013a). In these presentations, Freud put forward an idea that he had, until then, only conjectured in his "Psychology". We refer to the hypothesis that states that the nature of the experiences which caused the disposition to the neuro-psychoses and that determined the operation of repression would be not only *sexual* but also *infantile.* For example, in the presentation on October 21, Freud said: "When one examines the distressing causal impressions (of hysteria) it can be observed that they all include sexual content" (Anonymous, 1895a, p. 335). One week later, he completed that argument by referencing childhood: "As far as could be determined, in hysteria it was always possible to find ideas corresponding to sexuality, and the first repressions had always taken place in the period prior to puberty" (Anonymous, 1895b, p. 349). Also, in that lecture on hysteria, another element appeared that ended up playing a central role in the theory he developed in depth the following year. We refer to the possibility of the therapy modifying not only the symptoms but also the disposition to develop the illness:

> If one considers, therefore, just how limited the conditions for the emergence of repression are: of sexual nature, originated in the period prior to puberty, the linking of new symptoms to the repressions originated in childhood; the hope that if the first repression were to be found and annulled then the source of the later symptoms obtured in a long-lasting manner, is justified.
>
> (Anonymous, 1895b, pp. 350–351)

For the *Neurotica* to be complete, Freud only needed to make explicit what he had already imagined on October 8: the *distinct and specific* aetiological factor that would cause each clinical picture. It did not take long for this element to be featured in a publication.

3.1.4 The Neurotica: An Aetiological Theory That Explained Repression

The three papers in which Freud made his *Neurotica* public were written and published in 1896:

- "Heredity and the Aetiology of the Neuroses" (Freud, 1896a). Published in French in *Revue Neurologique* on March 30 and sent for editing on February 5.
- "Further Remarks on the Neuro-Psychoses of Defence" (Freud, 1896b). Published in the journal *Neurologisches Zentralblatt* on May 15 and sent for editing on February 5.

- "The Aetiology of Hysteria" (Freud, 1896c). Published in the journal *Wiener Klinische Rundschau* between May 31 and June 28, based on a lecture on April 21 for the Society of Psychiatry and Neurology.

As can be seen, the reference to aetiology was explicit in the title of two of these papers. In the other paper, the problem of aetiology was central, although its title did not announce it. As we stated at the beginning of the chapter, "Further Remarks" allowed Freud to return to his first paper on "The Neuro-Psychoses of Defence" to justify better the supposed existence of a disposition that was not hereditary. If his *Neurotica* were sustainable, the zero point could then be found in "the posthumous operation of a sexual trauma in childhood" (Freud, 1896b, p. 167). Repression and neurosis in adult life could only occur in people who had lived through this type of experience in their childhood. At this point, Freud believed he had achieved what he longed for: an alternative aetiological theory for hysteria and obsessional neurosis.

At the same time, it is possible to trace in different passages of the publications of 1896 the relationship of this theory with the "Project's" purpose of explaining defence. The main argument did not differ very much from the one presented in that manuscript. Freud recognised that it would be logical to assume that an event should generate a greater effect of excitation than a memory. However, a sexual experience in childhood would produce "little or no effect at the time" (Freud, 1896a, p. 154), given the subject's biological immaturity and lack of symbolic resources to comprehend what had happened. At that time, Freud did not yet conceive infantile sexuality as universal; rather, that a child was to go through a sexual experience was considered a contingency that left a predisposing mark. If the memory of the experience is awakened during or after puberty, it "will operate as though it were a contemporary event" (Freud, 1896a, p. 154), or rather, it will produce the "inversion of relative effectiveness. *The traumas of childhood operate in a deferred fashion as though they were fresh experiences; but they do so unconsciously*" (Freud, 1896b, p. 167, n.2; italics in original). For Freud, repression only operates if this unique circumstance (a memory producing greater unpleasure than an experience) were to take place. Furthermore, the latter could only occur in those who had gone through a sexual experience during childhood. This line of argument used the temporality previously presented in the "Project", regarding Emma's case study.

Many explicit references can be found in the papers of 1896 regarding what Freud aimed to solve with his *Neurotica*. "Heredity and the Aetiology of the Neuroses" was directed at "the disciples of J.-M. Charcot", who considered heredity to be "the sole true and indispensable cause of neurotic affections" (Freud, 1896a, p. 143). Thus, the psychoanalyst made explicit his attempt to distance himself from the French hereditary tradition (Freud, 1896a, pp. 143–145).[6] First, he affirmed that certain illnesses, which were considered nervous and hereditary, were actually post-infectious. Second, he objected to drawing a sharp line between neuropathic families and families without nervous predisposition since the facts would question this distinction. Third, he highlighted Fournier and Erb's theories (regarding the aetiological role of syphilis) to point out the influence of external aetiological factors in the development of diseases that heredity alone could not cause. Fourth, he stated that certain nervous disorders, such as neurasthenia, would occur in people lacking a predisposition to the illness. Lastly, he criticised *dissimilar* heredity, that is, the belief that any type of functional and organic nervous disorder that a person's predecessors suffered (and even certain habits such as alcoholism, living a licentious life, etc.) would cause a different type of nervous illness in the following generations. For Freud, "the theory of dissimilar heredity does not tell us why one person tolerates the same hereditary load without succumbing to it or why another person, who is sick, should choose this particular nervous affection (…) instead of choosing another one" (Freud, 1896a, p. 145).

That said, the Viennese doctor believed he was in a position to present his solution to the fundamental aetiological problem: not only "why do some fall ill while others do not?" but also "why do patients suffer from a certain illness and not from another?" As in his response to Löwenfeld regarding anxiety neurosis, Freud once again emphasised the importance of splitting aetiological influences into three classes: preconditions, concurrent causes and specific causes. Only the specific causes could determine the choice of neurosis. Heredity, fulfilling the role of a precondition, also seemed to be indispensable. Nevertheless, it would be possible to come upon "cases of neurosis in which we shall look in vain for any appreciable degree of hereditary disposition, provided that what is lacking is made up for by a powerful specific influence" (Freud, 1896a, pp. 147–148). This influence should always be the same for each type of neurosis. Otherwise, if different factors were present in different cases of the same illness, then "the explanation that hysterics" and all other neurotic people are "peculiarly constituted creatures – probably on account of some hereditary disposition or degenerative atrophy –" (Freud, 1896c, p. 201) would be valid. In order to dethrone heredity, Freud needed to find for each neurosis a single aetiological factor that could function as a specific cause. A factor that explained both the repression and the choice of neurosis, and that made it possible to construct a complete and comprehensive nosography of the entire domain of neurotic illness. That specific aetiological factor was the missing piece of this intricate puzzle.

On this crucial point, in the publications of 1896, Freud remained faithful to what he had anticipated to Fliess in the letter from October 8 of the previous year. For hysteria, the specific cause would be found in

> *infantile* experiences -which- are once more *sexual* in content, but they are of a far more uniform kind than the scenes at puberty that had been discovered earlier (…) It is (…) a question of (…) sexual experiences affecting the subject's own body – of *sexual intercourse* (in the wider sense).
>
> (Freud, 1896c, p. 203, italics in original)

"*with actual excitement of the genitals, resulting from sexual abuse committed by another person*" (Freud, 1896a, p. 152; italics in original).[7] Those experiences could range from a "brutal assault" to a "seduction less rapid and less repulsive" but they would always leave the person in a "passive sexual" position (Freud, 1896a, pp. 152–153). In turn,

> The obsessional neurosis arises from a specific cause very analogous to that of hysteria. Here too we find a precocious sexual event, occurring before puberty (…) There is only one difference which seems capital (…) In obsessional neurosis it is a question (…) of an event which has given pleasure.
>
> (Freud, 1896a, p. 155)

"a question of (…) acts of aggression carried out with pleasure and of pleasurable participation in sexual acts – that is to say, of sexual activity" (Freud, 1896b, p. 168), even when this activity could be traced back to "a scene of sexual passivity that preceded the pleasurable action" (Freud, 1896b, p. 169).

With these sexual factors acting as the specific cause of the neuro-psychoses of defence, Freud believed he could: displace heredity; explain repression and the choice of neurosis; construct a complete nosography (of the two neuro-psychoses and the two "actual" neuroses) whose clinical pictures were also differentiated by the differential aetiology; and, he even believed to have found a therapy capable of curing the neuroses "*in general* (…) not just individual symptoms but the neurotic disposition itself" (Masson, 1985, p. 145, letter of 16/10/95). Perhaps this allows us to better understand why the Vienesse psychoanalyst confessed to feeling "a kind of faint joy – for having lived some forty years not quite in vain -" (Masson, 1985, p. 145) or why he wrote that his theory was "an important finding, the discovery of a *caput Nili* in neuropathology" (Freud, 1896c, p. 203).

However, these displays of joy did not imply that the certainty regarding his revolutionary discovery had always been present. The correspondence with Fliess allows us to clearly see the speed with which these events unfolded and the weight of the expectations placed upon his *Neurotica*; but it also reveals the doubts and insecurities provoked in the author by his theory. In the same epistle in which he stated to have not lived in vain due to his new discovery, he acknowledged still being "all mixed up", and he described "the feverish work of these last few weeks" in terms of "enticing hopes and disappointments" (Masson, 1985, p. 145; letter of 16/10/95). Three weeks after announcing his discovery to his friend, Freud wrote: "I have begun to have doubts about the pleasure-pain explanation of hysteria and obsessional neurosis" (Masson, 1985, p. 148; letter of 31/10/95). However, he immediately added that "one of the cases" – the first to be mentioned regarding this matter – had given him what he "expected (sexual shock – that is, infantile abuse in male hysteria!)" (Masson, 1985, p. 149, letter of 02/11/95). Three months later, in the first extensive development of his *Neurotica* known as "Draft K" and titled by Freud as "A Christmas Fairy Tale", the Vienesse doctor still wondered about "the origin of the unpleasure which seems to be released by premature sexual stimulation and without which, after all, a repression cannot be explained" (Masson, 1985,

p. 163, letter of 01/01/96). The author ruled out that the unpleasure provoked by sexuality stemmed from disgust or morality. He hypothesised that "there must be an independent source for the release of unpleasure in sexual life: once that source is present, it can activate sensations of disgust, lend force to morality, and so on" (Masson, 1985, p. 164). As he himself clarified, on this point he held to "the model of anxiety neurosis in adults, where a quantity deriving from sexual life similarly causes a disturbance in the psychic sphere" (Masson, 1985, p. 164). His doubts regarding the origin of the unpleasure generated by sexuality show that the question of the reasons behind repression remained unanswered despite his *Neurotica*. In addition, the reference to a quantity introduces a feature that will accompany the Freudian notion of trauma: its oscillation *between the dynamic, representative dimension, and the economic, quantitative dimension.* Although at the beginning of 1896 the problem did not seem resolved entirely, on February 6 of that same year, he sent the first two articles of his new theory for publishing. In these, he affirmed to have "been able to carry out a complete psycho-analysis in thirteen cases of hysteria" and that "in none of these cases was an event" of infantile traumatism missing (Freud, 1896a, p. 152). On May 31, the final paper of his aetiological trilogy was published, in which he celebrated having solved the more-than-thousand-year-old problem of the origin of the neuroses (Freud, 1896c, pp. 202–203). But, paradoxical as it may seem, the day before he had confessed to his friend that he was still working on his theory and that "As the fruit of some tormenting reflections" he had reached "the following solution to the etiology of the psychoneuroses, *which still awaits confirmation* from individual analyses" (Masson, 1985, p. 187, letter of 30/5/96; italics added). Much later, he confessed that he had never completed a case, that he was always missing an essential piece and that "as long as no case has been clarified and seen through to the end, I do not feel sure and I cannot be content" (Masson, 1985, p. 218, letter of 17/12/96).

Was Freud lying, as some historians have claimed? There is no evidence in the letters to Fliess that allows us to conclude that he was aware of his deception. We believe, rather, that he was *deceiving himself*; that, as he himself affirmed, he became trapped by the "enticing hopes" of an integral solution to the problem of the neuroses; that he rushed to make public a revolutionary discovery that he believed to have come across; that he searched for evidence in his patients that confirmed his theory; that he ran into "disappointments" over and over again until he confessed to Fliess: "I no longer believe in my *neurotica*" (Masson, 1985, p. 264, letter of 21/09/97). Nevertheless, even after this, he still longed for it to work. On November 14, 1897, he conceived the idea that if the childhood sexual experiences had affected the genitals, then their later activation would produce libido. On the other hand, if they had affected the anus, the mouth, etc., their activation during maturity would produce disgust and, as a result of this, symptoms (Masson, 1985, p. 281, letter of 14/11/97). The fragment reveals, once again, that Freud needed certain scenes to exist to be able to explain (by not recurring to heredity) why people fell ill.

In 2004, Hall Triplett analysed the process by which, in the 1950s, this moment of Freud's theory acquired the name it is best known by: Seduction Theory. Said historian proposed that this new and erroneous denomination implied the substitution of the term "sexual abuse" for "seduction". The former would refer to real, traumatic events. The latter would be more compatible with later Freudian ideas regarding the role of oedipal phantasies in the genesis of neuroses and the production of patients' narratives. This substitution would conceal the fact that in 1896, Freud was referring to experiences of abuse (Triplett, 2004, pp. 647–665). However, was this truly forgotten? As we will analyse later, it is true that the different Freudian versions and those of traditional historiography of psychoanalysis obscure many aspects of what happened between 1895 and 1897; but the fact that the so-called seductions were originally thought of as experiences of abuse that actually occurred was always borne in mind.

For our part, we believe that the main transformation was another. "Seduction Theory" replaced the name Freud had given it: "*Neurotica*". Due to this substitution, what was omitted and forgotten is that his *Neurotica* was not a cry that denounced the horror of abuse within the household, but the missing piece and the great hope for a complete explanation of the neuroses. With the fall of this theory, the Vienesse doctor had to make a renunciation. But not, as Masson suggests, the renunciation of criticising the morality of the bourgeois home and the oppression of women. The true Freudian renunciation was of the aspiration to elaborate a definitive solution to the enigma of the aetiology of the neuroses which would definitively overthrow heredity.[8]

3.2 A Nachträglich Trauma

In the United States, a few years before Masson's book became a best-seller, the demands of the Vietnam veterans for the recognition of the psychological effects of war combined with the denunciations of the existence and frequency of infantile sexual abuse and its psychological impact (Borch- Jacobsen, 1996; Hacking, 1995; Hermann, 1992). Both movements shook public opinion, took up important space in the media, and achieved diverse institutional backing. To a large extent, as an effect of these struggles, two nosographic categories that focused on the problem of psychical trauma were admitted into the DSM: post-traumatic stress disorder (PTSD) and multiple personality disorder (MPD). At the time, it was assumed that the latter's cause was linked to the posthumous psychological consequences of a traumatic sexual experience that occurred in childhood, which caused a dissociation in consciousness, eventually leading to the multiplication of personalities. It is true that MPD was not included in the following versions of the Manual. However, the belief that childhood sexual abuse would necessarily be traumatic, cause illness and require therapy remains in force in many "Psy" practitioners and the common sense of much of Western culture.

The implicit conceptual configuration of trauma in a category such as MPD could be represented by a schema such as the following.

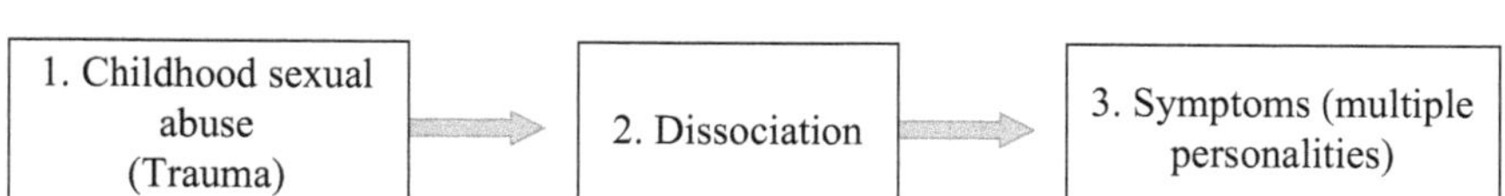

This schematic picture begins with the existence of a trauma that occurred in childhood and links it to the symptoms, thus hypothesising the mechanism that could lead from the cause to its effect. The relationship between the two is direct and, taking this reasoning to the extreme, it could be assumed that this event would not only constitute a particularly painful and violent crime but that it would also be pathological in itself and in all cases. In other words, the experience would always be traumatic regardless of the particularities of the person who lived through it and their ability to process it. It would also be independent of the response given by the child or by their caregivers in the face of the event. We have here a *prospective* approach, which begins with a childhood event and aims to predict or explain its future consequences.

If we observe this matter from the point of view of the clinician who treats an adult patient or if we follow the process of elaboration of these pathological theories, we will verify that the path is the opposite. First, the symptoms that the patient presents are verified; then, perhaps the link between these phenomena and certain memories arises; therefore, maybe a hypothesis is put forward regarding the mechanisms that link the latter with the former; and finally, it can be affirmed that the ultimate cause of the pathological phenomena is the experience of abuse as a child.

This seems to be the path followed by Freud, not only with each of his patients in the period of his *Neurotica*, but also in the construction of his theory between 1893 and 1896. In each analytical treatment, as in the course of his theoretical elucubration, Freud began his exploration starting with the symptoms until reaching the specific cause. In the article written in French, he describes the process that led him towards the notion of childhood trauma in the following way:

> By means of that procedure (…) hysterical symptoms are traced back to their origin (…) Travelling backwards into the patient's past, step by step, and always guided by the organic train of symptoms and of memories and thoughts aroused, I finally reached the starting-point of the pathological process; and I was obliged to see that at the bottom the same thing was present in all the cases submitted to analysis – the action of an agent which must be accepted as the specific cause of hysteria (…): *a precocious experience of sexual relations with actual excitement of the genitals, resulting from sexual abuse committed by another person* (…) before the child has reached sexual maturity.
>
> (Freud, 1896a, pp. 151–152; italics in original)

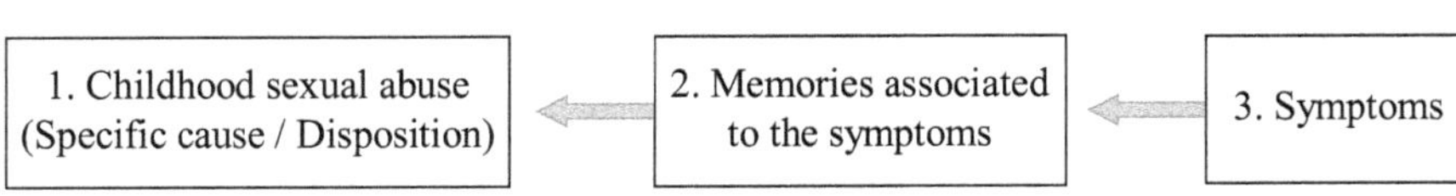

Unlike the previous one, this schematic picture is *retrospective*: the first element to appear is the most recent (the symptom needing to be interpreted) and the last is the oldest (that which would function as a specific cause and that determined the disposition to fall ill).

Although their directionalities are opposed, both schematic pictures share a trait: the linear nature of their temporality. Either it begins from a past event and moves towards the future until reaching the present, or it starts from the present and goes back to its origin.

However, neither of these schematic pictures describe well the temporality that Freud associated with trauma in his *Neurotica*. Both in "Further Remarks on the Neuro-Psychoses of Defence" and in "The Aetiology of Hysteria", Freud retrieves the postulates from his first work on these illnesses and reaffirms the validity of supposing that the origin of the illness comes before the onset of the symptoms. He suggests this origin be the moment in which the conflict occurs (M1), which leads to repression (R). In his words, "the outbreak of hysteria may almost invariably be traced to a *psychical conflict* arising through an incompatible idea setting in action a *defence* on the part of the ego and calling up a demand for repression" (Freud, 1896c, pp. 210–211; italics in original). Once the defence has acted, a period of "apparent health" (Freud, 1896b, p. 169) or latency (M2) begins, the end of which coincides with the onset of the symptoms, that is, with the disfigured return of the repressed (M3).

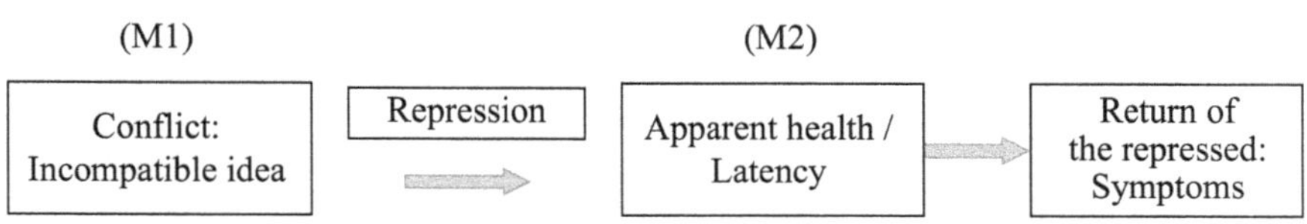

If the explanation were to stop here, Freud would continue to leave unsolved the problem posed in 1894: why are there "people who, under the same psychical influences, remain healthy" (Freud, 1894, p. 48), while others who have no confidence in their power to "resolve the contradiction between that incompatible idea and (…) – their – ego by means of thought-activity" (Freud, 1894, p. 47) repress and develop neuroses?

In other words, from the Freudian perspective, *a conflict is not necessarily traumatic,* nor does it lead in all cases to the repression of the incompatible ideas. For this reason, the field of trauma is sensibly limited. At the same time, it becomes necessary to postulate the existence of a particular disposition in which the emergence of a conflict produces a pathological resolution. As we have seen, for the Viennese psychoanalyst, the predisposing role traditionally given to heredity "can now be taken (…) by the posthumous operation of a sexual trauma in childhood" (Freud, 1896b, p. 166). In other words, only those people who lived through a scene of seduction in their childhood, of which a trace remains, and who, in adulthood, are confronted with an idea that "can be brought into logical or associative connection with an infantile experience of that kind" (Freud, 1896c, p. 211), will become neurotic. For someone to fall ill, a previous moment is needed (M0), the mark of disposition (or fixation point), which generates the conditions for the moments of the development of the illness to occur. This zero point is what Freud considered to be the specific cause of the illness.

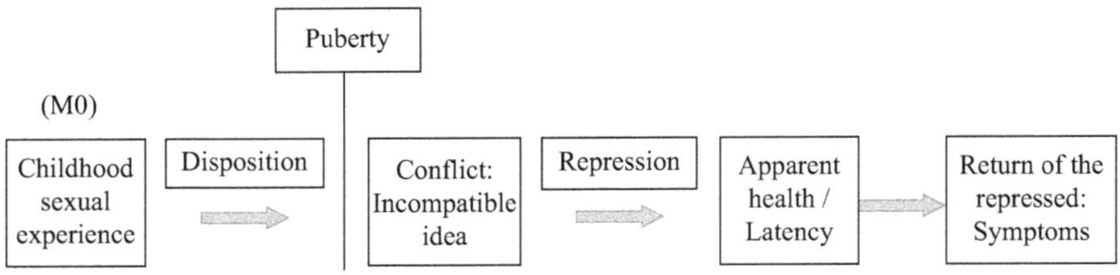

However, if we stopped our reasoning at this point, we would repeat the first of the schematic pictures. We would be conceiving a prospective schematic picture that indicates a causal, linear and unidirectional relationship between past child abuse and present illness. The temporal distance between childhood and adulthood would merely be a separation between both poles of personal development, with puberty representing the limit between them. In this sense, the following statement could be erroneously interpreted: "*The traumas of childhood operate in a deferred fashion*" (Freud, 1896b, p. 167 n.2; italics in original). At the same time, if childhood experiences were completely decisive on their own and we focused solely on the traumatic event, then we would be once again putting forward an *image* of the traumatised person as a totally passive victim: *the abused* and *asexual child*, to whom another person would externally impose sexuality.

However, the temporality of trauma is more complex in Freud's works. He questions the significance of experiences and defines another *image* of the traumatised person. Essentially, the German word *nachträglich* is itself ambiguous. In Sandra Berta's doctoral thesis, she references Luiz Hanns' *Diccionario comentado do alemão de Freud* to address the different meanings denoted by the term (Hanns, 1996, cited in Berta, 2014, pp. 21–23). For both authors, in the uses that Freud gave to the adjective *nachträglich*, two different meanings are present, implying two opposite temporal directionalities. On the one hand, the idea of an event having consequences that only later become manifest: the "deferred action". On the other hand, the idea of a return from the present to the past; an element that is transformed "*a posteriori*" (Berta, 2014, p. 23).

We believe that it is possible to find both meanings in the texts that make up the *Neurotica*. Thus, Freud never proposed a merely prospective schema that linked childhood sexual traumas and symptoms via a linear causal relationship. From his perspective, the power of childhood experiences was relativised by the idea that these produce "little or no effect at the time" (Freud, 1896a, p. 153) and that they could "after all only exert a psychical effect through their *memory-traces*" (Freud, 1896c, p. 202; italics in original). In other words, Freud made a distinction between events and traces. The importance of the events was determined by the *marks* they left on the psyche. The experiences themselves were lost; but a *trace* of some of them was preserved, acting as a fixation point that determined the ordering of the subsequent points. Given this mark, the subsequent neurosis (the possibility of repression and also the logical framework of the illness' symptoms) was structured around the text of that infantile scene.

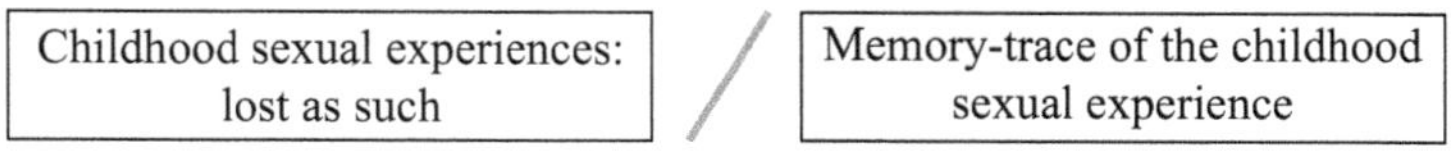

At this point, Freud clearly expressed that "it is not the experiences themselves which act traumatically but their revival as a memory" (Freud, 1896b, p. 164). This apparently simple phrase supposes a complexity that we want to make explicit. We have already relativised the significance of the event; now, we need to address the importance of the trace. The latter also is not traumatic due to its mere presence; it is simply the mark of a disposition. For it to *become* traumatic, it needs to be awakened at a later moment: that of the present conflict. Therefore, the trauma only occurs *a posteriori*: when in adulthood, an idea manages to be linked with the trace of the childhood scene, thus reviving it. In that moment, the past mark becomes a *present memory* (a *current past*), which comes into conflict with the ideas that make up the ego. This conflict occurs because puberty has allowed for a process of resignification of what was lived in childhood and, at the same time, has produced an increase in the quantity. Two related but different issues would be at play here: the activation of the memory (even if it does not become conscious) and the increase of the trace's levels of affect.

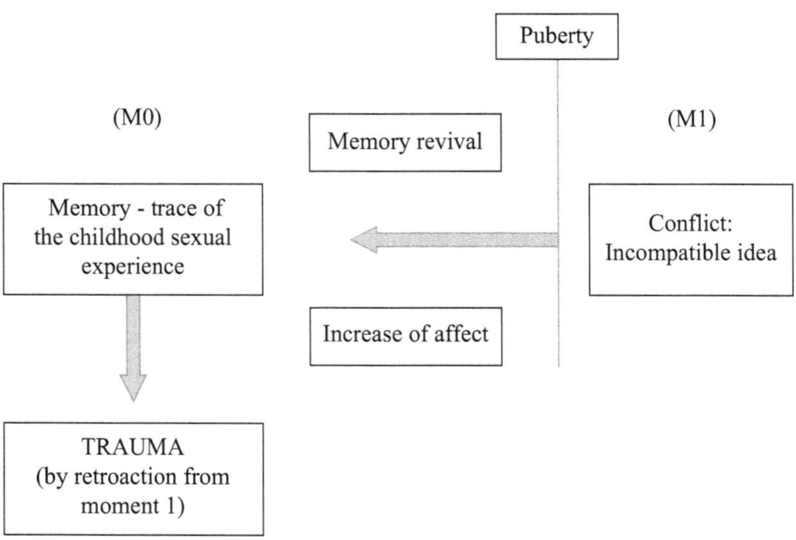

This *retroactive* directionality was emphasised by many psychoanalysts, especially those of a Lacanian orientation. As Omar Acha points out, *nachträglich* temporality has usually been translated, read and interpreted "following the temporal figure of the *après coup*" (Acha, 2010, p. 271). We believe that if this bias in the interpretation of the German term is not problematised it could produce a series of problems. First, we would run the risk of denying the importance that Freud gave to the traces of the past. Without those experiences that left traces, there would be no trauma nor anything to resignify. Therefore, Freud defended the existence of a prospective directionality, by which the past modifies or conditions the present. In fact, the content of a current idea cannot by itself explain the conflict that leads to repression. This idea can have a trivial or apparently traumatic meaning. In any case, for Freud, this idea will be repressed only in the presence of past traces that act as predisposing factors. Thus, the infantile scene determines the later neurosis.

However, despite the importance attributed to the infantile scene, disposition is not synonymous with necessity; the past experiences merely generate the illness' conditions of possibility. A *retroaction* is also required for the illness to be developed: the reactivation of the past trace in the present. This operation gives the trace a traumatic value because it introduces a new meaning to past events and produces an increase in the quantity.

Moreover, if only the retroactive movement is taken into account, two elements that are different for Freud would be equated: the *memory-trace* and the *idea*. The latter is always inserted in a set, in a series of links that make up webs of ideas with multiple mutual connections. Each idea's position in those webs depends on the relationship between those ideas. For example, an idea *incompatible* with those that make up part of the ego will be split off from these. The memory-trace, on the other hand, is not necessarily linked to others; it does not constitute webs. It can remain isolated, although it is also possible for it to change this characteristic when associated with a current idea (as we have just seen in the *Neurotica's* schema). In addition, the trace is linked in a much more direct way to the event: it is the mark left by an experience that affected the body. The trace marks a boundary, the border between an event (supposedly external) and the psyche (supposedly internal). At the same time, ideas and memory-traces have different relationships with the quantitative component. Freud admitted that an idea can provoke affects and that the webs of ideas attempt to process the quantities of excitation by displacing them until they are discharged. However, the relationship between the memory-trace and the affects is much more intense. Only the memory-trace can "lead to a release of affect" (Freud, 1896b, p. 166) that will trigger repression and, subsequently, neurosis. In short, the notion of memory-traces established a triply two-sided structure in Freud's writings. The notion marks the border between the exterior and the interior of the psychical apparatus. It can be associated with ideas and thus be included in the webs that make up the story of a person's life; but it also maintains a close link with the quantities of affect whose emergence disturbs the idea's normal functioning. It is linked to the past but can be reactivated and produce effects in the present.

It is also necessary to explain the notion of *memory* that appeared in the texts of 1896. It can be understood as the result of an operation that relates two heterogeneous elements: the memory-trace and the idea. When both are associated, the memory emerges, thus activating the trace. However, after the awakening of the memory of the childhood experience, the "memory-trace of these traumas in childhood (...) do not thereupon become conscious but lead to a release of affect and to repression" (Freud, 1896b, p. 166). This phrase introduces the possibility of conceiving a type of memory that is measured by its effects, even when the memory is not consciously remembered.[9] That is, a memory that is not limited to recollection: its recall can be missing, but even so, the memory operates, enabling another (unconscious) mode of remembering. Furthermore, in the last text of those published in 1896, the fact that the memory remained unconscious despite being reactivated in the present, became a condition for repression and illness, and a key factor for the orientation of the treatment. According to the author, people who remembered (as a conscious recollection) those childhood experiences "*ought not to be* hysterical *at all* (…) With our patients, those memories are never conscious; but *we cure them of their hysteria by transforming their unconscious memories of the infantile scenes into conscious ones*" (Freud, 1896c, p. 211; italics added). At the same time, if remembering (via conscious recall) cures, the illness would be a different form of remembering. For Freud, the symptoms were "mnemic symbols" which preserve the patient's memory of the past in a distorted way (Freud, 1896c, p. 193). The symptoms hide, while simultaneously preserving, the traces of a previous moment that could not be recalled and became traumatic. Lastly, as discussed in the previous chapter, the task of remembering this infantile trauma is not simple. The analytic procedure works "against an enormous resistance", which must be overcome to make it possible to remember (Freud, 1896a, p. 153).

In short, *nachträglich* temporality introduced a non-linear relationship between past and present into the field of trauma. What occurs in the past leaves marks that condition the present. The significance of a current experience depends partly on its connection with past traces. However, the past does not entirely determine the present, not even in the case of the return of the repressed via symptoms or repetition. Furthermore, each present moment gives the past new significance and can even make an experience become traumatic that, at the time, was not. At the same time, if the memory linked to this type of temporality supposes the efficacy and persistence of the past (independent of its conscious recollection), to recall would imply modifying the conflictive relationship of the present with the past, that is, to work through the resistances that sustain the forgotten memory. Thus, this *image* of the traumatised neurotic is not, for Freud, equivalent to that of the child who is a victim of abuse. The neurotic is an adult who, in order to overcome their neurosis, must change their subjective position with respect to their past marks. They are not guilty of what happened to them in the past, but they are responsible for how it affects them in the present.

As we will discuss in the final section of this chapter, Freud abandoned his *Neurotica* shortly after announcing it with great fanfare. However, this version of the trauma and temporality remained in force in many parts of the Freudian work. For example, the case history of the "Wolf Man" is structured according to *nachträglich* temporality. Successive subsequent experiences, such as a dream with wolves at the age of four (M1), "brought into deferred operation his observation of intercourse at the age of one and a half" (Freud, 1918, p. 109), which serves as a disposition/fixation for his future neurosis (M0). This experience fueled the dream's formation. However, this prospective directionality must be complemented by retroaction: the dream activates the scene, which "thanks to the advance in his intellectual development, he was now able to understand", acquiring a new meaning and operating "not only like a fresh event, but like a new trauma" (Freud, 1918, p. 109). This process by which the past becomes present and the present modifies the past leads to repression and the development of a phobia (as a form of the return of the repressed). This return, which is always distorted, again implies the presence of the repressed past in the present and a new alteration of the past influenced by the present.

Even in later writings, such as the one dedicated to Moses and monotheism (Freud, 1939), Freud once again made use of *nachträglich* temporality to account for the way in which certain traumatic experiences were unconsciously transmitted throughout different generations. Precisely, the problem of the transgenerational transmission of trauma will be one of the main objects of inquiry in the fifth chapter of this book.

We will now work on one of the central questions of this chapter dedicated to Freud's *Neurotica* and its different versions.

3.3 Reality or Phantasy?

In the preceding chapters, we observed the process of psychologisation of trauma. During this transformation, the determinism attributed to the event decreased as the importance attached to predisposition and "internal" psychological processes increased. Authors such as Page, Charcot and Janet conceived traumatic experience as a combination between past and present, between objective and subjective conditions. These three physicians distanced themselves from the most extreme positions that only took into account the role of one of the poles of these dichotomies (either objective *or* subjective; either determined by the past *or* determined by the present).

Did Freud, with his *Neurotica*, re-introduce the idea that the past event (in this case, infantile sexual abuse) would be traumatic in itself and cause all the symptoms single-handedly? From what has been said so far, it is possible to affirm that his *Neurotica* denies this interpretation. Nevertheless, the abandonment of this theory did not make phantasies the only cause of neuroses. Reality and phantasy are not two antagonistic terms: the first being objective and external; the second, subjective and internal. Many historical interpretations of Seduction Theory are based on this opposition. However, in order to understand the theoretical elaboration of 1896 (and even many of Freud's later ideas), we consider it necessary to abandon the exclusive dichotomies that separate: reality from phantasy, the objective from the subjective, the external from the internal, the past from the present, truth from falsehood.

Freud himself indeed contributed to emphasising these oppositions, above all due to the successive versions that he elaborated to account for what happened in 1896. We will now analyse some of them.

3.3.1 Versions from the 20s and 30s

Perhaps one of the most well-known narratives about Freud's *Neurotica* and its abandonment can be found in his conference on femininity:

> In the period in which the main interest was directed to discovering infantile sexual traumas, almost all my women patients told me that they had been seduced by their father. I was driven to recognize in the end that these reports were *untrue* and so came to understand that hysterical symptoms *are derived from phantasies and not from real occurrences*. It was only later that I was able to recognize in this phantasy of being seduced by the father the expression of the typical Oedipus complex in women.
>
> (Freud, 1933, p. 120; italics added)

This fragment merits several comments. The first of these concerns an aspect to which we have already referred. In this text, as in several of the historical accounts from the 1910s onwards, Freud affirmed that his first patients "told" him stories of seduction. This way of describing the facts leads one to believe that the patients spontaneously recounted those supposed memories. In the writings from 1896, Freud absolutely denied this possibility (Freud, 1896a, p. 153): they only reproduced the scenes due to "the strongest compulsion of the treatment" and, when they did, they "still attempt to withhold belief from them, by emphasizing the fact that (…) they have no feeling of remembering the scenes" (Freud, 1896c, p. 204).

The second comment that we would like to make refers to the relationship that Freud established between his interest in discovering childhood sexual traumas and the profusion with which his patients supposedly recounted these events. Was there any relation between what Freud was looking for and what he found in the stories of his analysands? Phrases like these are what have led some historians to point out the suggestive nature of the Freudian procedure (Borch-Jacobsen, 1996). However, as we have already pointed out, they could also account for the way in which Freud deceived himself with his findings due to his enormous interest in finding a more-than-thousand-year-old solution.

The quote mentioned above from 1933 calls for a third comment. In it, Freud affirmed that his female patients of 1896 frequently accused their fathers of committing sexual attacks and that these stories would be nothing more than the expression of the oedipal phantasy. These ideas surely would have been entirely plausible at the time they were written, given the central role that the Oedipus Complex had come to play in psychoanalytic theory. However, this interpretation of the events had not been formulated in the previous versions of his *Neurotica*. On the one hand, until well into the 20s, even when these stories were already thought of as phantasies, they were not directly linked to the Oedipus complex. On the other hand, in the papers published in 1896, it was never mentioned that the culprit of the scenes of abuse was the patient's father. There, the seducers were other people: strangers, domestic servants, governesses, teachers, older brothers… at most a close relative, but never the father (Freud, 1896a, p. 152, 1896b, p. 164, 1896c, p. 208). It could be thought that Freud knew that the fathers were to blame, but did not dare to publicly acknowledge it because of the scandal that this accusation would have produced. Strachey repeatedly mentions this interpretation in the footnotes of the Standard Edition of the Complete Psychological Works.[10] If this were true, it could not be understood why Freud did not mention that the abuser was the father in the letters to Fliess prior to or contemporaneous with the publication of these texts (since in this intimate and close epistolary relationship he dared to openly mention all types of concerns). The first indication of the father being the seducer only occurred several months after the three articles that make up his *Neurotica* were published. It appeared in a letter in which the psychoanalyst found new arguments in favour of displacing heredity (Masson, 1985, p. 212, letter of 6/12/96).[11]

Fourth, we wish to underline that this fragment clearly established a division between reality and phantasy: the narratives of seduction always referred to phantasies, never to real events, and were therefore considered false, since there would be no correspondence between the statements and the events that actually took place. However, at the same time, phantasies for Freud were not mere inventions; rather, they were expressions of something that he, at that point, considered real and universal: the Oedipus complex. Although the text enunciated by the patient did not *exactly* reflect an event that took place, it did express something real in a *distorted* way. The latter could only be known through this phantastic narrative. For these reasons, the exclusive opposition between reality and phantasy, between truth and falsehood, should be relativised.

A few years earlier, in 1925, Freud offered another version of what had occurred during the development of his *Neurotica*. This version had many similarities with the testimony from 1933, although there were also some differences. We will quote extensively the passage that we are interested in analysing:

> Before going further into the question of infantile sexuality I must mention an *error* into which I fell for a while and which might well have had fatal consequences for the whole of my work. *Under the influence of the technical procedure which I used at that time, the majority of my patients reproduced from their childhood scenes in which they were sexually seduced* by some grown-up person. With female patients the part of seducer was almost always assigned to their father. I believed these stories, and consequently supposed that I had discovered the roots of the subsequent neurosis in these experiences of sexual seduction in childhood. (…) When, however, I was at last obliged to recognize that these scenes of seduction had never taken place, and that *they were only phantasies which my patients had made up or which I myself had perhaps forced on them*, I was for some time completely at a loss. (…) When I had pulled myself together, I was able to draw the *right conclusions* from my discovery: *namely, that the neurotic symptoms were not related directly to actual events but to wishful phantasies,* and that as far as the neurosis was

> concerned psychical reality was of more importance than material reality. I do not believe even now that I forced the seduction-phantasies on my patients, that I 'suggested' them. I had in fact stumbled for the first time upon the Oedipus complex, which was later to assume such an overwhelming importance, but which I did not recognize as yet in its disguise of phantasy. Moreover, *seduction during childhood retained a certain share*, though a humbler one, *in the aetiology of neuroses*.
>
> (Freud, 1925, pp. 33–35; italics added)

In this fragment, he once again classified his theory of 1896 as an "error", one which was overcome by the emergence of a new explanation (the Oedipus complex). It is striking that an author who, in his theory and practice, resorts to a non-linear or progressive temporality, presents the history of the psychoanalytic movement as a development tending towards progress. Nevertheless, this form of historical narrative is most often the canonical way of describing the course of the *Neurotica* and even psychoanalysis in general.

On another note, there were two new elements in this passage. First, the suspicion (which was quickly discarded) of having been responsible for instilling those memories in the patients' minds. Second, and more importantly, the acceptance of the possibility that the seductions in childhood could have existed. At the beginning of the quote, by affirming that the scenes were mere phantasies with no correlation to reality, the creator of psychoanalysis seemed to be heading towards the blunt opposition that he would go on to defend a few years later. However, this initial statement was not entirely consistent with the affirmation that closed the fragment, which admitted the possibility that, in some cases, these attacks had actually existed and that they would be capable of producing neurosis.

This same tendency to relativise or weaken the presumed mutual exclusion between reality and phantasy can be found in a footnote, which the author added in 1924 with the re-edition of the 1896 texts. There, Freud explicitly stated that the fact that the majority of experiences were phantasies did not imply ruling out the possibility that, in certain cases, the attacks had effectively existed and played a role in aetiology. Let us read, for example, the following footnote to "Further Remarks on the Neuro-Psychoses of Defence":

> This section is dominated by an error which I have since repeatedly acknowledged and corrected. At that time I was not yet able to distinguish between my patients' phantasies about their childhood years and their real recollections. As a result, *I attributed to the aetiological factor of seduction a significance and universality which it does not possess*. When this error had been overcome, it became possible to obtain an insight into the spontaneous manifestations of the sexuality of children (…) Nevertheless, we need not reject everything written in the text above. Seduction retains a certain aetiological importance (…).
>
> (Freud, 1896b, p. 168, n.1; italics added)

It is clear that in this text, more than in others, Freud emphasised that his error was not have considered the narratives of seduction to be real, but rather to have assumed that in *all* cases of neurosis, episodes of childhood sexual abuse had occurred and that these were the cause of the illness. In other words, the problem of his *Neurotica* was the *universalisation* of this aetiological factor. But, logically, recognising that *not all* these events actually took place did not imply affirming that none of them did.

3.3.2 The Versions from the First Two Decades of the Twentieth Century

Continuing the revision of Freud's path in reverse chronological order (from the latest versions to the texts of 1896), and leaving aside, for the moment, a reference to seduction found in the 23rd "Introductory Lecture on Psycho-Analysis" (Freud, 1916–1917), we wish to now dwell upon a fragment of "On the History of the Psycho-Analytic Movement" (Freud, 1914a). This paper, written at the same time as his estrangement with Carl Jung, was the first in which he affirmed that *all* stories of seduction in childhood were phantasies and would, therefore, not be true.

> Influenced by Charcot's view of the traumatic origin of hysteria, one was readily inclined to *accept as true and aetiologically significant* the statements made by patients in which they ascribed their symptoms to passive sexual experiences in the first years of childhood – to put it bluntly, to seduction. When this aetiology broke down under the weight of its own improbability and contradiction in definitely ascertainable circumstances, the result at first was helpless bewilderment. Analysis had led back to these infantile sexual traumas by the right path, and yet *they were not true*. The firm ground of reality was gone (…) If hysterical subjects trace back their symptoms to traumas that are fictitious, then the new fact which emerges is precisely that *they create such scenes in phantasy, and this psychical reality requires to be taken into account alongside practical reality*. This reflection was soon followed by the discovery that these phantasies were intended to *cover up the auto-erotic activity* of the first years of childhood, *to embellish it* and raise it to a higher plane.
>
> (Freud, 1914a, pp. 17–18; italics added)

Once again, we come across a universalisation of the *realness* of the narratives (while he believed in his *Neurotica*) as opposed to their phantastic nature (when he abandoned it). We also find that reality and truth are equated: the narrative was considered true if it referred to an event that occurred; if not, it was false. However, a different idea also appeared, forcing us to relativise these statements. Although the phantasies of seduction did not faithfully reproduce the events of a scene of abuse that occurred, they could refer to an event considered *real*: the auto-erotic activity of early childhood. The phantasies were considered distortions of this activity, covering it up but also signalling its existence. They could be considered a text destined to hide said activity while at the same time marking something real that would otherwise escape remembrance.

Just a few lines down from the quoted paragraph, Freud affirmed that K. Abraham had "the last word on the subject of traumatic aetiology" for having pointed out that "the sexual constitution which is peculiar to children is precisely calculated to provoke sexual experiences of a particular kind – namely traumas" (Freud, 1914a, p. 18). In other words, not only could traumatic sexual experiences occur in childhood, but also the congenital constitution of the child could provoke them.

In any case, the praises of Abraham's work were problematic, as other authors have already pointed out (Good, 1995; Masson, 1984). The actual content of the praised publication (Abraham, 1907) presented serious contradictions with the version Freud embraced in 1914 on the topic of seduction. First, according to Abraham, the childhood sexual attacks reported by adult patients were always real (not phantasised) events, the reason for which the Freudian *Neurotica* would conserve certain validity. However, for Abraham, childhood sexual abuse did not cause neurosis. On the contrary, he considered that certain children, by being predisposed to neurosis, unconsciously sought or induced sexual attacks from adults (Abraham, 1907). Second, the sexual impulses thought to be at the root of these incitements were the exclusive domain of those children who, due to their abnormal sexual constitution, were more prone to developing neurosis. While in 1914 Freud was trying to link phantasies to a supposedly universal characteristic of childhood sexuality (the auto-erotic activity), Abraham was affirming that the scenes of seduction were not phantasies and that they were dependent on a sexual element that appeared only in certain children with pathological constitutional traits. Freud probably supported Abraham's hypotheses not so much because he agreed with his ideas but because of his distance from Jung.

As can be seen, the different versions analysed so far seem to have in common the attempt to define the narratives of childhood seduction scenes as phantasies. However, at the same time, all the versions attempted to link phantasies to a particular sexual element whose realness was supposed by Freud: be it abuse that actually occurred (an option which could not be ruled out in any case), be it the development and resolution of the Oedipus Complex, be it infantile auto-erotic activity. Why did Freud insist so much on anchoring the narrative of a phantasy to a real event, while at the same time seemingly affirming that the patient's discourse did not strictly coincide with reality? To answer this crucial question we need to, first of all, continue investigating the different versions regarding his *Neurotica* until we reach the year 1896 once again; second of all, we need to analyse some aspects of the debate that caused Freud and Jung to part ways in the mid-1910s.

In 1905, Freud wrote two of the first versions destined to be published on the abandonment of his *Neurotica*:

> I cannot admit that in my paper on the 'The Aetiology of Hysteria' I exaggerated the frequency or importance of that influence -the effects of seduction-, though I did not then know that persons who remain normal may have had the

> same experiences in their childhood, and though I consequently overrated the importance of seduction in comparison with the factors of sexual constitution and development.
>
> (Freud, 1905, p. 190)

As can be seen, there were no traces of him considering that the narratives of seduction could have been phantasies; rather, his error would have been not considering that other people who were abused in childhood remained healthy despite these events. He, therefore, continued to support the possibility that the ultimate cause of neurosis was not rooted in those traumas but in the inherited sexual constitution.

In the second paper, written in 1905 but published one year later, his argument is noticeably different:

> At that time my material was still scanty, and it happened by chance to include a disproportionately large number of cases in which sexual seduction by an adult or by older children played the chief part in the history of the patient's childhood. I thus over-estimated the frequency of such events (though in other respects *they were not open to doubt*). Moreover, I was at that period *unable to distinguish* with certainty between falsifications made by hysterics in their memories of childhood and traces of real events. Since then I have learned to explain a number of *phantasies* of seduction as attempts at fending off memories of the subject's own sexual activity (infantile masturbation). When this point had been clarified, the 'traumatic' element in the sexual experiences of childhood lost its importance (…).
>
> (Freud, 1906, p. 274; italics added)

In this case, he did not claim that all stories of seduction referred to real events, but neither did he claim them all to be phantasies. Freud admitted here both possibilities. However, he seemed to have "over-estimated the frequency of such events". It is true, his argument does not add up: the papers of 1896 were based on only 13 or 18 case studies. Nevertheless, this limited number of cases did not lead him to suppose a high frequency of sexual seduction; rather, he raised a significantly different point: that seduction was a universal trait in all cases of neuro-psychoses. This universality was not derived from the number of cases studied but from the starting premises. As we have seen, these childhood experiences were the missing piece to an aetiological, clinical, psychological and physiological puzzle. Freud's certainty regarding the presence of these experiences in all cases of neurosis was rooted in the vital role they played in his theory at that time.

Furthermore, we wish to highlight that in this paragraph, Freud, for the first time, publicly admitted the difficulties he encountered when trying to distinguish narratives that referred to real events from those that did not, thus recognising the possibility of them being phantasies. To say that they can be phantasies did not imply that they all are (as he claimed in 1914 and 1933), but it did mean admitting that some of these discursive pieces of analysis did not refer to experiences of seduction but rather that they served to mask infantile masturbation.[12] Once again, phantasy was understood as a text that, although it did not remit to what its content explicitly affirmed (a case of infantile sexual abuse that actually occurred), it did denote a *real* episode (in this case, the child's auto-erotic activity) in a *distorted* fashion. Phantasy, therefore, would not be a false text but one to be *interpreted.* A text which revealed and, at the same time, concealed something *real.*

3.3.3 The Original Versions

As we have mentioned, "The Aetiology of Hysteria", the final paper of the trilogy, was published between May and June 1896. It was partially based on a lecture with the same title delivered by Freud on April 21 before the *Verein für Psychiatrie und Neurologie*. In the author's words, his presentation "was given an icy reception by the asses and a strange evaluation by Krafft-Ebing: 'It sounds like a scientific fairy tale'" (Masson, 1985, p. 184, letter of 26/04/96). The epistle itself did not clarify what was specifically criticised by Krafft-Ebing, but the published paper offers some clues in this regard. Especially because, in this paper, we find Freud eagerly attempting to counter two possible objections to his thesis: "that the physician forces such scenes upon his docile patients, alleging that they are memories,[13] or else that the patients tell the physician things which they have deliberately invented or have imagined" (Freud, 1896c, p. 204). Faced with the possibility that the narratives of childhood sexual abuse were considered *responses to suggestion* or *patients' phantasies*, Freud gave various arguments to convince his readers of the realness of those scenes.

The same problem had already appeared in "Heredity and the Aetiology of the Neuroses". In this paper, Freud introduced the following question: "How is it possible to remain convinced of the reality of these analytic confessions which claim to be memories preserved from the earliest childhood?" (Freud, 1896a, p. 153). Following on from this question, one of the phrases we quoted at the beginning of this chapter appears, where the author explicitly states that the patients never spontaneously recounted these stories. It was thanks to "the most energetic pressure of the analytic procedure" that the "resistance" could be overcome, allowing for the scenes to appear, although not in their totality but "piece by piece" (Freud, 1896a, p. 153). After completing this process, the patients became the "prey to an emotion which (...) would be hard to counterfeit" (Freud, 1896a, p. 153). These details do not seem to play in Freud's favour in his attempt to justify the realness of the scenes reported by his patients. Nevertheless, although his arguments are not entirely convincing, they allow us to see the element that guided the Vienesse psychoanalyst. The patient's *resistance* seemed to convince Freud that the memory he was searching for was hidden behind it. From his point of view, if those scenes were not based on real experiences, they would neither produce resistance to admit them nor "an emotion which (...) would be hard to counterfeit".

After providing those arguments, the author added two further reasons to support the realness of the seductions. First, a practical reason: "the therapeutic effect of the analysis lags behind if one has not penetrated so far" (Freud, 1896a, p. 153). The reverse side of this phrase was the assertion that neurotics could be completely cured of their illness if the memory of the traumatic scenes that functioned as the specific cause of the illness could be accessed.

Second, he argued that the "symptoms" and other "special features" of the cases could only be explained by the existence of the experiences. In this sense, the scenes of seduction appeared as a necessary part of "the intrinsic structure of the neurosis" (Freud, 1896a, p. 153). This relationship between the different symptoms (and the complete structure of the neurosis) with a scene will be an idea maintained by Freud throughout his entire work. The pathological phenomena were thus considered to be structured around a single script: the text of a scene central to a subject's life. As we pointed out a few pages back, the "Wolf Man" case served as a good example of the validity of some of the ideas developed around Freud's *Neurotica*. This case history was structured entirely around a scene whose realness Freud tried to justify. However, certain doubts can be found here and there: is it not possible for the scene that seems to structure the entirety of the pathogenic material to merely be a phantasy? As we will see, the way in which the founder of psychoanalysis responded to this question will allow us to substantially relativise the opposition between reality and phantasy.

But before that, we wish to return to the 1896 article "The Aetiology of Hysteria". In this article, the arguments raised in the text written in French were repeated and developed at greater length. Once again, Freud compared his method with that of the archaeologist. Just as the latter finds ruins and, from these, reconstructs the history of an entire culture, he could, from the symptoms, reconstruct "the history of the origin of the illness" until arriving at the "traumatically operative scenes" that determined these symptoms (Freud, 1896c, p. 193). In turn, only by accessing these scenes could the symptoms be understood and eliminated. Once again, the existence of the scenes of seduction was justified by the idea that only these would allow for the (logical and therapeutic) solution of a case.

In this paper, Freud allowed himself to be guided again by the resistance:

> Before they come for analysis the patients know nothing about these scenes (…) Only the strongest compulsion of the treatment can induce them to embark on a reproduction of them. While they are recalling these infantile experiences to consciousness, they suffer under the most violent sensations, of which they are ashamed and which they try to conceal; and, even after they have gone through them once more in such a convincing manner, they still attempt to withhold belief from them, by emphasizing the fact that, unlike what happens in the case of other forgotten material, they have no feeling of remembering the scenes.
>
> (Freud, 1896c, p. 204)

For Freud, this behaviour, far from calling into question the realness of the scenes, provided "conclusive proof", since he considered it "incompatible with the assumption that the scenes are anything else than a reality which is being felt with distress and reproduced with the greatest reluctance" (Freud, 1896c, p. 204). In this way, he intended to rule out the possibility that the scenes be considered products of suggestion or phantasies.

Perhaps the arguments in favour of the realness of the scenes were flimsy. Not in vain did he stop believing in his *Neurotica*. However, why was he so insistent on defending these arguments? The reasons for his emphasis must be looked for in the hopes he had placed on his aetiological theory. As we discussed in the first section of this chapter, Freud could only provide an answer to the question of disposition and thus displace heredity from its aetiological role if he could prove the existence of certain accidents that only some people had suffered (precisely, those who later fell ill). For the theory to fall apart, it was not necessary for all the narratives to be considered phantasies: it was enough for there to be one case in which the existence of the traumatic experience could not be verified for the heredity hypothesis to gain strength once again.

The efforts placed in displacing heredity could explain the need to defend the realness of the scenes of seduction, but this was where Freud's interest in the experience itself stopped. The entire conceptual framework of 1896 used to explain the neuroses implied establishing a very marked distance between the event and the symptoms. Years could pass between one and the other. It was also possible for the illness to never develop, leaving only the mark of a latent disposition. In addition, the *nachträglich* temporality further questions the importance given by Freud to the event itself. For this very reason, Freud did not need to conceive phantasies as being completely separated from reality to question the relevance given to the experiences when these were considered the absolute cause of the symptoms. As Schimek stated,

> internal psychological processes and transformations already play a central role in the seduction theory. Thus Freud's later shift of emphasis from reproductions of real events to fantasies (which contain at least fragments of actual past experience) did not represent such a radical break in the continuity of his thought.
>
> (Schimek, 1987, p. 939)

This idea becomes even more plausible when we analyse the letters to Fliess from the first appearance of the notion of phantasies to the announcement of his abandonment of the *Neurotica*. On April 6, 1897, Freud told his friend about

> the discovery of a different source, from which a new element of the product of the unconscious arises. What I have in mind -Freud continued- are hysterical fantasies which regularly, as I see it, go back to things that children overhear at an early age and understand only subsequently.
>
> (Masson, 1985, p. 234, letter of 6/4/97)

One month later, a new missive showed even more eloquently the way in which phantasies, far from being radically opposed to actual events, for Freud confirmed his *Neurotica.*

> I have gained a sure inkling of the structure of hysteria. Everything goes back to the reproduction of scenes. Some can be obtained directly, others always by way of fantasies set up in front of them. The fantasies *stem from things that have been heard* but understood subsequently, and all their material is of course *genuine.* They are *protective structures, sublimations of the facts, embellishments* of them.
>
> (Masson, 1985, p. 239, letter of 2/5/97; italics added)

In 1897, when Freud was beginning to conjecture about the function of phantasies, they were not considered to be the opposite of events; rather, they came from something real: something that was heard and could only subsequently be understood; and they expressed something real, although they did so with distortions that protected, sublimated, embellished the denoted facts. Therefore, the conjecture that phantasies might play a role in neurosis did not immediately lead to the assertion that the patients' narratives about their childhoods were false or that these stories had no connection with something that actually took place.

It is worth noting that in Draft L (which was sent in the same epistle from which we extracted the previous quote), the creator of psychoanalysis repeated the same ideas, although adding a hypothesis that would remain intact throughout his entire work. We refer to the idea that the text of a phantasy, formed by something that the person heard, could perhaps not be based on an experience that occurred in their personal life but on an event experienced by their ancestors. Phantasies, Freud stated, "are manufactured by means of things that are heard, and utilized subsequently, and thus combine things experienced and heard, past events (from the history of parents and ancestors), and things that have been seen by oneself" (Masson, 1985, p. 240). The opposition between phantasy and reality receives, in this way, a new blow. For Freud, there is no possibility for phantasies to not refer to something that was experienced: even if the event had not occurred in the subject's own life, Freud conceived the possibility of it being a part of their ancestral history that could be transmitted. It supposed a new conception of the role of heredity (and not an absolute rejection of the latter).

Finally, when the Viennese physician told his Berlin colleague about the abandonment of his *Neurotica,* he in no way stated that it was impossible for the reports of abuse to be experiences that actually occurred, nor did he affirm that they were all phantasies without any connection to real experiences (Masson, 1985, p. 240, letter of 21/9/97). As a matter of fact, Freud wrote something that, although it may sound similar to these ideas, was actually very different. According to his new insight: "there are no indications of reality in the unconscious, so that one cannot distinguish between truth and fiction that has been cathected with affect" (Masson, 1985, p. 264, letter of 21/9/97). It is true that with this statement, he admitted the probability that the patients' narratives did not refer to lived experiences. However, probability does not mean necessity: Freud did not exclude that child sexual abuse may have existed. Nevertheless, this affirmation did force him to give up his *Neurotica*, because although in some cases these types of experiences had actually occurred, his theory could only be sustained if *all* cases of neurosis presented one of these traumatic experiences. In short, the abandonment of the Seduction Theory did not imply the belief in a sharp opposition between reality and phantasy. It implied believing in the possibility that a testimony in analysis could say something more than or something different to what it seemed to refer to directly.

3.3.4 Reality and Phantasy at the Moment of Estrangement with Carl Gustav Jung

The intricate institutional and conceptual details that led to Sigmund Freud's estrangement from Carl Jung (who held the presidency of the International Psychoanalytic Association until April 20, 1914), have been addressed in numerous works (Acha, 2007; Jones, 1953–1957; Sherry, 2010; Solomon, 2003; Sulloway, 1991). On this occasion, we wish to focus solely on the form and the relevance that the problem of reality and phantasy took on during the course of that rupture.

As is known, in works such as *Totem and Taboo* (Freud, 1913), "On the History of the Psycho-Analytic Movement" (Freud, 1914a) and "On Narcissism: an Introduction" (Freud, 1914b), Freud accused Jung of trying to desexualise psychoanalytic theory. At the same time, he demonstrated his opposition to the theory of archetypes, with which the Swiss doctor sought to study the origin of religious phenomena, and which allowed for the interpretation of the phantasies and narratives of his patients without making any reference to real and historical events.

In this context, Freud constructed, with little time difference, two versions of his *Neurotica*. The first of them, included in his "...History of the Psycho-Analytic Movement", was analysed a few pages above. In that paper, he stated that all narratives of seduction remitted to phantasies, but that these, in turn, remitted to real episodes: the auto-erotic activity of early childhood, which was covered up, embellished and transformed by these phantasies. What Freud seemed to be defending with multiple (or even contradictory) arguments was the need for a historical, real and sexual basis for phantasies and neurotic phenomena.

The second version appeared published shortly afterwards, in Lecture XXIII of his "Introductory Lectures on Psycho-Analysis" (Freud, 1916–1917). There, the Vienesse psychoanalyst gave an extensive argument intended to show that the division between (material) truth and phantasy did not make much sense since both elements are combined in many cases. Furthermore, the reason for the relative uselessness of that separation would be even more robust due to the conclusion reached by Freud. He stated that, concerning the resulting neurosis, the effect of both elements was the same, regardless if the scene was something actually experienced by the subject or something phantasised.

As expected, this idea was not developed without surprises or apparent contradictions. When Freud introduced the topic by stating that "in the majority of cases" the recounted events from childhood were not true, everything seemed to indicate that he was preparing the later versions (Freud, 1916–1917, p. 367). But he immediately changed his course: "the position can be shown to be that the childhood experiences constructed or remembered in analysis are sometimes indisputably false and sometimes equally certainly correct, and *in most cases compounded of truth and falsehood*" (Freud, 1916–1917, p. 367; italics added).

The Viennese psychoanalyst then went on to specifically address the scenes of seduction. Thus, he introduced several very different ideas to those from the later versions reviewed above. In Freud's words, "Phantasies of being seduced are of particular interest, because so *often they are not phantasies but real memories*. Fortunately, however, they are nevertheless not real as often as seemed at first to be shown by the findings of analysis" (Freud, 1916–1917, p. 370; italics added). According to the versions after 1920, the source of the phantasies was the Oedipus complex. In this lecture, the phantasies were tied to the same element as in the 1914 text:

> A phantasy of being seduced when no seduction has occurred is usually employed by a child to screen the auto-erotic period of his sexual activity. He spares himself shame about masturbation by retrospectively phantasying a desired object into these earliest times.
>
> (Freud, 1916–1917, p. 370)

This clarification was substantial: it was not that the child felt erotic impulses towards his parents and, for that reason, created such phantasies; instead, the bond with an object, present in the scene of seduction, was *retrospectively* allocated into an early period (that of auto-erotism), a period in which, according to Freud, the object was absent. Therefore, the true event that would be hidden behind the phantasies was the auto-erotic activity: drives that try to obtain satisfaction from different erogenous zones, with the libido not yet being able to find an object which would allow for an at least partial synthesis of these drives (Freud, 1914b).

All these arguments led to a proposition regarding the necessity of certain content in the narratives of the childhood events told by patients: seduction, the threat of being castrated and the observation of parental intercourse. According to Freud:

> The only impression we gain is that these events of childhood are somehow demanded as a necessity, that they are among the essential elements of a neurosis. If they have occurred in reality, so much to the good; but if they have been withheld by reality, they are put together from hints and supplemented by phantasy. *The outcome is the same, and up to the present we have not succeeded in pointing to any difference in the consequences, whether phantasy or reality has had the greater share in these events of childhood.*
>
> (Freud, 1916–1917, p. 370; italics added)

The last statement is surely shocking to common sense and opposed to any theory that attempts to highlight the pathological potential that events that actually occurred could have. When taken to an extreme, it is difficult to conceive that the outcome of a phantasised seduction is the same as that of child sexual abuse. However, the entire paragraph highlighted a feature that was crucial to psychoanalytic theory and practice, which had been present since the days of the *Neurotica*. In the patients' narratives (especially those that refer to the distant past), distinguishing between reality and phantasy would be neither so simple nor so important. In both cases, the stories could be *true* if these scenes made up part of the structure of the neurosis.

Freud's indifference towards determining the real or phantastic nature of the narratives was based on his certainty that the phantasies were not totally invented. For him, instead, they find their origin in historical experiences, even when these had not taken place in the subject's lifetime:

> Whence comes the need for these phantasies and the material for them? There can be no doubt that their sources lie in the instincts; but it has still to be explained why the same phantasies with the same content are created on every occasion (…) I believe these *primal phantasies* (…) are a phylogenetic endowment. In them the individual reaches beyond his own experience into primaeval experiences at points where his own experience has been too rudimentary. It seems to me quite possible that all the things that are told to us to-day in analysis as phantasy -the seduction of children, the inflaming of sexual excitement by observing parental intercourse, the threat of castration (or rather castration itself)- were once real occurrences in the primaeval times of the human family, and that children in their phantasies are simply filling in the gaps in individual truth with prehistoric truth.
>
> (Freud, 1916–1917, p. 371; italics in original)

In his view, reality and phantasy, again, showed a complex interplay and not mutual exclusion. Phantasies can only be derived from real events; at the same time, we can only access these events thanks to the phantasies. Freud considered them the distorted narratives of episodes that have occurred, either in a person's individual history, or humanity's history. Like scars from a remote past, they would grant access to a prehistoric truth, which is not part of the explicit narratives but is preserved in phylogenetic memory. The "'traumatic' element" (Freud, 1906, p. 274), which seemed to have lost its importance along with Seduction Theory, recovered its relevance in Freudian theory within the framework of a new problem: how would these traumas be transmitted from one generation the next? We shall deal with this problem in Chapter 5.

However, this was not the only way in which the notion of trauma regained importance in Freud's work. The First World War brought traumatic neuroses back to the fore. In this context, Freud developed a new conception of trauma based on an economic point of view. In this way, a trauma would no longer refer to a scene capable of being recounted even when there could be doubts regarding its real or phantasist nature; rather, this notion began to be conceived at the limits of representation. We will deal with these issues linked to the war neuroses in the following chapter.

Notes

1 *Neurotica*" was the name Freud used in his letters to Fliess to refer to his theory of the traumatic origin of neurosis.
2 Freud also contributed to the idea of resistance to psychoanalysis due to its affirmation of infantile sexuality in his "An Autobiographical Study": "Few of the findings of psycho-analysis have met with such universal contradiction or have aroused such an outburst of indignation as the assertion that the sexual function starts at the beginning of life and reveals its presence by important signs even in childhood" (Freud, 1925, p. 32). However, various historians have underlined the prevalence of ideas about sexuality and, in particular, about infantile masturbation in times before the rise of psychoanalysis. Known are Foucault's theses on the masturbating child as an object of medical practices and knowledge (Foucault, 1978, 1999). We would also like to mention Bonomi's work that supports the existence of paediatric theories on the pathogenic influence of infantile masturbation and the proposal for preventive castrations, which Freud had opposed (Bonomi, 1994).
3 This idea was supported by Freud when referring to his *Neurotica*: it would be "the solution of a more-than-thousand-year-old problem, a *caput Nili*!". These expressions are found in the same letter in which he told Fliess his grief occasioned by the poor acceptance of the lecture he gave on his aetiological theory (on April 21, 1896), in front of the members of the Vienna Society for Psychiatry and Neurology.
4 This was the name by which Freud habitually referred to his Project in the letters to Fliess since its first mention on March 28, 1895 (Masson, 1985, p. 123, letter of 28/03/1895).
5 These theses were known as the "principle of neuronal inertia" and "principle of constancy", respectively.
6 It is true, as M. Vallejo argued in his doctoral thesis and in his book *La seducción freudiana* (Vallejo, 2011, 2012), that it would be possible to establish continuities between the French hereditary tradition and the totality of Freud's work. Nevertheless, the Freudian shift of 1896 was the most important and explicit attempt to displace heredity and move away from that tradition.
7 In "Further Remarks on the Neuro-Psychoses of Defence" he used a phrase almost identical to the one found in "The Aetiology of Hysteria": "their content must consist of an actual irritation of the genitals (of processes resembling copulation)" (Freud, 1896b, p. 163).
8 Freud made this point explicitly. He made the following statement, after acknowledging that he could not lead the analyses to their definitive conclusion, that he was beginning to suspect the frequency with which the father appeared as a seducer, and that he had difficulties in differentiating the narratives that referred to facts from those that are "fiction that has been cathected with affect": "I was so far influenced (by this) that I was ready to give up two things: the complete resolution of a neurosis and the certain knowledge of its etiology in childhood" (Masson, 1985, pp. 264–265, letter of 21/9/97).
9 The *model* on which this psychical conception of memory is based seems to be that of *physiological and biological memory*, which was present in evolutionary thinking at the end of the nineteenth century.
10 For example, in Freud (1896b, p. 164, n.2).

11 In his book on Seduction, Mauro Vallejo puts forward an interesting hypothesis about the reasons why Freud would have replaced the caregivers with the father. If the latter were the seducer, it would be easier to replace heredity with *another form of family determination of the illness*: paternal seduction (Vallejo, 2012, pp. 80–95).

12 We disagree on this point with Triplett, who stated that in this text "Freud clearly failed to claim that his patients of 1896 had fooled him with fictional stories" and that he would only "take that step in his next revision in 1914" (Triplett, 2004, p. 657). Our dissent is twofold. First, because Freud never said that he was "fooled" by his patients; in any case, that he was fooling *himself* with their narratives and with his own theory. Second, because in 1906 he was already introducing the possibility that these stories were phantasies, although not in all cases.

13 Borch-Jacobsen was the first to conjecture that the criticism that Freud's contemporary colleagues directed at him was not motivated by the supposed scandal that the affirmation of the existence of child sexual abuse would generate. Authors like Krafft-Ebing had also made reference to these types of attacks. The objections would, in actuality, have been focused on the possibility that the patient's narratives were produced by the use of hypnosis and the probable suggestive influence exercised by Freud (consciously or not) when searching for the key to such an important problem (Borch-Jacobsen, 1996, pp. 22–24). The historian's hypothesis becomes even more plausible when it is noted that Freud himself recognised the possibility of such a critique and went to such lengths to refute it.

References

Abraham, K. (1907). La experimentación de traumas sexuales como una forma de actividad sexual. In K. Abraham (Ed.), *Psicoanálisis clínico* (pp. 35–47). Buenos Aires: Hormé, 1980.

Acha, O. (2007). *Freud y el problema de la historia.* Buenos Aires: Prometeo.

Acha, O. (2010). No todo es historia. Lacan y los entretiempos freudianos. In Acha, O. & Vallejo, M. (Comp.), *Inconsciente e historia después de Freud. Cruces entre filosofía, psicoanálisis e historiografía* (pp. 267–282). Buenos Aires: Prometeo.

Anonymous (1895a). S. Freud: Über Hysterie. Wiener klinische Rundschau. In Freud, S. (Ed.), *Gesammelte Werke. nachtragsband. Texte aus den Jahren 1885–1938* (pp. 328–341). Frankfurt am Main: Fischer.

Anonymous (1895b). S. Freud: Über Hysterie. Wiener medizinische Presse. In Freud, S. (Ed.), *Gesammelte Werke. nachtragsband. Texte aus den Jahren 1885–1938* (pp. 342–351). Frankfurt am Main: Fischer.

Berta, S. (2014). *Escribir el trauma, de Freud a Lacan.* Buenos Aires: Letra Viva.

Bonomi, C. (1994). Why have we ignored Freud the 'paediatrician'? The relevance of Freud's paediatric Training for the Origins of Psychoanalysis. In Haynal, A. & Falzeder, E. (Eds.), *100 Years of Psychoanalysis: Contribution to the Hystory of Psychoanalysis* (pp. 55–99). London: Karnac.

Borch-Jacobsen, M. (1996). Neurotica: Freud and the seduction theory. *October*, *76*, 15–42.

Breuer, J. & Freud, S. (1893). On the physical mechanism of hysterical phenomena: preliminary communication. In Freud, S. (1955) (Ed.), *The Standard Edition of the Complete Psychological Works of Sigmund Freud, Vol. II: Studies on Hysteria* (pp. 3–47). London: The Hogarth Press and the Institute of Psycho-Analysis.

Breuer, J. & Freud, S. (1895). Studies on hysteria, 1893–1895. In Freud, S. (1955) (Ed.), *The Standard Edition of the Complete Psychological Works of Sigmund Freud, Vol. II: Studies on Hysteria.* London: The Hogarth Press and the Institute of Psycho-Analysis.

Carter, C. (1980). Germ theory, hysteria, and Freud's early work in psychopathology. *Medical History, 24*, 259–274.

Charcot, J.M. (1894). *Poliklinische Vorträge von Prof. J. M. Charcot. Ubersetzt von Dr. Sigm. Freud. I. Band Schuljahr 1887–1888.* Vienna: Franz Deuticke.

Esterson, A. (1993). *Seductive mirage. An exploration of the Work of Sigmund Freud.* Chicago, IL: Open Court.

Esterson, A. (2001). The mythologizong of psychoanalytic history: Deception and self-deception in Freud's accounts of the seduction theory episode. *Hystory of Psychiatry, 12*, 329–352.

Foucault, M. (1978). *The History of Sexuality, Volume 1: An Introduction.* New York: Pantheon Books.

Foucault, M. (1999). *Los Anormales. Curso en el Collège de France, 1973–1974.* Buenos Aires: F.C.E.

Freud, S. ([1888a] 1966). Hysteria. In S. Freud (Ed.), *The Standard Edition of the Complete Psychological Works of Sigmund Freud, Vol. I: Pre- Psycho-Analytic Publications and Unpublished Drafts* (pp. 37–59). London: The Hogarth Press and the Institute of Psycho-Analysis.

Freud, S. ([1892–1893] 1966). A case of successful treatment by hypnotism. In S. Freud (Ed.), *The Standard Edition of the Complete Psychological Works of Sigmund Freud, Vol. I: Pre-Psycho-Analytic Publications and Unpublished Drafts* (pp. 115–128). London: The Hogarth Press and the Institute of Psycho-Analysis.

Freud, S. ([1892–1894] 1966). Preface and footnotes to Charcot's Tuesday lectures. In S. Freud (Ed.), *The Standard Edition of the Complete Psychological Works of Sigmund Freud, Vol. I: Pre-Psycho-Analytic Publications and Unpublished Drafts* (pp. 130–143). London: The Hogarth Press and the Institute of Psycho-Analysis.

Freud, S. ([1893] 1962). On the psychical mechanism of hysterical phenomena: A lecture. In S. Freud (Ed.), *The Standard Edition of the Complete Psychological Works of Sigmund Freud, Vol. III: Early Psycho-Analytic Publications* (pp. 25–39). London: The Hogarth Press and the Institute of Psycho-Analysis.

Freud, S. ([1894] 1962). The neuro-psychoses of defence. In S. Freud (Ed.), *The Standard Edition of the Complete Psychological Works of Sigmund Freud, Vol. III: Early Psycho-Analytic Publications* (pp. 41–68). London: The Hogarth Press and the Institute of Psycho- Analysis.

Freud, S. (1895a). Obsessions and phobias: Their psychical mechanism and their aetiology. In S. Freud (1962) (Ed.), *The Standard Edition of the Complete Psychological Works of Sigmund Freud, Vol. III: Early Psycho-Analytic Publications* (pp. 69–84). London: The Hogarth Press and the Institute of Psycho- Analysis.

Freud, S. ([1895b] 1962). On the grounds for detaching a particular syndrome from neurasthenia under the description 'anxiety neurosis'. In S. Freud (Ed.), *The Standard Edition of the Complete Psychological Works of Sigmund Freud, Vol. III: Early Psycho-Analytic Publications* (pp. 85–117). London: The Hogarth Press and the Institute of Psycho-Analysis.

Freud, S. ([1895c] 1962). A reply to criticisms of my paper on anxiety neurosis. In S. Freud (Ed.), *The Standard Edition of the Complete Psychological Works of Sigmund Freud, Vol. III: Early Psycho-Analytic Publications* (pp. 119–139). London: The Hogarth Press and the Institute of Psycho-Analysis.

Freud, S. ([1895d] 1966). Project for a scientific psychology. In S. Freud (Ed.), *The Standard Edition of the Complete Psychological Works of Sigmund Freud, Vol. I:*

Pre-Psycho-Analytic Publications and Unpublished Drafts (pp. 283–394). London: The Hogarth Press and the Institute of Psycho-Analysis.

Freud, S. ([1896a] 1962). Heredity and the aetiology of the neuroses. In S. Freud (Ed.), *The Standard Edition of the Complete Psychological Works of Sigmund Freud, Vol. III: Early Psycho-Analytic Publications* (pp. 141–156). London: The Hogarth Press and the Institute of Psycho-Analysis.

Freud, S. ([1896b] 1962). Further remarks on the neuro- psychoses of defence. In S. Freud (Ed.), *The Standard Edition of the Complete Psychological Works of Sigmund Freud, Vol. III: Early Psycho-Analytic Publications* (pp. 157–185). London: The Hogarth Press and the Institute of Psycho- Analysis.

Freud, S. ([1896c] 1962). The aetiology of hysteria. In S. Freud (Ed.), *The Standard Edition of the Complete Psychological Works of Sigmund Freud, Vol. III: Early Psycho-Analytic Publications* (pp. 187–221). London: The Hogarth Press and the Institute of Psycho-Analysis.

Freud, S. ([1905] 1953). Three essays on the teory of sexuality. In S. Freud (Ed.), *The Standard Edition of the Complete Psychological Works of Sigmund Freud, Vol. VII: A Case of Hysteria, Three Essays on Sexuality and Other Works* (pp. 124–243). London: The Hogarth Press and the Institute of Psycho-Analysis.

Freud, S. ([1906] 1953). My views on the part played by sexuality in the aetiology of the neuroses. In S. Freud (Ed.), *The Standard Edition of the Complete Psychological Works of Sigmund Freud, Vol. VII: A Case of Hysteria, Three Essays on Sexuality and Other Works* (pp. 271–279). London: The Hogarth Press and the Institute of Psycho-Analysis.

Freud, S. ([1913] 1955). Totem and taboo. In S. Freud (Ed.), *The Standard Edition of the Complete Psychological Works of Sigmund Freud, Vol. XIII: Totem and Taboo and Other Works* (pp. 1–164). London: The Hogarth Press and the Institute of Psycho-Analysis.

Freud, S. ([1914a] 1957). On the history of the psycho-analitic movement. In S. Freud (Ed.), *The Standard Edition of the Complete Psychological Works of Sigmund Freud, Vol. XIV: On the History of the Psycho- Analytic Movement, Papers on Metapsychology and Other Works* (pp. 1–66). London: The Hogarth Press and the Institute of Psycho-Analysis.

Freud, S. ([1914b] 1957). On narcissism: And introduction. In S. Freud (Ed.), *The Standard Edition of the Complete Psychological Works of Sigmund Freud, Vol. XIV: On the History of the Psycho- Analytic Movement, Papers on Metapsychology and Other Works* (pp. 67–102). London: The Hogarth Press and the Institute of Psycho- Analysis.

Freud, S. ([1916–1917] 1963). Lecture XXIII. The paths to the formation of symptoms. In S. Freud (Ed.), *The Standard Edition of the Complete Psychological Works of Sigmund Freud, Vol. XVI: Introductory Lectures on Psycho- Analysis (Part III)* (pp. 358–377). London: The Hogarth Press and the Institute of Psycho-Analysis.

Freud, S. ([1918] 1955). From the history of an infantile neurosis. In S. Freud (Ed.), *The Standard Edition of the Complete Psychological Works of Sigmund Freud, Vol. XVII: An Infantile Neurosis and Other Works* (pp. 1–123). London: The Hogarth Press and the Institute of Psycho-Analysis.

Freud, S. ([1925] 1959). An autobiographical study. In S. Freud (Ed.), *The Standard Edition of the Complete Psychological Works of Sigmund Freud, Vol. XX: An Autobiographical Study. Inhibitions, Symptoms and Anxiety. The Question of Lay Analysis and Other Works* (pp. 1–70). London: The Hogarth Press and the Institute of Psycho-Analysis.

Freud, S. ([1933] 1964). Lecture XXXIII. Femininity. In S. Freud (Ed.), *The Standard Edition of the Complete Psychological Works of Sigmund Freud, Vol. XXII: New Introductory,*

Lectures on Psycho-Analysis and Other Works (pp. 112–135). London: The Hogarth Press and the Institute of Psycho-Analysis.
Freud, S. ([1939] 1964). Moses and monotheism: three essays. In S. Freud (Ed.), *The Standard Edition of the Complete Psychological Works of Sigmund Freud, Vol. XXIII: Moses and Monotheism, an Outline of Psycho- Analysis and Other Works* (pp. 1–137). London: The Hogarth Press and the Institute of Psycho-Analysis.
Gelfand, T. (1989). Charcot's response to Freud's rebellion. *Journal of the History of Ideas, 50* (2), 293–307.
Good, M. (1995) Karl Abraham, Sigmund Freud, and the fate of the seduction theory. *Journal of the American Psychoanalytic Association, 43* (4), 1137–1167.
Hacking, J. (1995). *Rewriting the Soul: Multiple Personality and the Sciences of Memory.* Princeton, NJ: Princeton University Press.
Hanns, L. (1996). *Dicionario comentado do alemão de Freud.* Río de Janeiro: Imago Ed.
Hermann, J. (1992). *Trauma and Recovery.* New York: Basic Books.
Israel, H. & Schatzman, M. (1993). The seduction theory. *History of Psychiatry, 4,* 23–59.
Jones, E. (1953–57). *The Life and Work of Sigmund Freud: Volume I, II and III.* New York: Basic Books.
Masson, J.M. (1984). *The Assault on Truth: Freud's Suppression of the Seduction Theory.* New York: Penguin Press.
Masson, J.M. (1985). *The Complete Letters of Sigmund Freud to WIlhelm Fliess, 1887–1904.* Cambridge, MA and London: The Belknap Press of Harvard University Press.
Sanfelippo, L. & Vallejo, M. (2013a). Orígenes de la Teoría de la Seducción. Etiología y herencia en los primeros escritos de Sigmund Freud. *Revista de la Sociedad Argentina de Psicoanálisis, 17,* 257–276.
Schimek, J. (1987). Fact and fantasy in the seduction theory: A historical review. *Journal of the American Psychoanalytic Association, 35* (4), 937–965.
Sherry, J. (2010). *Carl Gustav Jung. Avant-Garde Conservative.* New York: Palgrave Macmillan.
Solomon, H.M. (2003). Freud and Jung: An incomplete encounter. *Journal of Analytical Psychology, 48,* 553–569.
Sulloway, F. (1991). Reassessing Freud's case histories: The social construction of psychoanalysis. *Isis, 82,* 245–275.
Triplett, H. (2004). The Misnomer of Freud's "seduction theory". *Journal of the History of Ideas, 65* (4), 647–655.
Vallejo, M. (2011). Teorías hereditarias del siglo XIX y el problema de la transmisión intergeneracional. Psicoanálisis y Biopolítica. Doctoral thesis. UNLP.
Vallejo, M. (2012). *La seducción freudiana (1895–1897). Un ensayo de genética textual.* Buenos Aires: Letra Viva.

Chapter 4

The War Neuroses and a New Economic Conception of Trauma (1914–1920)

In this chapter, we intend to study some of the conceptual, technical and ethical problems that emerged during the First World War regarding the category of *war neurosis.* The first thing we wish to state is that this major armed conflict, and the nosographic category associated with it, generated debates about the nature of trauma and about its treatment. These debates acquired such relevance, extension and even urgency that had not been seen since the nineteenth century's final decades. As we mentioned in Chapter 1, immediately before the turn of the century, the appearance of difficult-to-diagnose cases linked to railway accidents, the development of systematic research on hysteria and the controversies about the nature of hypnosis and suggestion promoted theoretical debates and practical innovations in the medical world. However, these topics also transcended the closed and minor field of specialists. The pension claims, the possibility of crimes being induced beyond the author's will by means of suggestion, and the mysterious illnesses that developed without leaving an anatomical mark on the body, captured the attention of doctors, public officials, judges, journalists, novelists and the general public, who followed these "modern" debates carefully via the written press. Through these (epistemic, clinical, judicial, literary) paths, the notion of trauma underwent different transformations: it moved to areas other than the medical-surgical domain, it was applied to a greater number of situations even when these did not imply a mechanical action affecting the organism, it acquired psychological characteristics, it transformed its most common meaning. However, this great wave of "trauma" subsided over time. As more attention was paid to the psychological processes capable of producing symptoms, less interest was sparked by the notion of trauma.

In Germany, very early on, Oppenheim's ideas encountered fierce opposition from the medical establishment installed in public institutions. In the face of his "traumatic neurosis", a nosographical category that supposed the existence of a specific type of organic illness caused entirely by the accident, the doctors in universities defended the importance of hereditary predisposition and psychological factors such as "wish complexes" and "imaginative desires" (*Begehrungsvorstellungen*, a term coined by Strümpell in 1895). The determining role of the accident thus ended up being questioned since it was assumed that imaginative desires were set in motion when there existed the possibility of obtaining an exemption from

DOI: 10.4324/9781003380016-5

obligations or some type of pecuniary benefit for the accident suffered (Micale & Lerner, 2001, p. 14). Because of this, Oppenheim and his category were accused of promoting an epidemic of "pension neurosis". In this manner, the German neurologist's loss of prestige and the consolidation of psychological hypotheses about the mechanism of neurotic symptoms caused a loss of interest regarding the accident (and, by extension, the trauma). At the same time, this process contributed to producing distrust in patients' complaints regarding their suffering.

As we have seen, in the Parisian tradition, the panorama seemed different. During the 1880s, trauma and psychological factors were not considered mutually exclusive; rather, the old anatomical notion had acquired psychological attributes. Charcot's teaching made it possible to conceive that intense emotions and ideas introduced during altered states of consciousness could have traumatic effects. However, after Charcot's death, the interest in trauma and his conception of hysteria as a nervous illness slowly began to lose validity. We have already seen how Janet affirmed himself more decidedly in the field of psychology without taking away heredity's preponderant causal role. If the hereditarily determined weakening of the ability for synthesis was the pathogenic key of hysteria and other neuroses, then the trauma (physical or psychical) could not play a central role in his conceptualisations or in his therapeutic approach.

As Edelman argues, "Charcot's neurophysiological interpretation backed away until it disappeared: hysteria became a psychical illness" (Edelman, 2003, p. 263). This psychologisation of hysteria should not be solely attributed to Bernheim's influence. It is clear that this author interpreted hysterical phenomena as "cultural" phenomena based on suggestion (Bernheim, 1903, p. 218; cited in Edelman, 2003, pp. 272–273). Hysteria thus not only lost its neurological character but also risked not being considered a medical illness. At the same time, the idea of trauma had no importance whatsoever at Nancy. However, other doctors played an important role. They were neurologists and part of the hospital system. Their proposals ended up expelling hysteria from the neurological domain and contributed to delineating in France the frontiers of a new field: the psychotherapies.

One of them was Joseph Jules Dejerine. Trained at *L'hôpital de Bicêtre*, he obtained a position at the Salpêtrière in 1895 and, in a few years, managed to obtain Charcot's position in his service and his chair (Edelman, 2003, pp. 265, 281). Hysteria was, from his point of view, a "psychoneurosis" produced by the action of an "emotion" capable of dissociating an organ or a part of the psychical centres on which its functioning depended (Dejerine & Gauckler, 1911, p. 380; cited in Edelman, 2003, pp. 266–267). Edelman argues that the importance attributed to emotional shock seems to bring his conception closer to "Charcot's *nervous shock*" (Edelman, 2003, p. 267). However, unlike Bernheim, Charcot or Janet, this author downplayed suggestion, which in this case also meant that he was not interested in the ideas that made up the experience in which the emotion arose. From his point of view, the "forgetting" that characterised hysterical accidents did not refer to the event that supposedly caused the symptom: what was forgotten was merely the part of the body that stopped working (Edelman, 2003, p. 267). The recalling of the trauma obviously had no place in his psychotherapeutic proposal. Neither did suggestion. The treatment consisted of isolation (similar to the old moral treatment) and "persuasion" therapy (Edelman, 2003, pp. 268–269; Swain, 1994, p. 14). Seeking to move away from the passivity in which the subject was subsumed in hypnosis, he attempted to get them to participate more actively. Through reasoning (instead of suggestions), the therapy sought to persuade the subject that "he does not have an injured nervous system, that the condition from which he suffers is not serious and that he will surely be cured" (Dejerine, 1904, p. 170; cited in Edelman, 2003, p. 269). However, as Gladys Swain (1994, p. 17) points out, this rationalism had a "blind spot" that once again brought it closer to suggestion. Dejerine himself admitted that

> one does not cure a hysteric, one does not cure a neurasthenic, one cannot change their mental state with reasoning, with syllogisms. We can only cure them when they manage to believe in us. In fact, psychotherapy can act only when the one on whom we exercise it has confessed his entire life to us, that is, when he has absolute trust in us.
>
> (Dejerine & Gauckler, 1911, p. IX; cited in Edelman, 2003, p. 271; Swain, 1994, p. 18)

To cure the disease, the patient must surrender entirely to the doctor's influence. Furthermore, if that act of surrendering does not occur, "the doctor should exercise an act of authority" until reaching the point where they could "restore the patient's freedom, the power of his intellectual control" (Edelman, 2003, p. 271). Just like moral treatment, this rationalist perspective, which sought to escape from the dangers of suggestion, could turn into authoritarianism in the name of the patient's well-being.

The second neurologist who brought hysteria into the field of psychotherapies was Joseph Babinski. He had been Head of clinic in Charcot's Service between 1885 and 1887 (that is, at the time of maximum research on traumatic hysteria), before obtaining a medical position at the Hôpital de la Pitié in 1890 (Edelman, 2003, p. 271). From 1901 onwards, this doctor tried to distance himself from Charcot's teachings and proposed a new name for the old illness: *pithiatism* (Baños Orellana, 2013, p. 271; Edelman, 2003, p. 272). In his writings, hysteria ceased to be understood neurologically and even ceased to be considered an illness: "Hysteria is a psychic state in which the subject is prone to autosuggestion" (Babinski, 1901, p. 1075; cited in Edelman, 2003, p. 272), though this did not eliminate the possibility of being suggested by others. According to this author, pithiatism was completely curable through persuasion. Both perspectives (Dejerine's and Babinski's), although different, led to a treatment that did not take into account the issue of trauma and attempted to rectify via persuasion the psychical element that produced the illness (the emotion or the suggestion, respectively). They both also led to the problem of those patients who, despite being persuaded, remained ill: from then on, persuasion could give rise to the use of authority or violence, a central problem during the war.

In the English-speaking context, around the turn of the century, there was also an increase in psychological hypotheses and decreased interest regarding traumatic experiences. As we saw in Chapter 1, in the United States, the first psychotherapeutic practices and the psychological hypotheses that relativised the determining power of trauma were disseminated by the surgeons of railway companies. These physicians relied on psychology to answer to the medical and legal repercussions Erichsen's book's initial reception had provoked. Across the Atlantic, "hysteria and neurasthenia were staple topics for discussion in the pre-war British medical press" (Loughran, 2008, p. 27). In a recent article, Tracey Loughran took an in-depth look at the state of British medicine prior to the beginning of the war. Contrary to what is usually affirmed, she concluded that "the shift from a predominantly somatic to a psychological paradigm" in the approach to both clinical pictures "was in evidence before World War I" (Loughran, 2008, p. 28). At the same time, heredity was still the most important factor regarding aetiology. In this way, the question of "'neurotic temperament'" was "linked to discourses of nation and race" (Loughran, 2008, p. 28). As in Germany and France, the relevance given to psychological factors regarding the mechanisms of the illnesses was not incompatible with a somatic conception of heredity. In addition, psychology and heredity contributed to displacing the issue of trauma from the central role it had obtained due to the railway accidents.

If we shift our gaze and focus on the more limited context of Freud's work, we can also observe similar displacements. Until 1896, the Viennese psychoanalyst proposed an extension of the concept of traumatic hysteria and tried to establish trauma as the ultimate cause of the neuroses. However, later on, the questioning of his Neurotica made "the 'traumatic' element in childhood sexual experiences lose its importance" (Freud, 1906, p. 274). The traditional history of psychoanalysis interpreted this change as substituting experiences for phantasies. As we tried to argue in the preceding chapter, these notions did not imply mutual exclusion or a lack of consideration of events that actually took place. However, after the abandonment of the Seduction Theory, another series of consequences did occur. First, heredity regained importance in aetiology. Freud admitted this in the same letter in which he abandoned his *Neurotica* and confirmed it with the creation of the notions of "complemental series" (Freud, 1916–1917d, p. 362)[1] and "phylogenetic heritage" or "Prehistoric Experience" (Freud, 1916–1917d, p. 362, 1918, p. 97).

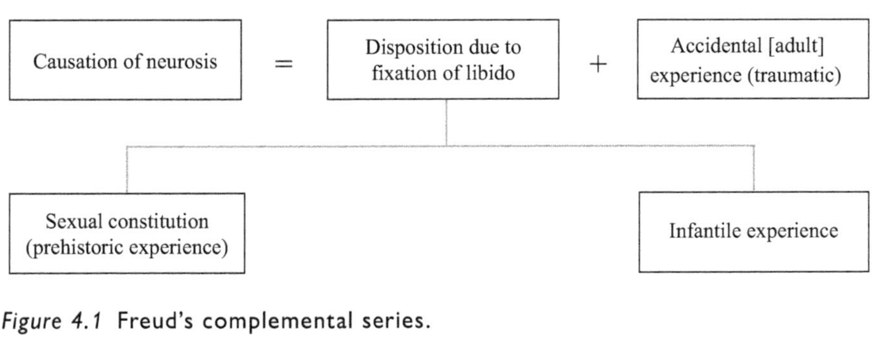

Figure 4.1 Freud's complemental series.

Second, infantile sexuality ceased to be a contingent element (reduced only to those subjects who suffered abuse), and it became a factor of universal occurrence. At the same time, the *image* of the child, which Freud derived from the analysis of adults, was also transformed. If in his *Neurotica* the child was considered to be asexual and received sexuality from an external source (by means of a seducer), in his *Three Essays on the Theory of Sexuality*, the child became polymorphously perverse (Freud, 1905). Lastly, the idea of a psychical conflict, which had originally been closely related to the notion of trauma, was separated from the latter. In 1894 the instant in which the ego was faced with an incompatible idea was called a "traumatic moment" (Freud, 1894, p. 50). In 1896, the conflict that led to repression and neurosis only occurred if the person had suffered sexual traumas in childhood. However, after the abandonment of the Seduction Theory, Freud was able to consider a conflict at the core of neurosis without needing to resort to "trauma". In other words, *not all trauma gives rise to neurosis, nor does every neurosis require the existence of a trauma in order to develop* since the conflict that leads to repression can just as well take place without the occurrence of traumatic experiences. In turn, the terms used to describe the conflict also changed. It was no longer a question of incompatibility between ideas but of the subject's "conflict between their libido and their sexual repression" (Freud, 1906, p. 277) or "between the ego-instincts and the sexual instincts" (Freud, 1916–1917f, p. 412).

The panorama developed thus far could be summarised in the following way. During the final two decades of the nineteenth century, the psychologisation of trauma was produced by the confluence of different processes. The anatomical trauma implied that illness depended solely on the mechanical and objective force of the impact. Instead, the psychical trauma included subjective elements, such as the previous particularities of the person or the subject's response to the event. Furthermore, if in the face of a trauma that caused a serious material injury – such as the tearing of the spinal nervous tissue – the person could only be compensated for the damage suffered but no treatment could be carried out, the psychological trauma opened the door to the possibility of therapy.

This trend was modified in the first decade and a half of the new century. During this period, the use of a psychological framework to address neuroses and mental illness was consolidated. At the same time, the number of psychotherapeutic orientations multiplied. Said consolidation and multiplication decreased interest in trauma, even when it was understood in psychological terms. The "psychologisation" seems to have functioned as an "interiorisation": the pathological processes were searched for within the psyche. Those who held the most extreme positions could come to believe that a person's lived experiences did not influence the development of psychical illness.

The beginning of the First World War and the virtual epidemic of cases of war neurosis forced everything to be rethought. The war helped consolidate the idea that psychological factors participate in the production of mental illness and that the latter can be treated through different types of therapeutic approaches, many of them psychical in nature. However, during the war, psychologisation and trauma were again reunited.

This chapter has been divided into two main parts. In the first, we will attempt to address the main conceptual, technical and ethical debates that arose around the war neuroses in the different national contexts. Here the ideas held by psychoanalysts were included in a broader domain, where other discourses and therapeutic orientations occupied the dominant positions in those debates during much of the war. It could even be thought that this historical event served as a privileged occasion for the psychoanalytic movement. Because of the movement's marginality with respect to the European medical and psychiatric establishment, the war allowed it to gain greater visibility and for its members to become recognised and summoned to work for government agencies; without this implying, however, a massive acceptance or a definitive consecration of psychoanalysis. This first part of the chapter has three sections, organised around three questions that dominated the debates on the war neuroses: What characterised war traumas and the illness associated with them? What roles did the experience of war and the subjective particularities of those affected play in developing the illness? Which were the chosen methods of treatment, and by which principles were these governed?

The second part of the chapter involves a modification of our analysis perspective since we will solely address the impact of the war on the work of Sigmund Freud from 1920 onward. This part is also divided into two sections: one referring to the ethical implications linked to the stance taken by the Viennese psychoanalyst regarding the use of electrotherapy; the other will be devoted to analysing the conceptual implications of certain clinical phenomena (in particular, dreams that repeat traumatic experiences) which contributed to the construction of a new conception of trauma.

4.1 Part I: Debates on the War Neuroses

The First World War extended throughout a good part of the European territory the impact of the industrial and technological advancements on the old art of war. Similar to the railway, but in a much more atrocious way, it allowed humanity to observe the shadows produced by the lights of reason and its progress. We want to avoid dwelling here on the collective cultural effects of a technical deployment capable of producing mass killings in a short period. Instead, we intend to focus on how the subjective consequences of the war were thought about and treated. It is worth clarifying that, as we shall see, not all the doctors or authors who dealt with these problems coincided in that the neuroses that arose *during* the war were war neuroses (different from those that arose in times of peace) or that they were *consequences of* the war (and not the effect of other factors unrelated to the armed conflict).

We now intend to address the main debates on the neurotic illnesses of soldiers, basing our analysis on the three questions posed in this chapter's introduction.

4.1.1 Characterisation of the War Neuroses

4.1.1.1 Somatic Damage?

In a Foucauldian-inspired book entitled "Governing the Soul. The Shaping of the Private Self", Nikolas Rose devoted a section to "The Psychology of War" (Rose, 1999, pp. 15–21). In it, he stated that since the start of the First World War, there had been a large number of desertions in the English army associated with shell shock: "7 to 10 per cent of officer casualties and 3 to 4 per cent of casualties from other ranks came into this category" (Rose, 1999, p. 20). According to this author, these were basically "individuals with well developed psychiatric symptoms, yet whose background was apparently normal" (Rose, 1999, p. 20). This situation led, on the one hand, to the rejection of the approaches that considered these cases to be "of organic origin and untreatable" and, on the other hand, to the acceptance of "a dynamic conception of psychological processes, with such characteristics as an unconscious and repression", which at the same time disproved the Freudian argument for a specific sexual aetiology of mental disturbance (Rose, 1999, pp. 20–21). This succinct description of the consequences of the war in the field of neurotic illness suggests that there was a broad consensus among the medical specialists of that time on the following four points: (1) the minor importance of antecedents in the development of the symptoms; (2) the psychological and curable nature of the illness; (3) the presence of unconscious dynamic processes; and (4) the low influence of sexual factors in the war neuroses. We believe that Rose's description should be relativised, because although it points out a trend that gradually prevailed during the war, a more detailed analysis quickly reveals the controversies and disagreements on these four points.

At the beginning of the war, the assumption that the soldier's symptoms (which varied between deep amnesia and the intrusive repetition of war images, between anaesthesia and hyperaesthesia, between mutism and the compulsive need to recount the lived scenes) were caused by an organic alteration was still widespread. In the article entitled "Why Are They Not Cured? British Shellshock Treatment During the Great War", Peter Leese argued that in Britain, alongside other more psychological or even psychoanalytic trends, there was a group of doctors during the war that leaned towards a somatic interpretation of the illness, focusing "on physical shock, concussion, and hereditary causes" (Leese, 2001, p. 217). As suggested by the literal meaning of the expression most used in English-speaking mass media when referring to war pathologies, "shell shock" seemed to be caused by the shockwave of an explosion which produced a lesion in the nervous system.

This was clearly Oppenheim's hypothesis in the German context. As we have stated, before the war, for most German neurologists and psychiatrists, the diagnosis of "traumatic neurosis" had been largely forgotten after having been associated with an "epidemic of pension neurosis" (Micale & Lerner, 2001, p. 154). However, the enormous number of soldiers who developed neurotic symptoms during the war seemed to open up a new opportunity for Oppenheim to confirm his theories. He got the opportunity to do so when he was appointed head of a makeshift military hospital with 200 beds in what was at the time the Berlin Museum of Applied Arts (Brunner, 2000, pp. 297–298; Micale & Lerner, 2001, p. 154). Although the German neurologist came to admit the role of emotional factors, from his perspective, the cases of war neurosis were explained by the fact that the explosions caused "an acoustic stimulus" that sent "an overwhelming, and hence traumatic, wave of excitation" into the brain, which damaged the nervous tissue or provoked molecular damage (Oppenheim, 1916, p. 228; cited in Brunner, 2000, p. 299).

Also, in France, there was a group of neurologists who, despite being the minority, held a somatic interpretation of the illness. The most representative figure of the organic interpretation was probably Paul Sollier. He had been a disciple of Charcot during the 1880s and later developed both an institutional and private medical practice, eventually being appointed head of the Lyon neurological centre during the war (Roudebush, 2001, p. 258). Sollier thought of "the psychological and emotional symptoms of hysteria as epiphenomena of their physiological cause: *engourdissement* (numbness or somnolence) of the brain" (Roudebush, 2001, p. 258). And although he "played the role of a father-confessor to his patients" and attempted to impose the doctor's superiority over them, he interpreted said task in materialistic terms: "I do not need to make a single suggestion, or to dissect psychologically a single idea or a single emotion. I limit myself simply to awakening the cerebral sensibility, and this sometimes by strictly mechanical means" (Sollier, 1901, p. 170; cited in Roudebush, 2001, pp. 258–259).

Very quickly, however, these somatic conceptions were called into question in the French, German and English-speaking contexts. As we will see, far from there being a consensus, different psychological conceptions of illness and trauma appeared under tension. Within these debates, the voices of some psychoanalysts began to emerge, first in a marginal way and then, towards the end of the war, with greater institutional recognition.

4.1.1.2 French Criticisms of Organicist Conceptions: Pithiatism and Simulation

Sollier's ideas about the war neuroses were opposed to the more widespread view, generally inspired by Babinski's ideas regarding "pithiatism", which, as we saw, was considered to be caused by suggestion cured by persuasion (Edelman, 2003, p. 272). This view, which in appearance surpassed the Charcotian conception of hysteria (considered a neurological illness common to both sexes) constituted a return to more traditional perspectives since it converted said illness into a more *moral* problem (similar to the alienist's conceptions from the previous century) rather than a *psychological* one (in the sense that Freud or Janet might use that term). This interpretation of hysteria linked the symptoms suffered by soldiers with a process of *feminisation*, with *individual interests* that were opposed to the needs of the nation and with *suspicions* regarding the motivations behind the pathological phenomena. Ultimately, war hysteria ended up being a clinical picture of effeminate, selfish, simulators.

Perhaps the book by Maxime Laignel-Lavastine and Paul Carbon, *Les Accidentés de la guerre: leurs ésprit, leurs réactions, leur traitement*, best exemplifies the most widespread view of the war neuroses in France (Laignel-Lavastine & Carbon, 1919; cited in Roudebush, 2001). As Marc Roudebush recounts, these authors compared the neurotic soldier with the insured worker who obtained benefits from prolonging their illness or was expecting compensation for their damage. That is why they designated these cases as "sinistrosis", a term coined by Brissaud to designate the insured workers' fraudulent pathologies (Roudebush, 2001, p. 265). While soldiers were expected to respond to the "collective mentality" and become actors ready to perform on the stage of history, neurotics would, in contrast, return to their individuality, thus becoming mere spectators, like most civilians (Roudebush, 2001, p. 266). In turn, the authors recommended that women should not take part in the treatment of psychoneurotics, as their presence was thought to make it more difficult for the patients to reconquer their lost virility of character (Roudebush, 2001, p. 266).

In this way, certain traits that had always been attributed to hysteria (especially its link to femininity and simulation), were once again assigned to the ill soldiers. On top of this, they were morally reproached and accused of working against the country's best interests. In this sense, most doctors that dealt with the treatment of war neuroses seemed to ignore the first and most essential hypothesis of Janet's work, namely, the existence of automatic psychological elements that imposed themselves beyond the subject's will and, therefore, that should be differentiated from simulation or fraud.

4.1.1.3 The Psychological Hypotheses in Germany and the Austro-Hungarian Empire

By the time Oppenheim published the book *Die Neurosen infloge von Kriegsverletzungen*, in 1916, his somatic conceptions had already been strongly questioned by much of the medical establishment at a War Congress of German psychiatrists and neurologists held in Munich in September of the same year (Brunner, 2000, pp. 298–299; Lerner, 2001, pp. 156–168). This scientific meeting was attended by more than 300 specialists and high-ranking members of the German army, such as representatives from the Prussian Ministry of War, and the psychiatrist Karl Moeli, who called for a psychiatric consensus regarding war-time matters for the benefit of military policy (Lerner, 2001, p. 163). Criteria for psychiatric unity on these issues were quickly reached (Lerner, 2001, pp. 142 and 163): in opposition to Oppenheim's traumatic neuroses, the diagnosis of hysteria was imposed; psychological hypotheses proliferated against a somatic conception of the illness; the subject's predisposition and their expectations of obtaining future benefits were considered more important than the severity of the current event; finally, different types of therapies were disseminated, instead of disability pensions.

The arguments used to reject the validity of traumatic neuroses had been accumulating since the beginning of the war and even before the Congress took place.

One of these arose from the systematic study on prisoners of war, which confirmed the low incidence of war neuroses among these prisoners, who were excluded from receiving pensions and other compensatory benefits due to illness. A second argument used against the category of traumatic neuroses was the rarity of neurotic symptoms among those who had suffered severe physical wounds (Lerner, 2001, p. 159). A third source of information that weakened Oppenheim's conceptions was the large number of people who had never been on the battlefield but who, regardless, presented neurotic symptoms (Lerner, 2001, p. 160). Lastly, the treatment success rates of suggestive and psychical therapies reinforced the idea of the functional nature of the illness (Lerner, 2001, p. 161).

During the Congress, after Oppenheim's presentation, the doctor Max Nonne demonstrated his hypnotic abilities by quickly suppressing neurotic symptoms in several soldiers (Brunner, 2000, p. 300; Lerner, 2001, p. 164). Nonne was a neurologist from Hamburg who, prior to this scientific event, had been putting forward a psychogenic interpretation of the neuroses and proposing hypnotic therapy as the main treatment for these illnesses. His performance in the Congress was as consecrating for him as it was devastating for his opponent. If the symptoms could be eliminated via psychical means, they could, therefore, not have a somatic basis. At the same time, he was opposed to viewing them as signs of a neurosis specific to traumatic situations; rather, he interpreted the symptoms as the manifestation of at least two different nosological categories: hysteria or neurasthenia in which traumatic experiences did not always influence their development (Brunner, 2000, p. 300).

In his proposal, Nonne split the cases of war neuroses into two large groups. On the one hand, there were cases in which the experience of war did acquire a traumatic character for the person and led to symptom production, but these could be dealt with "quickly and completely" with hypnotic and suggestive therapies (Nonne, 1915, p. 850; cited in Brunner, 2000, p. 300). Given their "curable" nature, these cases did not present major inconveniences in the war-time context, since these soldiers could quickly return to the battlefield without claiming pensions. On the other hand, certain patients presented symptoms that returned after the therapy had concluded or had not been suppressed in the first place (Brunner, 2000, pp. 300–301). Nonne explained this resistance to hypnotic therapy by claiming the presence of often unconscious (but in a certain way immoral and selfish) desires, since those *begehrungsvorstellungen* were aimed at obtaining a personal benefit (a pension, escape from active duty, etc.) which went against their obligation and the collective interests (Brunner, 2000, p. 301; Micale & Lerner, 2001, p. 14). In this way, the illness was described as an escape from obligations and a source of potential benefits. Nonne's explanation, centred on desire complexes and the diagnosis of hysteria (a point that was also defended by other renowned psychiatrists, such as Robert Gaupp),[2] managed to displace Oppenheim's ideas and impose itself onto most German-speaking specialists (Lerner, 2001, pp. 164–165).

These references to unconscious desires and to the illness as a form of escaping and gaining benefits, together with the use of psychical means in therapy, opened a door through which some psychoanalytical ideas entered the debate. This opening occurred at the same time that the need for medical human resources during the war made it possible for some psychoanalysts to begin holding positions in state or military organisations, thus moving away from their traditional private practice. With the exception of Sigmund Freud, who was not drafted into the army due to his age, and Ernest Jones, who lived in England and did not hold a position in the military, most of the psychoanalysts who wrote about the war neuroses and who belonged to the narrow Freudian circle served as doctors on the side of the Central Powers: Karl Abraham, Max Eitingon, Sandor Ferenczi and Victor Tausk.

In *Psicoanalistas en el frente de batalla*, one of the few books devoted entirely to this subject, Ramirez Ortiz (2007) states that all these psychoanalysts agreed with the assigned task of promoting the prompt return of soldiers to the front but that in addition, they assigned themselves "another task, corresponding to their own cause: that of providing proof of the high efficacy of their psychoanalytically inspired methods for the treatment of war neurosis" (Ramirez Ortiz, 2007, p. 7).

In 1916, the Hungarian psychoanalyst Sandor Ferenczi was appointed "chief physician of the Hospital Department for Nervous Diseases" based in the Maria Valeria military hospital in Budapest (Brunner, 2000, p. 308). That same year, based on the observation of 200 cases, he gave an exposition to the doctors of that hospital at a congress, which was published one year later under the title "Two Types of War Neuroses" (Ferenczi, 1916–1917). The article began with the admission that the severity of the symptoms (tremors, weakness, paralysis, etc.) and the narrations of many patients blaming their symptoms on a shell explosion, at first lead him to believe these were caused by an "organic injury to the brain or spinal cord" (Ferenczi, 1916–1917, p. 125). But later, after making a finer semiological observation (reminiscent of the diagnostic work and rhetorical strategy of Page and Charcot), he found the presence of "extraordinarily variable and usual disturbances of innervation" that, from his perspective, "were powerful arguments against an organic, even if only a 'molecular' or 'micro-organic' change in the nervous reticulum" (Ferenczi, 1916–1917, p. 126). In this way, Ferenczi joined in on the criticism that Oppenheim's ideas were receiving in Germany at that very moment.

The paper's main thesis was that the cases of war neurosis he observed could have been included in the Freudian nosographic categories of "conversion hysteria" and "anxiety hysteria". In other words, the war did not bring about a completely new illness, even if there were difficulties in establishing the role of sexuality in its development (as we will specifically address later). He reached the diagnosis of "conversion hysterias in the sense of Breuer and Freud" by observing "mono-symptomatic" patients, whose contractures and paralyses reproduced "*the innervation predominating at the moment of the concussion (of the shock)*"; at the same time, that shock was not remembered by the patient (Ferenczi, 1916–1917, p. 128; italics in original). The "*trauma*" for Ferenczi was caused by "the sudden affect that could not be psychically controlled (the shock); (...) undischarged parts of the affective impulses are still active in the unconscious" even when the patient "does not consciously think of it any longer" (Ferenczi, 1916–1917, p. 129). In other words, the suddenly aroused and undischarged affect was displaced to a bodily innervation thus producing the symptom as a substitute for the forgotten memory and caused a "petrification" of the subject in the attitude adopted at the moment of the accident (Ferenczi, 1916–1917, p. 129). This explanation of the diagnosis and of the mechanism that produces the symptoms contained a detail which was not highlighted by Ferenczi nor by Ramirez Ortiz (2007) in his detailed commentary on the article by the Hungarian psychoanalyst, which deserves to be highlighted. The symptom, according to Freud, understood as a substitute of the forgotten memory and as a compromise between the repressed material and the repressive agencies, implied the *distorted* return of that which had been forgotten. This distortion was not present in these cases since the symptoms seemed to reproduce the traumatic moment exactly, as if the symbolic work had been made impossible or, at least, made difficult by the suddenness and intensity of the affect.

This "economic" dimension was reinforced by the explanation of the cases of "anxiety hysteria", which characteristically presented generalised tremors, palpitations, sweating, hyperaesthesia and terrifying dreams that repeated the situations experienced on the battlefield (Ferenczi, 1916–1917, pp. 132 and 135). Since the tremors and the most intense symptoms did not appear while the patients were in bed but at the moment they were about to walk, Ferenczi interpreted that they functioned as a phobia, where the anxiety associated with walking served as a way of preventing the subject being exposed to a situation analogous to the shock that they experienced (Ferenczi, 1916–1917). As in the cases that received the diagnosis of conversion hysteria, there was also a reference to the sudden nature of the experience and the absence of organic damage, features that, according to Ferenczi himself, had already been highlighted by Freud:

> We must adopt the following assumption of Freud in explanation of this symptom. If one is prepared for a shock, for the approach of a danger, then the attention excitations mobilized by the expectation are able to localize the stimulus of the shock and to prevent the development of those remote effects which we see in the *traumatic neuroses*. Another means of localizing the effects of shock is – according to Freud – a severe, actual, physical injury proportionate to the psychic shock occurring with the traumatic incident. In the cases here shown of traumatic *anxiety hysteria* none of these conditions are fulfilled; we are dealing with a sudden, mostly unexpected shock without a serious bodily injury. But even in the cases in which the approach of the danger was noticed, the expectation excitation may not have been proportionate to the actual stimulus force of the shock and so was unable to prevent the discharge of the excitement along abnormal channels.
>
> (Ferenczi, 1916–1917, pp. 138–139; italics in original)

These economic considerations highlighted the importance of preparation in order to avoid pathological consequences and introduced the idea of a sum of excitation that cannot be processed through "normal channels". Freud introduced this perspective in some of his "Introductory Lectures on Psycho-Analysis". In Lecture XXV, devoted to anxiety, Freud for the first time introduced the difference between this affect and "fright". The latter highlights the subjective consequences of the lack of preparation in the face of danger, while the former limits the intensity of stimuli (and of unpleasure) and functions as an expectant "preparedness", as a "signal" that prepares the subject to face the dangerous element (Freud, 1916–1917e, pp. 394–395). However, it is above all in Lecture XVIII, "Fixation to Traumas – The Unconscious", where the Viennese psychoanalyst puts forward an economic conception of trauma and the neuroses associated with the latter, that is very similar to the developments of Ferenczi in the cited article:

> The traumatic neuroses give a clear indication that a fixation to the moment of the traumatic accident lies at their root. These patients regularly repeat the traumatic situation in their dreams; where hysteriform attacks occur that admit of an analysis, we find that the attack corresponds to a complete transplanting of the patient into the traumatic situation. It is as though these patients had not finished with the traumatic situation, as though they were still faced by it as an immediate task which has not been dealt with; and we take this view quite seriously. It shows us the way to what we may call an economic view of mental processes. Indeed, the term 'traumatic' has no other sense than an economic one. We apply it to an experience which within a short period of time presents the mind with an increase of stimulus too powerful to be dealt with or worked off in the normal way, and this must result in permanent disturbances of the manner in which the energy operates.
>
> (Freud, 1916–1917a, pp. 274–275)

We consider it important to underline several elements of this excerpt. First, the relationship that Freud establishes between the notion of trauma and the concepts of fixation and repetition. Going through a traumatic situation seems to leave a mark on the subject that could function as a fixation and *force the repetition* of that situation in dreams or attacks. The entire paragraph underlined the affective, instinctual, drive-based, quantitative component of this process. Mnemic functioning is thus altered: the past trace functions as an experience that is still present, persisting as a pending exigency, which the subject returns to again and again. Second, if the emphasis was not placed on the representative content of the situation but on its compulsive nature, then it can be understood that an economic perspective is required to address it. The trauma is characterised by a quantitative "increase". This increase is not absolute but relative to two variables. On the one hand, relative to the length of time the psychical apparatus is exposed to the magnitude of stimuli: an equal amount of excitation distributed over longer time intervals might not be traumatic. On the other hand, relative to "the normal way" in which the subject attempts to deal with or work off the stimuli that they encounter. In other words, the trauma also depends on certain particularities of the person who went through the experience and not only on the latter's characteristics. Third, the trauma leaves lasting consequences on the economic functioning of the psyche. Therefore, it does not act like a *scar* (like the healed mark from a past time) but like an *open wound* that continues to demand work from the psychical apparatus, although the latter cannot completely process it.[3]

In 1918, Ferenczi once again addressed the topic of war neuroses at the Fifth International Psycho-Analytical Congress held in Budapest. Although it was not as well-attended or as important as the Munich Congress mentioned above, many government delegates and military officers from the German and Austro-Hungarian Empires also took part in it, which could be interpreted as a growing official recognition of psychoanalysis in the context of the war and of war neuroses (Brunner, 2000, p. 306; Falzeder, 2002, p. 405; Jones, 1953–1957, t. 2, p. 210). The Hungarian psychoanalyst was one of the three speakers who explicitly referred to the topic of war neuroses (the other two being Karl Abraham and Ernst Simmel). One year later, the respective presentations of the three psychoanalysts were published in the book *Psycho-Analysis and the War Neuroses* (VVAA, 1919), which also included an introduction written by Freud (1919) and a paper by Ernest Jones (1919).[4]

In his presentation, Ferenczi once again insisted that "the mass-experiment of the war" confirmed the insufficiency of organic perspectives, such as Oppenheim's, in explaining the development of certain cases of neuroses (Ferenczi, 1919, p. 6). He then immediately presented a good summary of the state of the art of the psychological conceptions of the war neuroses in the German-speaking sphere. He considered Strümpell to be one of the first to oppose the somatic position and to support the idea that the symptoms were not caused directly by the traumatic experience but rather by an "interest in being able to prove an injury as caused by the trauma", in order to obtain financial compensation (as in the cases of railway accidents) or to free themselves from the military authorities (as in war) (Ferenczi, 1919, p. 8). On this point, he attempted to separate himself from his German colleague, since he considered that these ideas led to the fact that "the sufferers (…) were treated not much better than if they were malingerers" (Ferenczi, 1919, p. 8). He also considered that the "affective side" and the "unconscious" aspect of the psychical processes involved in the pathogenic experience were ignored by his German colleague (Ferenczi, 1919, p. 9). After this, he continued to enumerate arguments in favour of the psychogenic nature of the war neuroses; for example, the low incidence of this illness in prisoners of war – which was pointed out by Mörchen and Bonhöffer – or the disproportion between the trauma and the severity of the neurotic symptoms – noted by Schuster and Singer (Ferenczi, 1919, p. 9). He then included Nonne among the authors who contributed to consolidating the idea of the psychical nature of the war neuroses, not only by categorising them as "hysteria" but also by proving that it was possible to eliminate their symptoms via suggestion (Ferenczi, 1919, p. 10). Afterwards, he went on to enumerate authors who defended psychogenic conceptions of the war neuroses (Gaupp, Bonhoeffer, Birnbaum, Vogt, Liepmann, Schuster, etc.) and he added that many of them were near to psychoanalysis "without knowing it" (Ferenczi, 1919, p. 15), since they used terms and concepts previously developed by Freud (such as psychical conflicts, unconscious, fixations, abreaction).

Finally, Ferenczi addressed two other issues: on the one hand, the role of sexuality and narcissism in the war neuroses; on the other hand, the debate on whether predisposition or the experience of war had a greater impact on the development of the illness. Both problems were also discussed by other psychoanalysts, such as Tausk, Abraham, Jones and Freud himself, so we prefer to specifically deal with them further on.

Before that, we wish to move on to the British context in order to analyse some of the psychological hypotheses regarding the war neuroses that were developed there, as well as investigate the insertion of psychoanalytic ideas in that region.

4.1.1.4 The War Neuroses in the United Kingdom

In the article cited above, Peter Leese argued that there were "three main schools of thought" in Great Britain regarding shell shock: the first held a somatic explanation of the illness; the other two schools shared a psychological explanation, but only the least widespread of these two groups was influenced by psychoanalytic ideas (Leese, 2001, pp. 217–218). At the same time, there was no consensus in these English-speaking countries on the diagnostic category that should be applied to cases of war neuroses. Leese points out that in the National Hospital in Queens Square, London, a referral hospital during the war, the doctors used a wide variety of notions to define patients affected by the war: neurasthenia, mutism, hysterical mutism, shell shock (understood as physical concussion), hysterical monoplegia, traumatic neurasthenia (Leese, 2001, p. 217). If these factors are taken into account, it is clear that although the popularity of psychological hypotheses had increased, they could still coexist with somatic hypotheses.

The debates on the war neuroses very quickly transcended the closed sphere of specialists and began to be depicted in the daily press. For example, an influential newspaper such as *The Times*, in 1914 and 1915, devoted successive instalments to the description of war hospitals and to the treatment of "Battle Shock" (Leese, 2001, p. 206; n.3). According to Leese, this early diffusion had generated a consensus in the public opinion about the legitimacy of the war neuroses,[5] unlike what happened in France and Germany, where the soldiers who left the battlefront were much more frequently accused of malingering. In this context, the story of the British anti-war poet Siegfried Sassoon became known, who left the battlefront and was treated at the Craiglockhart War Hospital by the psychiatrist W.H.R. Rivers (Leese, 2001, p. 206; Robinson, 2005).[6]

Rivers is an extraordinary example of the reception of psychoanalytic ideas in the British sphere outside of the circle closest to the movement led by Freud. After carrying out activities as an anthropologist in Australia, he returned to Great Britain in March 1915 to join the aforementioned Scottish hospital. Throughout the war, he gave several presentations that all had in common the purpose of recovering and transmitting certain Freudian hypotheses in a medical environment that ignored

Freud's work. Thus, on March 7, he delivered a lecture at the Edinburgh Pathological Club, in which he presented "Freud's Psychology of the Unconscious" as a theory that had been underestimated by his contemporaries due to "prejudice and misunderstanding", but which deserved to be dealt with "dispassionately" (Rivers, 1920, p. 159). A short time later, on December 4 of that same year, he gave a presentation at the Royal Society of Medicine entitled "The Repression of War Experience" (Rivers, 1920, pp. 185–204). In this presentation, he intended to warn about the pathological risks that the attempt to make soldiers forget ("banish") their war experience could entail (Rivers, 1920, p. 188). In other words, he understood that the development of neurotic symptoms did not solely depend on the lived events but on the subjective repressive stance taken on their memories. From his perspective, the only way to overcome the neurosis was to face the memories of the war experiences and try to make them more "tolerable" (Rivers, 1920, p. 189). Finally, in 1920 he published a book, *Instinct and the Unconscious: A Contribution to a Biological Theory of the Psycho-Neuroses*, in which he aimed to give "a biological view of the psycho-neuroses" and where he also compiled several of the lectures he delivered during war-time (Rivers, 1920, p. 1). Concepts and notions linked to the clinic of the neuroses in general and psychoanalysis in particular (such as the unconscious, instincts, inhibition, dissociation, complexes, suggestion, sublimation, etc.) were reread from an original evolutionary framework. As Caroline Cox points out, for Rivers "the instinct of self-preservation was more powerful and basic than Freud's theories of sexual instinct" (Cox, 2001, p. 289). That is to say, although Rivers admitted the existence of both kinds of instincts or drives,[7] like many of his contemporaries, he minimised the role of sexuality when thinking about the pathologies of war and gave more importance to the vicissitudes of the instinct of self-preservation. In particular, he warned of the harmful consequences of trying to suppress soldiers' most basic biological reactions to danger, such as pain and fear (Rivers, 1920, p. 60).

Montague David Eder was an author closer to Freud, although without being part of the inner Freudian circle. He translated into English several psychoanalytic texts such as Sigmund Freud's *On Dreams* and Carl Jung's *Diagnostic Association Studies* and *The Theory of Psychoanalysis*. During the war, he held the position of Medical Officer in charge of the neurological department in Malta, enabling him to carry out an investigation based on 100 cases of war neuroses. This research was published in a book entitled *War-Shock. The Psycho-Neuroses in War Psychology and Treatment* (Eder, 1917). Like Ferenczi and many other authors, he criticised Oppenheim for his somatic approach and for believing that war or accidents could create new and specific diseases (Eder, 1917, p. 1). The nosographic categories that he used to classify his patients stemmed from psychoanalysis and French psychopathology: of the 100 observed and treated cases, 77 were diagnosed as Conversion-Hysteria, 17 as Anxiety-Hysteria and 6 as Psychasthenia – as Janet understood it (Eder, 1917, p. 9). Nevertheless, this traditional approach did not prevent him from recognising that "a psycho-neurosis can be produced by stress of external conditions", since "in war-shock the external psychic factor is overwhelmingly greater than (…) the predisposition" (Eder, 1917, pp. 1–2). As we can see in the section specifically dedicated to treatment methods, his therapeutic techniques were fundamentally based on suggestion (Eder, 1917, pp. 128–133).

Finally, we wish to mention Ernest Jones. Unlike Rivers and Eder, Jones was one of the Vienesse psychoanalyst's closest disciples. The English psychoanalyst's paper in *Psycho-Analysis and the War Neuroses* was, in fact, the transcription of a lecture that he had delivered on April 9, 1918. This exposition was given to the same audience that – one year earlier – had listened to River's presentation on repression, that is, the Royal Society of Medicine (Ramirez Ortiz, 2007, p. 52). The article's title marked his Freudian affiliation: "War Shock and Freud's Theory of the Neuroses" (Jones, 1919). We wish to include some of its central ideas here. First, Jones rejected the idea that the strain of war conditions could be in themselves enough to create neurotic symptoms without the existence of a previous disposition prior to the war experience (Ramirez Ortiz, 2007, p. 56). To support his thesis, he invoked the fact that the percentage of individuals who fell ill was always much lower than the amount of people who participated in the war (Jones, 1919, pp. 44–45). Second, he believed that

> although some symptoms – e.g., dread of shells – assume a form that is coloured by war experiences, no symptom (…) occurs in war neuroses that is not to be met with in the neuroses of peace, a fact which in itself would suggest that fundamentally very similar agents must be at work to produce the neurosis in both cases.
>
> (Jones, 1919, pp. 46–47)

However, these claims do not imply that Jones denied that war could lead to changes in the psyche. On the contrary, according to him, the circumstances of war encourage humankind

> to commit deeds and witness sights that are profoundly revolting to our aesthetic and moral disposition. All sorts of previously forbidden and buried impulses, cruel, sadistic murderous and so on, are stirred to greater activity, and the old intrapsychical conflicts (…) are now reinforced, and the person compelled to deal with them afresh under totally different circumstances.
>
> (Jones, 1919, p. 48)

In other words, for Jones, the war altered the former balances, the long-standing forms of conflict resolution between the "aggressive and sexual drives" and "the demands of civilisation" (Ramirez Ortiz, 2007, p. 57). It did so by dragging everyone involved into repulsive situations (determined as such by their own and the collectively shared representations) and by reinforcing cruel impulses that the ego had already managed to master. However, these elements introduced by the armed conflict were not completely new: in times of peace, those same components also exist, although in a repressed or sublimated state. Third, if there were no such radical differences between the neuroses of peace and the war neuroses, then the aetiological factors that produce both pathologies would be the same: a combination of personal antecedents and the current situation. These factors could be expressed in terms similar to those used by Freud:

> a specific hereditary predisposition; secondly an unresolved infantile conflict which means that the person has not satisfactorily developed past a given stage of individual evolution – in other words, that he has been subjected to what is called an 'infantile fixation' at a given point in development, and thirdly the current difficulty.
>
> (Jones, 1919, p. 54)

Finally, he addressed the question of "real fear" (Jones, 1919, p. 56), which seems self-evident in a situation like war. It could be believed that fear is an adequate, normal response in this context and that it differs from what occurs in the neuroses of peace, where "morbid anxiety" was considered "a defensive reaction of the ego against the claims of unrecognised 'sexual hunger' (Libido), which it projects on to the outside world – e.g., in the form of phobias – and treats as if it were an external object" (Jones, 1919, pp. 56–57). However, Jones was opposed to this differentiation between realistic and neurotic fear: for him, "even in situations of real danger" a percentage of the dread experienced depends on neurotic mechanisms.[8] Except that, in these circumstances, the dread is not derived from "the repressed sexual hunger that is directed towards external objects, as is the case with morbid anxiety of the peace neuroses, but from the narcissistic part of the sexual hunger that is attached to the ego" (Jones, 1919, pp. 57–58). Immediately afterwards, Jones ventures "to suggest that we may here have" – that is, in narcissism – "the key to the states of terror in which we are so familiar in the war neuroses" (Jones, 1919, p. 58).

At this point, the English psychoanalyst was not putting forward an original argument; rather, like many of his contemporary colleagues, he found in the notion of narcissism the way to refute the criticisms towards the psychoanalytic theory that stemmed from the widely held hypothesis about sexuality playing no role in the war neuroses. We will address these issues below.

4.1.1.5 Narcissism and Sexuality in the Aetiology of the War Neuroses

The role of sexuality in the development of war neuroses was one of the great issues that psychoanalysts attempted to prove in those years. If it were true that, as much of the medical establishment claimed, sexual elements played no role in the development of these illnesses, then there were two possibilities: either these neuroses were radically different to the neuroses of peace, and therefore psychoanalysis, designed for the latter, could not be applied to war neuroses; or the war neuroses were identical to those that developed in times of peace and, therefore, in the common neuroses, sexuality would not have the importance that Freud attributed to it. For this reason, these psychoanalysts who were close to Freud attempted to argue in favour of the sexual nature of the war neuroses. Like Jones' case, the fulcrum for most of these interventions on this problematic issue was "narcissism" (Brunner, 2000; Ramirez Ortiz, 2007). Given the importance that this category acquired within the context of these debates and in the subsequent transformations of the notion of trauma, we consider it necessary to present some of its main characteristics.

The notion of narcissism, which had already been mentioned in the analysis of President Schreber's memoirs (Freud, 1911), was formally introduced into the psychoanalytic theory three years later (Freud, 1914). The complex article from 1914, which was written in the heat (and the corresponding urgencies) of his estrangement with Carl Jung, presented many ideas and situations which revolved around the problem of the allocation of the libido in the ego. Here we would like to highlight the points which were linked to the debates on the war neuroses and to the transformations of the notion of trauma.

First, narcissism was linked to the constitution of the ego and conceived as a regular phase of development which occurs between auto-erotism (a period in which there is not yet "a unity comparable to the ego") and object-love (Freud, 1914, p. 77). It consists, precisely, of the ego being taken as the object of libidinal cathexis. Only after this "primary narcissism" has taken place, the "libidinal cathexis of the ego" can be "later given off to objects" (Freud, 1914, p. 75). According to Freud, narcissism leaves marks (fixations) like any process that involves the libido. On the one hand, the original libidinal cathexis of the ego is never completely abandoned: it acts like "the body of an amoeba" in relation to "the pseudopodia which it puts out" (Freud, 1914, p. 75); on the other hand, the subject can also return to narcissism via regression (the libido withdrawn from objects returning to the ego).

Second, the notion of narcissism led to a transformation of his drive theory. By adopting the assumption that the ego can be cathected by the libido, Freud was forced to modify the former theory of drive dualism (which implied a conflict between the sexual drives and the self-preservative or "ego" drives). This modification introduced a new "antithesis between ego-libido and object-libido" (Freud, 1914, p. 76). Thus, the characteristics of the "ego" are not necessarily opposed to those of "sexuality".

Third, narcissism was also associated with serious clinical phenomena and nosographic pictures, such as paraphrenia and hypochondria, which are characterised by "a damming-up of ego-libido" (Freud, 1914, pp. 84–85). Two relevant issues arise from this last idea. On the one hand, the birth of a new nosographic classification, which opposed the transference psychoneuroses (suited for classic analytic treatment) to the "narcissistic" psychoneuroses (which made the therapeutic process run into obstacles) (Freud, 1914). Among the narcissistic neuroses, Freud included schizophrenia, paranoia and, from 1917 onwards, melancholia.

The link between narcissism and these three clinical pictures further complicates the nature of this notion. Because although it could refer to the constitution of the ego as a unified and unifying agency, it could also denote serious disturbances of that unity. In schizophrenia, once detached from its objects, the libido regresses to auto-erotism, the phase prior to the ego's constitution, causing a decomposition of the bodily unit (Freud, 1911, p. 76). In paranoia, the regression only extends to narcissism, meaning the ego is newly cathected by the libido. This process is manifested clinically in the form of megalomania (Freud, 1911, p. 77). Lastly, in melancholia, after the object cathexis is brought to an end, the libido is also withdrawn into the ego, where it serves to establish an "identification of the ego with the abandoned object", thus leading to "a cleavage between the critical activity of the ego and the ego as altered by identification" (Freud, 1917, p. 249). From the above, we can conjecture that it is not narcissism alone that determines either the constitution of the ego or its decomposition, aggrandisement or splitting; rather, the decisive factor in one case or the other is the magnitude of the libidinal cathexis attached to the ego.[9]

This last idea leads to the second issue that we wanted to highlight. The "ego-libido", which in certain circumstances can become "dammed-up", constitutes an *economic* problem linked to severe disturbances in the economy of the libido and is comparable to the new economic definition of trauma that, as we have seen, Freud was beginning to develop in those years (Freud, 1916–1917a, p. 275).

If the notion of narcissism made it possible to tie together problems linked to the ego, sexuality and the economic point of view, then it also seemed adequate for dealing with the war neuroses and trauma. Thus, narcissism reconciled the psychoanalytic hypotheses about the libido as an aetiological factor in the neuroses with the danger for the ego and self-preservation, as highlighted by most non-analytic authors. In other words, narcissism seemed to be the key to refuting the criticisms that questioned the role of sexuality in the development of war neuroses and that reduced this matter to the subject's life being at risk.

On January 19, 1916, the Slovakian psychoanalyst Victor Tausk participated in the Second Conference of Medical Officers in Lublin, where he presented an article entitled "Diagnostic Considerations Concerning Symptomatology of the So-Called War Psychoses" (Tausk, 1916). His lecture began with a nosographic critique: from his viewpoint, there was no such thing as specific war psychoses; these were the usual clinical pictures of melancholia and paranoia that, at most, could contain war-themed delusional ideas without implying any essential nosographic difference (Ramirez Ortiz, 2007, pp. 42–43). He then put forward an original argument, which sought to tie a war-time particularity with the assertion of the sexual nature of those psychotic clinical pictures:

> Let us assume, in accordance with psychoanalysis, that paranoia is a defense against the break-through of the unconscious homosexual-narcissistic component, as demonstrated by Freud in the Schreber case. *The army provides all the*

> *conditions for mobilizing this component, in particular the close and exclusive contact with individuals of the same sex on active service.*
>
> (Tausk, 1916, p. 395; italics added)

From his perspective, war's influence on the development of the illness does not depend on the mechanical action of the bombs that impact the soldiers' bodies, nor on the horror brought about by the experience of war, but on the conditions of permanent proximity to people of the same sex which awakened homosexual and narcissistic aspects of the libido, thus propitiating the outbreak of psychoses. As Ramirez Ortiz proposed, "if we are to speak of trauma" within the framework of Tausk's conception of the war psychoses, "it does not arise from the actions of war, but from an aspect of sexuality put into play in the forced coexistence between men in the army" (Ramirez Ortiz, 2007, p. 50). However, we consider it important to highlight that Tausk's perspective seems to ignore the fact that in prisons and military training camps, men were also forced to live with members of the same sex, without this producing the same amount of cases of illness as those reported during the war.

As we had anticipated, Ferenczi also attempted to place the concept of narcissism at the centre of the psychoanalytic interpretation of the war neuroses (Brunner, 2000, p. 308). By basing his arguments on this notion, he believed he was in a position to respond to those who claimed that "Freud's idea of the almost exclusively sexual foundation of hysteria has been conclusively disproved during the war" (Ferenczi, 1919, p. 17). At the Budapest Congress of 1918, he argued that

> the war neuroses, according to psycho-analysis, belong to a group of neuroses in which not only is the genital sexuality affected, as in ordinary hysteria, but also its precursor, the so-called narcissism, self-love, just as in dementia praecox and paranoia.
>
> (Ferenczi, 1919, p. 17)

This statement implied a change in the attitude that he himself had adopted regarding the diagnosis of these illnesses. In the text of 1917, he maintained, like many German, French and English doctors, that most war neuroses could be understood as cases of hysteria. One year later, he brought the category of war neuroses closer to that of narcissistic neuroses, pointing out clinical and metapsychological reasons for this nosographic shift. He suggested that the predominant symptoms of the condition in the psychical sphere (that is, apart from paralysis or other motor and sensory abnormalities) were: "hypochondriacal depression, terror, anxiousness, and a high degree of irritability with a tendency to outbursts of anger" (Ferenczi, 1919, p. 18). These semiological characteristics could be traced back to an "*increased ego-sensitiveness*" (Ferenczi, 1919, p. 18; italics in original).

In fact, despite the diagnostic shift, Ferenczi had already made a similar statement in his previous paper by indicating that some of his patients "carried their estimation, perhaps their over-estimation, of self pretty far" (Ferenczi, 1916–1917, p. 136). The encounter of these same patients with an experience that had a "shattering effect upon their self-confidence" resulted in a *regression* to the first year of life (Ferenczi, 1916–1917, p. 137). At the Congress in Budapest, the Hungarian psychoanalyst added some conceptual precisions to his description of the symptom-producing mechanism: "in consequence of the shock (…) the interest and sexual hunger (libido) of the patients is withdrawn from the object into the ego" (Ferenczi, 1919, p. 18). This withdrawal of the libido from the objects of the external world towards the ego explains, according to his point of view, the "hypochondriacal organic sensations and over-sensitiveness" as well as the "diminution of object-love" and of "genital potency", which would give the clinical picture a desexualised appearance, when in reality it was not (Ferenczi, 1919, p. 18). As Ramirez Ortiz points out, by giving this explanation, Ferenczi was describing "a process analogous to the Freudian explanation of mourning and melancholia, and to the processes of loss of reality in the neuroses and the psychoses" (2007, p. 85).

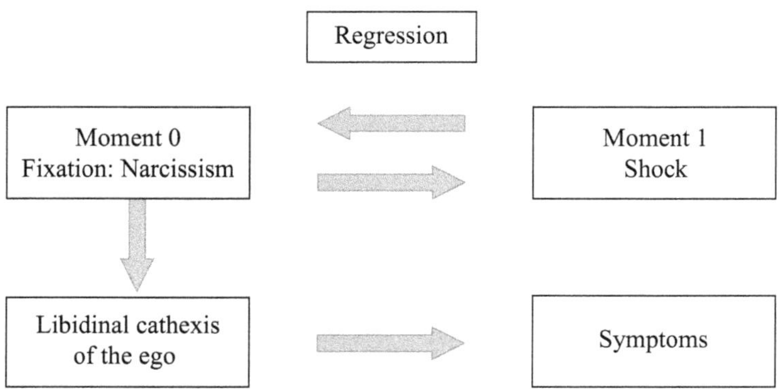

Karl Abraham was another speaker at the Fifth International Psychoanalytic Congress. Since the beginning of the war, he had participated as an army surgeon, first in Berlin and from 1915 onwards in Allenstein, East Prussia, where he became head of the psychiatric clinic of the XX Army Corps of the Austrian-Hungarian Empire (Brunner, 2000, p. 307; Ramirez Ortiz, 2007, p. 9). At the beginning of his exposition, he made clear his objective of addressing "the unconscious and sexual" factors of the war neuroses, and not only "the manifest expressions of the neurosis" and "the reactions of the ego impulses to the trauma" as the "academic neurologists" did (Abraham, 1919, p. 22; Ramirez Ortiz, 2007, pp. 91 and 105). The influence of these unconscious and sexual factors, which are central to any psychoanalytic conception, was justified, once again, based on the notion of narcissism. The German psychoanalyst admitted in the following terms that he "fully coincides" with what his Hungarian counterpart had communicated on that point: "The trauma acts on the sexuality of many persons in the sense that it gives the impulse to a regressive alteration which endeavours to reach narcissism" (Abraham,

1919, p. 23). However, as we see in the following paragraphs, a difference immediately appears between the two colleagues due to Abraham's greater emphasis on predisposition, which led him to believe that "the war neurotics already before the trauma were labile people (…) and especially so as regards their sexuality" (Abraham, 1919, p. 23).

Finally, we wish to mention that Freud himself also believed that with narcissism he had found a way of thinking about the war neuroses that allowed him to tie the idea of a conflict in the *ego* with the notion of *libido* and with an *economic* view of trauma. The introduction to the book *Psycho-Analysis and the War Neuroses* began with the admission that due to certain special characteristics, the war neuroses can be distinguished from the "ordinary neuroses of peace-time" (Freud, 1919, p. 208), bringing them nosographically closer to "traumatic neuroses, which (…) occur in peace-time too after frightening experiences or severe accidents" (Freud, 1919, p. 209). Freud then immediately alluded to an issue that, in war neuroses, concerns the ego. From his point of view, the splitting of this psychical agency is neither due to the consequences suffered by the ego when exposed to an objectively life-risking situation that arouses fright nor the ego's interest in obtaining a benefit (such as a pension or desertion). Instead, it is due to the internal presence of a *conflict* "between the soldier's old peaceful ego and his new warlike one" (Freud, 1919, p. 209). In a letter sent to Jones on February 18, 1919 (prior to the publication of this introduction and the book on the war neuroses), Freud highlighted the unconscious and refractory nature of this conflictual situation, stating that "war neurosis is a case of narcissistic conflict in the ego, somewhat analogous to the mechanism of melancholia" (Paskauskas, 2001, p. 396). The latter clinical picture is one in which the ego is split into two parts, one that identifies itself with the object whose cathexis was resigned, and another critical part, which denigrates the former part, thus obtaining a "sadistic satisfaction" from its suffering (Freud, 1917, p. 251).

With these references, Freud complexified the relationship and limits between the external world and the psyche, between the real-objective danger and the internal danger:

> It would be equally true to say that the old ego is protecting itself from a mortal danger by taking flight into a traumatic neurosis or to say that it is defending itself against the new ego which it sees is threatening its life.
>
> (Freud, 1919, p. 209)[10]

Towards the end of the short introduction, he insisted on this point. It could be thought that in the transference neuroses, what is feared by the ego are the demands of the libido, while in the war neuroses, the danger stems from "external violence"; however, for Freud, in the latter, "what is feared is nevertheless an internal enemy" (Freud, 1919, p. 210).

Here, narcissism came to bridge the gap between ego-conflict and libido and between the war neuroses and the neuroses of peace-time. Freud knew there were hypotheses denying sexuality's role in the causality of war pathologies. However, he affirmed that in this aspect, "the emergence of the war neuroses could not introduce any new factor" since it was also difficult to apply the libido theory to the "narcissistic" neuroses: *dementia praecox*, paranoia and melancholia (Freud, 1919, p. 209). For their part, "the traumatic neuroses of peace-time" were "the most refractory material" in his attempts to demonstrate the libido's pathogenic influence in the development of symptoms (Freud, 1919, p. 209). However, Freud considered that there was a way to include all these clinical pictures in the same conception:

"It only became possible to extend the libido theory to the narcissistic neuroses after the concept of a "narcissistic libido" had been put forward and applied – a concept, that is, of an amount of sexual energy attached to the ego itself and finding, satisfaction in the ego just as satisfaction is usually found only in objects (...) The traumatic neuroses of peace will also fit into the scheme as soon as a successful outcome has been reached of our investigations into the relations which undoubtedly exist between fright, anxiety and narcissistic libido" (Freud, 1919, pp. 209–210).

As we anticipated, the notion of narcissism was the conceptual support that linked *the dangers to the ego* (and a *dynamic* conception of the conflict) to *the dangers of the libido* (and an *economic* conception, attentive to the increases in quantity whose subjective correlates are fright and anxiety). At the same time, it allowed for the influence of sexuality to be conceived in all the neuroses. In this way, "the theoretical difficulties" that stood in the way of a "unifying hypothesis" (of all the neuroses being structured around the libido) did no longer "seem insuperable" to Freud (Freud, 1919, p. 210).

This shift had its counterpart. If the libido were present in the traumatic neuroses and not only in the transference neuroses, then the trauma would also play its part in the transference neuroses. Freud concluded his article with the following statement: "after all, we have a perfect right to describe repression, which lies at the basis of every neurosis, as a reaction to a trauma – as an elementary traumatic neurosis" (Freud, 1919, p. 210).

In short, for some psychoanalysts, the traumas brought to the fore by the war did not question the thesis regarding the sexual origin of the neuroses. However, they did allow for the notion of trauma to once again occupy an important role in psychoanalytic theory, thanks to the theoretical support provided by the concepts of narcissism and ego-libido. However, a new conceptual turn would take place very shortly thereafter, a turn that displaced the problem of narcissism from the centre of the scene (although, as we will see, that did not completely eliminate it) and that led to the conception of trauma being established as an economic disturbance. In the final section of this chapter, we will address this conceptual transformation in the Freudian work, which also involved a rereading of certain elements already present in the first Freudian texts and those dedicated to narcissism. Before that, we wish to address the other two questions that, together with the issue of the nature of the war neuroses, were part of the most pressing clinical debates of the time.

4.1.2 Objective Conditions or Subjective Particularities?

In the previous section, we attempted to present the different somatic and psychological hypotheses about the nature of the clinical pictures that arose during the First World War. Now we intend to analyse a different problem: can the war neuroses be understood as a consequence of the events of the war? Or, arising in this context, do they depend on certain characteristics of the person who developed the symptoms? In statistical terms, the arguments are not conclusive because although it is true that during the war, more cases of neurosis came about (or were made visible) than in times of peace, it is also true that many more people participated in combat than those who ended up ill. The debates on these issues concern a central problem related to trauma, which we have been addressing since the introduction of this book: does trauma depend on the objective and external pole of the experience or the subjective and internal pole of it?

In the somatic conceptions of the war neuroses, such as those held by Oppenheim or Sollier, we came across a causal and deterministic schema similar to the one we had attributed to Erichsen: the subject becoming a passive victim of a completely external and determining event. Therefore, in these types of conceptions, any consideration of the subjective responsibility regarding the development of the symptoms is excluded. The neurotic soldier also seemed to represent the *image of a victim* whose suffering solely depended on the event they had to go through.

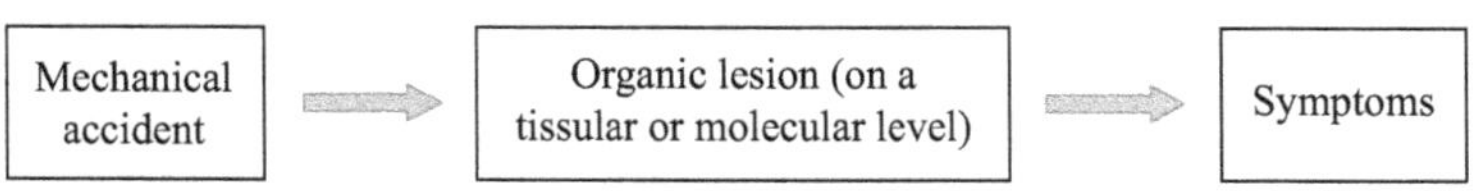

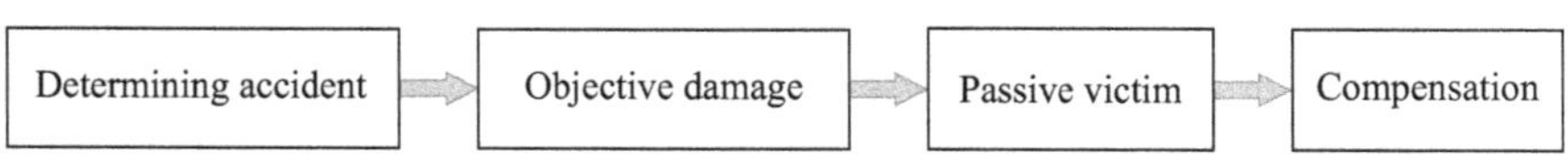

Marc Roudebush established a close relationship between this type of approach to the problem of the neuroses and the private nature of the practice of those physicians who adhered to it (Roudebush, 2001). In France, the *physiological* pole of the neurological profession (opposed to the *moral* pole, which was much more widespread)

> was especially attractive to practitioners who, like Sollier, had catered to private clients. By objectifying hysteria and defining its treatment in purely medical terms, this approach absolved the patient of responsibility for his or her condition, and affirmed the relevance of the neurologist's expertise.
>
> (Roudebush, 2001, p. 260)

Paul Lerner made a similar point regarding the German and Central European context. From his viewpoint, this context's psychiatrists and neurologists could be divided into two rough groups: university researchers and clinicians. Both groups differed "in terms of status, patient pools, and often ethnicity (Lerner, 2001, p. 147). The doctors in the most prestigious medical establishment often held positions in universities and the hospitals dependent on them, for which they were well paid. Thus, they were able to more freely engage in research programs than those clinicians – many of them of Jewish backgrounds – who depended economically on the patients they treated in their private practice. While the first group received patients who, in their vast majority, belonged to the working class, the second group attended mainly to a bourgeois clientele (Lerner, 2001, pp. 147–148). According to Lerner:

> Private clinicians were more likely to diagnose somatic disorders, while among their university counterparts in this period psychogenic theories were beginning to gain popularity. Significantly, somatic disorders lacked the stigma of mental illnesses. Doctors like Oppenheim had to face an increasingly competitive medical marketplace (...) and a clinician who told patients what they did not want to hear might have found his waiting rooms quickly deserted.
>
> (Lerner, 2001, p. 148)

However, this hasty correlation between somatic conceptions, the de-responsibilisation of subjects and private practice should be relativised. On the one hand, in the German-speaking context, the psychoanalytic movement was characterised by a therapeutic practice undertaken almost exclusively in the sphere of private practice. Nevertheless, this had not led to the proliferation of organic conceptions of illnesses or to their patients being assigned the role of passive victims of trauma, thus exempting them from any responsibility. On the other hand, in the United States, it was possible to consider that the war veterans suffering from symptoms were "psychoneurotics". That is, they were considered to be ill due to a disease (psychical in nature) that, however, did not arouse suspicion or the moral blame that was common in French and German medical circles. As Caroline Cox states, in that country, it was possible to publicly present "the war-neurotic veteran as a battle-scared hero" who therefore deserved to receive all the necessary benefits and treatments from the State (Cox, 2001, p. 281). To achieve this purpose, the lobby carried out by the veterans association "American Legion" was of vital importance, as well as the support provided by "the nation's top psychiatrists. While these men shared the Legion's goal of improving care for the psychoneurotic, their association with the Legion also helped to advance psychiatry from the confines of the insane asylum and into the public eye" (Cox, 2001, p. 281).

At the opposite end of the organicist positions and those held by the American Legion, the predominant conceptions in the French and German contexts are worth mentioning. These were characterised for granting greater aetiological significance to the affected person's particularities prior to the war or to certain psychical elements (suggestions, desires), which seemed to say more about the subject than about the experience they had gone through. Whether their hereditary traits had made them more susceptible to suggestions and effeminacy, or whether due to their constitution they had developed individual desires that were contrary to collective interests and moral obligation. In any case, the situations experienced during the war lost relevance in the conception of the pathological process. Most of the authors who studied these contexts agree that, regarding their theoretical consideration and their practical treatment, there did not seem to be many differences between the malingerer and the pithiatic, hysterical or neurasthenic patient (Brunner, 2000; Lerner, 2001; Roudebush, 2001). Understood in this way, the *image* of the neurotic soldier represented the *antithesis of the hero and a symbol of moral degeneracy.*

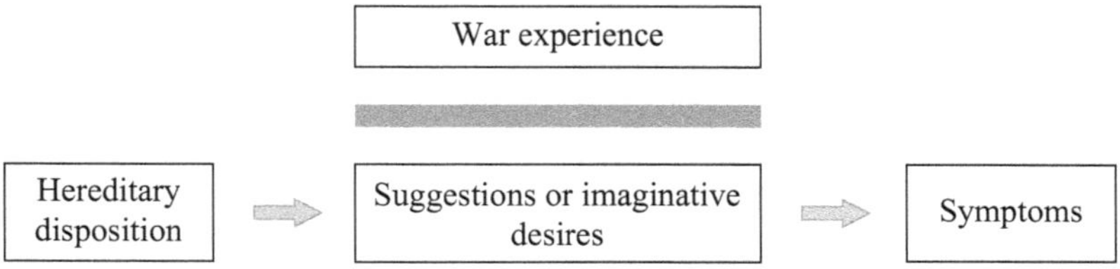

This type of perspective, inspired by Babinski, Strümpell or Nonne, left the interest in trauma aside, not only as a mechanical event but also as a contingent factor that could produce illness. As we mentioned in the previous section, the little importance given to the lived experience was usually justified by the observation that "very few severely physically injured soldiers and prisoners of war seemed to develop rigid nervous symptoms, even though tens or even hundreds of thousands of them had undergone severely traumatic experiences" (Brunner, 2000, p. 303). This argument was complemented by "the lack of a parallel or proportionality between the grimness of the trauma that had been suffered and the severity and rigidity of symptoms that emerged in response" (Brunner, 2000, p. 304). In other words, compared with the somatic approaches, these conceptions better explained why some people fell ill while others remained healthy even though they had gone through the same experiences. However, neither heredity nor the interest in obtaining benefits from the illness fully explained the development of such a large number of cases of neurosis during the war, nor the persistence of the symptoms despite the suffering they generated. If it was necessary to make improvised military hospitals to treat neurotics, if many non-specialist doctors ended up treating the mental illnesses of war, if so many soldiers seemed possessed by the desire to escape from their obligations, and if many of them forgot their experiences or could not stop remembering them, then it was therefore very likely that the events played a part in the development of the illness.

It seemed impossible for the two great opposing and exclusive positions that we have pointed out to think in a more balanced way about the relationship between objective experience and subjective particularities, between chance and determination and between accident and heredity. Most psychoanalysts who participated in the war conflict moved away from both extremes, although they did not adopt a homogeneous position.

In fact, in the writings of an author like Abraham, we again find a great emphasis put on the role of predisposition, analogous to what we observed in his hypothesis regarding scenes of child abuse (Abraham, 1907).[11] As we stated, the Berlin psychoanalyst thought that the war neurotics were already "labile people" prior to the trauma. We now wish to quote a paragraph that better reflects his viewpoint:

> Many of these men were unable to carry out their tasks in practical life, others (...) showed little initiative and manifested little impelling energy. In all of them sexual activity was diminished, their sexual hunger (libido) being checked through fixations; in many of them already before the campaign potency was weak or they were only potent under certain conditions. Their attitude towards the female sex was more or less disturbed through partial fixation of the sexual hunger (libido) in the developmental stage of narcissism. Their sexual and social capacity of functioning was dependent on their making certain concessions to their narcissism.
>
> (Abraham, 1919, pp. 23–24)

Incapable, impotent, narcissistic ... although Abraham was referring to unconscious characteristics at a psychoanalytic congress, it should not be forgotten that army officers were present at the event, in whom prejudices about war neurotics were commonplace. It could be thought that the psychoanalyst's assessments contributed to the consolidation of a degraded image of those who fell ill during the war. Even more so when, with psychoanalytic terminology, we come across some of the most widespread ideas in the German medical context. In war, according to Abraham, soldiers are required to be prepared for "unconditional self-sacrifice in favour of the mass", which implies "the renunciation of all narcissistic privileges": "the healthy person is able to accomplish such a complete suppression of his narcissism"; the neurotic, is not (Abraham, 1919, p. 24). It was also usually demanded of these soldiers to be prepared to perform "aggressive acts" and to endure being associated exclusively with men during the war. Once again, for Abraham, "the sexuality of the normal person takes no harm from this, but it is otherwise in men with strong narcissistic traits", even more so if "the connection between homosexuality and narcissism" is taken into account (Abraham, 1919, p. 24).

As can be seen, the significance that Abraham granted to the subject's characteristics prior to the war is greater than that of other psychoanalysts. Furthermore, in his view, the narcissistic fixation was linked to an "effeminate" disposition and was contrary to the collective demands of an "unconditional self-sacrifice"; thus, his conception did not seem very different from those held by many of the doctors from the Central Empires or from France (Abraham, 1919, p. 24). When reading these same passages, Ramirez Ortiz maintained that "the argument of sexual predisposition (...) was a sign of the times. (...) It was a way of explaining the non-encounter, the non-harmonious nature of the relationship between the sexes" (Ramirez Ortiz, 2007, p. 95). We make a different interpretation since we consider that the emphasis he put on the antecedents prior to the war experience does not seem to refer to a structural feature of human sexuality but to a characteristic of a person predisposed to illness.

Furthermore, Abraham also argued that many of the "neurotically disposed" people, "have supported themselves only through an illusion connected with their narcissism, namely, through the belief in their immortality and invulnerability" (Abraham, 1919, pp. 25–26). On this point, Abraham agreed with Ferenczi, who, in his 1917 article, had referred to the over-estimated self-image many war neurotics had before being deployed to the battlefield. From this point of view, this fragile imaginary support shattered when faced with the first explosions and war wounds, quickly giving rise to neurosis (Abraham, 1919, p. 26; Ferenczi, 1916/1917, p. 136).

In short, Abraham's ideas about the war neuroses, even when they referred to unconscious characteristics linked to narcissism, were similar to those most widespread among war doctors. They downplayed the importance of the horrors of war and gave more relevance to predisposition, thus painting the picture of an impotent, narcissistic and effeminate soldier. However, it is fair to say that Abraham did not derive a coercive therapeutic practice from this conception, as many of his non-psychoanalytic colleagues did.

We consider that, regarding these questions, Ferenczi's approach is different. When he addressed the issue of predisposition to illness, the Hungarian psychoanalyst stated that most authors gave contradictory answers. From his viewpoint, most of them maintained that war neurotics were already ill before the war: "the shock merely playing the part of the releasing factor" (Ferenczi, 1919, p. 13). Other authors, including Nonne, argued that "the deciding factor in falling a victim to war neuroses lies less in the personal constitution than in the nature of the operating injury" (Ferenczi, 1919, p. 13).

This description made by the Hungarian psychoanalyst well reflected the extreme positions of the long-standing dilemma regarding trauma: should the illness be attributed to the lived event (the objective, external pole of the trauma) or to the particularities of the person who experienced it (the subjective, internal pole)? Faced with this dilemma, Ferenczi argued that "Psycho-analysis takes a median position with regard to this question, which Freud has frequently and expressly stated" (Ferenczi, 1919, p. 13). This "median" position, which opposes the need to opt for one pole and reject the other, was explained with the following argument: "A trifling predisposition and severe shock can produce the same effects as an increased predisposition and a much lesser degree of shock" (Ferenczi, 1919, p. 13).

It could be thought that by claiming that neurotic soldiers were affected by a regression to the first year of life (Ferenczi, 1916/1917, pp. 136–137, 1919, p. 18), Ferenczi gives a childish quality to the *image* of the soldier, perhaps different from the attribution of feminine traits, but just as pejorative and moralising. This interpretation seems justified if we take into account that he described war neurotics in the following terms: "the patients would like to be pampered, cared for, and pitied like children" (Ferenczi, 1919, p. 18); "the entire personality of most of the victims of trauma corresponds therefore to the child who is fretting, whimpering, unrestrained and naughty in consequence of a fright" (Ferenczi, 1919, p. 19). However, we consider that this reading can be relativised. Although Ferenczi affirmed that there are men who are particularly "predisposed to narcissism", he also considered that "no one is entirely immune from it, since the stage of narcissism forms a significant fixation point in the development of the sexual hunger (libido) of every human being" (Ferenczi, 1919, pp. 18–19). This statement is in line with psychoanalysis' median position regarding the dilemma between predisposition and current experience. From Ferenczi's (and Freud's) point of view, narcissism is a necessary stage of human development and, therefore, a universal one, even though it can grant each person different degrees of fixation and predisposition. Along the same lines, the infantile characteristics are not an exclusive attribute of a few predisposed people, but a universal feature of human sexuality. Thus, the war neurotics were not men who were particularly childish *before* the traumatic experience but who regressed to a childish attitude *after* having suffered a shock. Ultimately, the possibility of undergoing such a regression depended on the combination of the degree of predisposition and the intensity of the experience.

In addition, according to Ferenczi, the regression to infancy was due to an unconscious process and not a deliberate intention to obtain a gain in the present moment. This is why he criticised Strümpell, who associated the neurotic soldier with the malingerer and considered that the illness was produced on account of an "actual gain (pension, compensation for injury, flight from the front)" (Ferenczi, 1919, p. 19). For Ferenczi, all these benefits are "secondary" in regards to the primary illness gain, that is: "the pleasure itself of remaining in the secure retreat of the childish situation" (Ferenczi, 1919, p. 19). This primary gain constitutes a paradoxical situation since although the neurotic is saved from having to face the conflict thanks to taking refuge in the illness, they end up paying the price of a satisfaction that can only be reached through suffering. Freud, two years earlier, in similar terms, had opposed himself to the perspectives that associated the patient with the simulator:

> Thus in traumatic neuroses, and particularly in those brought about by the horrors of war, we are unmistakably presented with a self-interested motive on the part of the ego, seeking for protection and advantage.
>
> (Freud, 1916–1917d, p. 382)

Nevertheless,

> ...the *ego puts up with the neurosis, which it cannot, after all, prevent*, and that it makes the best of it, *if anything can be made of it at all*. That is only one side of the business, the pleasant side, it is true. So far as the neurosis has advantages the ego no doubt accepts it; but it does not only have advantages. As a rule it soon turns out that the ego has made a bad bargain by letting itself in for the neurosis. *It has paid too dearly for an alleviation of the conflict*, and the sufferings

attached to the symptoms are perhaps an equivalent substitute for the torments of the conflict, but they probably involve an increase in unpleasure. *The ego would like to free itself from this unpleasure of the symptoms without giving up the gain from illness, and this is just what it cannot achieve.*

(Freud, 1916–1917d, pp. 383–384; italics added)

Furthermore, for Freud, the notion of complemental series accounted for the aetiology of all neuroses, meaning that it could also be applied to the problem of the causation of war neuroses. As we discussed in the previous section, Jones (1919, p. 54) agreed with this perspective. Heredity, childhood and current experience were all factors that seemed to combine and admit different degrees of participation in the development of war neurosis. As we will see in the second part of this chapter, the notion of trauma developed by Freud after the war necessarily takes into account the *relationship* between the objective conditions of the experience and the subjective particularities of the person, thus preventing the conceptualisation of these factors in mutually exclusive terms.

4.1.3 The War Neuroses and Their Diverse Treatments

In order to analyse the therapeutic practices carried out during the war, it is necessary first to discuss three features of the context in which they were carried out. These features probably determined the treatment procedures to a greater extent than the theoretical conceptualisations of the illnesses themselves. First, isolation, electrotherapy, hypnosis, suggestion therapies, persuasion, catharsis, and psychoanalysis: the same result was demanded of all these techniques, namely, for the soldier to return to the battlefront as quickly as possible (Brunner, 2000; Leese, 2001; Roudebush, 2001). Therefore, the pragmatic criterion of efficacy could often prevail over epistemic or moral considerations. Second, given the large number of cases, the treatments were usually carried out by non-specialist doctors, who were as close to the emergencies of the trenches as they were far from academic debates (Leese, 2001). Lastly, there was no direct relationship between how the illness was conceived (either somatically or psychically) and the type of therapeutic approach used to treat it: those who maintained that the symptoms were of a psychical origin could nevertheless still utilise a physically oriented therapy (Leese, 2001).

In this sense, electrotherapy seems to clearly illustrate the dilemmas involved in choosing a particular type of therapeutic technique. This approach was used in almost all of the countries that participated in the war and within the framework of different therapeutic conceptions. In France, where Babinski's ideas prevailed, and the hysterical soldier was perceived as a simulator, neurologists' use of "an amount of force proportional to the bad faith of their patients" was justified (Roudebush, 2001, p. 267). Marc Roudebush presented in detail Clovis Vincent's method of "intensive reeducation" (Roudebush, 2001, p. 268). Vincent was a former disciple of Babinski who took over the Neurological Center of Tours during the war. "Like Laignel-Lavastine" (who compared the hysterical soldier to the insured individual who expected to receive benefits for their illness), "he believed that the treatment of hysteria required physical strength and charismatic virility (…) Vincent prided himself on obtaining immediate results through a combination of accurate diagnosis, personal authority, and the unflinching use of high-intensity electrical currents" which allowed him to show his patients the illusory nature of their paralyses and alterations (Roudebush, 2001, p. 268). These practices, which would be easily critiqued from the lens of today's sensibility and legal frameworks, were not strange in his time. On the contrary, Roudebush clearly showed the extent to which Vincent was fully consistent with the general guidelines of his contemporaries, who saw his facility and his procedures as a benchmark for referring "psychoneurotics who have not responded to other treatments" (Roudebush, 2001, p. 268). Even neurologists such as Joseph Gasset, who criticised the equivalency of hysteria and simulation and argued that hysterics are ill people who deserve treatment, regularly referred patients to the Neurological Center of Tours. For most French doctors, the electrical current was not considered an "instrument of coercion" but an "agent of persuasion" (Gilles, 1917, p. 209; cited in Roudebush, 2001, p. 269). In other words, it was a mere technical tool that made up part of a larger therapeutic strategy generally accepted in France. As we have pointed out, persuasion therapy had displaced the use of suggestion, in favour of greater conscious participation of the patient in the healing process. However, in many cases, the persuasive methods seemed to contain disciplinary and authoritarian characteristics (Roudebush, 2001, p. 269).

In Germany, where hypnosis and suggestion were more prevalent than in France, the general therapeutic orientation was also marked by the assumption that the patient possessed an individual desire that was contrary to the will of the nation. It is thus understandable that Nonne's hypnotherapy could coexist with more aggressive methods, such as Fritz Kaufmann's "surprise-attack method" (Brunner, 2000, p. 305). This method encouraged his colleagues to "use every possible means in order to convince the patient that one is capable to impose on him one's own strong will" (Kaufmann, 1916, p. 803; cited in Brunner, 2000, p. 305). He also had no qualms about encouraging faradisation because, from his perspective, "the powerful impact of pain displaces all negative wishful ideas" (Kaufmann, 1916, p. 804; cited in Brunner, 2000, p. 305). José Brunner maintains that far from being criticised, this therapeutic approach was well received by Kaufmann's colleagues and was even considered more practical than Nonne's hypnotherapy since it did not require the expertise needed to perform hypnosis (Brunner, 2000, pp. 305–306). Therefore, the choice between one approach and the other did not depend on their underlying concepts nor on ethical considerations but on more pragmatic criteria, which led doctors like Nonne to use electricity to treat resistant patients (Brunner, 2000, p. 306).

Regarding this last point, a similar panorama can be found in the United Kingdom. As Peter Leese pointed out, "Electric shock therapy, faradization, was a potential technique within the wider therapeutic regime for both progressive and disciplinary medics, and in practice it was used in both ways" (Leese, 2001, p. 218). Although some came to denounce the use of electrical currents as an instrument of torture, especially after the war had finished, it is true that it was also defended in the name of its supposed effectiveness (Leese, 2001, p. 218). However, it was also common for soldiers who returned to the battlefield after being "cured" by these coercive methods to fall ill again very quickly once they reencountered the same type of war experiences. Many doctors, most likely motivated by the search for better therapeutic results, resorted to "psychotherapeutic techniques broadly derived from the work of Freud and Janet" (Rose, 1999, p. 20) or even from their predecessors. Within the English army, M.D. Eder used suggestion (with or without hypnosis) above all other treatment methods. With the help of this old technique, he claimed to have fully cured 79 of the 100 patients he mentioned in his book on war-shock (Eder, 1917, p. 128). Although he considered psychoanalysis to be "the only method for the radical treatment of the psycho-neuroses", he also thought that "it is inapplicable and unnecessary for the treatment of cases of war-shock (…) to use it here is to employ a Nasmyth hammer to crack a nut" (Eder, 1917, p. 133). In his view, the effectiveness of direct suggestion rested on two factors: first, on the assumption that "the soldier is peculiarly susceptible to suggestion" given that "the whole training and discipline make him respond to the authority of the Medical Officer" (Eder, 1917, p. 130) and second, on the fact that "the shock of battle is not an every-day affair", which therefore would require that the soldier's willpower be reinforced; suggestion under hypnotism could provide this reinforcement (Eder, 1917, p. 133).

For his part, also in the British context, Rivers adopted a therapeutic approach that was closer to classic psychoanalysis. He opposed those doctors who suggested that soldiers should ignore and repress their war experiences, and he encouraged his patients to talk to him about them (Rivers, 1920, p. 189). We want to underline two aspects of his therapeutic method. First, Rivers also dealt with a problem that we have worked on at length in Chapter 2. We refer to the affirmation that in order for a subject to be cured, it is not enough for them to recall the past. As was the case for Janet and Freud, Rivers believed "something else" was needed: in his view, to turn the memories into tolerable companions (Rivers, 1920, p. 189), or to find an aspect which would make the memories' contemplation more endurable (Rivers, 1920, p. 192), or to re-educate patients to give up the practice of repressing war experience (Rivers, 1920, pp. 200 and 204). In any case, it was clear to him that remembering could not be an end in itself and that "to dwell persistently upon painful memories" could be just as harmful as attempting to banish them from memory completely (Rivers, 1920, p. 203). Second, the English doctor interpreted the disappearance of symptoms following the cessation of voluntary repression as a form of "catharsis", through which "a suppressed or dissociated body of experience is brought to the surface so that it again becomes reintegrated with the ordinary personality" (Rivers, 1920, p. 199). This interpretation of catharsis emphasised the role of the memory being recalled and put into association with the rest of the ego's ideas. It was opposed to a different way of understanding the technique, emphasising the discharge of affect.

These two opposing readings of Breuer's technique were the subject of a debate in Great Britain immediately after the end of the war, a debate which Ruth Leys described and analysed. The controversy took place during the spring of 1920, and was published in the *British Journal of Medical Psychology* (Leys, 2000, p. 84). The protagonists, William Brown, C. S. Myers and William McDougall, had in common the fact that they had accumulated great amounts of experience in the treatment of war neuroses using the cathartic technique put forward by Breuer and Freud in the previous century. However, they differed in their conceptions about the determining factor of neurosis and the effectiveness of the technique. As Leys noted, "Brown argued that the characteristic signs of shell shock (…) were all bodily expressions of obstructed or 'repressed' emotions" (Leys, 2000, p. 84). On the other hand, Myers and McDougall did not put as much emphasis on the *emotional* elements: for them, the basis of the symptoms was not the repression of emotion, but of *memory*, that is, the ideas which were separated from conscious memory and therefore constituted a hole in that person's life narrative (Leys, 2000, p. 86). These different interpretations of the determining element in pathogenesis led to different readings about the foundations of therapeutic action. Whereas Brown held that the cathartic treatment essentially consisted of the emotional *reliving* of the traumatic scene, which would allow for the discharge of *affect*, Myers and McDougall argued that the method's essential core was the reintegration of the *forgotten memory* to a coherent *narrative* of the individual's past life (Leys, 2000, pp. 83–87).

Within this opposition, the two great psychological factors that, as we saw in Chapter 1, have been used to explain the neuroses and trauma since the end of the nineteenth century once again appeared opposingly: emotions or ideas, affects or representations. At the same time, there were two different ways of conceiving the treatment and the role of memory: a form of repetition that mobilised affects or a memory-based narrative that claimed to be free of gaps. From what we discussed in Chapter 2, both possibilities are probably too optimistic. On the one hand, the repetition of the traumatic experience, in the absence of any other type of modification, does not seem to guarantee the cessation of the traumatic effect and could even become symptomatic and compulsive. On the other hand, it also does not seem possible to fully and seamlessly integrate the traumatic experiences into a narrative devoid of gaps. In the second part of this chapter, we will address the transformations of the notion of trauma in Freud's work. We will attempt to identify the particular way in which these elements were combined throughout them (the webs of representations and the unbound sums of affect, the narrative of the past and the current irruption of an element that interrupts it).

Before that, we wish to finish addressing the question of the treatment of the war neuroses. In order to do so, we will move away from the British context and analyse some of the therapeutic approaches from the Central Empires, which were inspired by catharsis and psychoanalysis.

The third speaker at the Budapest Congress of 1918 was Ernst Simmel, whom we have yet to discuss. During the war, he worked for two years as the senior medical officer in charge of a field hospital for war neurotics in Posen (Brunner, 2000, p. 308). As a result of his work, at the beginning of 1918, he published a booklet entitled *War Neuroses and Psychic Trauma. Their Mutual Relations, Presented on the Basis of Studies in Psychoanalysis and Hypnosis* (Simmel, 1918; cited in Falzeder & Brabant, 2001, p. 124).[12] Immediately after reading it, Freud sent separate letters to Ferenczi and Abraham in which he asked them to read and review the booklet, and showed his enthusiasm for a text that "is grounded without reservation in psychoanalysis" (Falzeder & Brabant, 2001, p. 124), even if the method used by the author "takes essentially the cathartic standpoint" (Falzeder, 2002, p. 393). In both cases, he pointed out the German background of the author, which made him believe that "German War Medicine" had "bitten" the hook of psychoanalysis for the first time (Falzeder & Brabant, 2001). A few months later, the still unknown physician was invited to speak at the Budapest Congress.

Unlike the other lectures, his presentation was not focused on conceptual issues but on therapeutic problems. Simmel criticised both "forcible and restrictive methods", which would produce "new psychic injuries" as well as "the use of pure suggestion in the form of hypnosis when carried out indiscriminately as a blind technique" (Simmel, 1919, p. 30). In his view, "the removal of the symptom" without taking into account "the remaining psychic constellations of the patient" produced a new "general disturbance". From here, symptomatic relapses were a possibility due to the fact that these "palliative measures" did not modify "the root cause of the suffering", which could only be elucidated "by means of psychoanalysis" (Simmel, 1919, p. 30). That said, confronted with the need to shorten the duration of the treatment in the context of war, he used "a combination of analytical-cathartic hypnosis with analytical conversations during the waking state, and dream interpretation" which, according to his testimony, "on an average of two or three sittings brought about relief of the symptoms" (Simmel, 1919, p. 30). The use of hypnosis and catharsis was probably not only due to a pragmatic criterion of brevity. As Brunner suggests, unlike his colleagues, Simmel did not find in the notion of ego-libido the key to understanding the war neuroses (Brunner, 2000, p. 308); rather, he approached these illnesses with a conceptual framework reminiscent of that used by Breuer and Freud in the 1890s (or even of Charcot's ideas from the previous decade).[13] This framework justified his use of the cathartic method.

At the same Congress, Abraham (who, as we have seen, adopted a standpoint close to the German medical establishment due to the emphasis he put on predisposition and on desires contrary to collective interests) also criticised "'active' curative procedures, the best known of which is Kaufmann's" (Abraham, 1919, p. 28). His questioning was based less on ethical reasons than on certain criteria of effectiveness: he believed these methods led to "the rapid improvement of a great number of patients", but their therapeutic effects did not last and produced "certain unwished-for phenomena" due to their severity (Abraham, 1919, pp. 28–29).

According to his own words, in his medical station during the war, Abraham did not use "hypnosis and other suggestive means"; instead, he used "a kind of simplified psycho-analysis" through which he sought to make intelligible to his patients "the origin and nature of their suffering", by arousing in them "the feeling of being understood" (Abraham, 1919, p. 29). Although it is very difficult to know what his therapeutic practice on the battlefront actually consisted of and what its effects were, it is clear that its declared achievements contrasted enormously with the objectives pursued by a methodology such as Kaufmann's.

Finally, we also wish to mention the insights expressed by Freud regarding the treatment of war neuroses. As we have pointed out, the Vienesse psychoanalyst did not directly participate in the battlefront. Neither did he deal with any specific technical aspect that might be involved in the treatment of neurotic soldiers. However, we consider that his presentation at the Fifth International Psycho-Analytical Congress can only be understood in light of the debates caused by the issue of the war neuroses. The title of the exposition, "Lines of Advance in Psycho-Analytic Therapy" (Freud, 1919 [1918]), foreshadowed the axis of the discussion. Along these lines of advance, he highlighted "the one which Ferenczi (…) has lately termed 'activity' on the part of the analyst" (Freud, 1919 [1918], pp. 161–162). An activity that aims to provide help to overcome resistance and that seeks to modify external circumstances so that patients achieve their goals was, for Freud, "unobjectionable and entirely justified" (Freud, 1919 [1918], p. 162). Before continuing, let us remember that not only psychoanalysts from Freud's close circle participated in this congress but also officials and delegates from the Austro-Hungarian Empire. Faced with an audience with ties to the army and the State, which seemed willing to invest funds in the creation of psychoanalytically oriented clinics and which was eager to hear about techniques that would allow soldiers to be sent quickly back to the battlefront, the founder of psychoanalysis allowed himself to propose a more active (and directive) participation of whoever conducted the treatment. However, he immediately presented one of the most extended passages in his work on the principles of *abstinence* and *neutrality*. In this context, this presentation could be read as his stand against the most common therapeutic approaches to the war neuroses. Contrary to expectations, Freud suggested that the treatment should not bring the patient's suffering to a premature end. Otherwise, "the instinctual force impelling him towards recovery" would be diminished, and there would be a risk of the patient finding new substitutive satisfactions (in their personal life or in the transference relationship with the physician), which would be just as neurotic as the symptoms (because they had not yet modified their subjective position regarding the conflict) (Freud, 1919 [1918], p. 163). Said satisfactions were thought to diminish the energy necessary for the continuity of the analysis and for overcoming the resistance to making conscious the repressed elements which the neurotic does not want to know anything about (Freud, 1919 [1918], pp. 163–164). The physician was therefore expected to energetically oppose these substitutive satisfactions and seek to maintain the condition of privation during the treatment.

At the same time, he stated that those conducting the treatments should also hold up this condition of privation against themselves regarding a series of issues that pertain to the course of any treatment but which seemed to be particularly linked to war therapies.

> We refused most emphatically to turn a patient who puts himself into our hands in search of help into our private property, to decide his fate for him, to force our own ideals upon him, and with the pride of a Creator to form him in our own image and see that it is good.
>
> (Freud, 1919 [1918], p. 164)

This declaration of principles was made in a context in which direct suggestion and any type of coercive method were used to twist the patient's individual desires in pursuit of aligning them with the collective will of which the doctor seemed to be representative and guardian. Freud was indeed willing to face the task of "adapting our technique to the new conditions", even if that meant having to "alloy the pure gold of analysis freely with the copper of direct suggestion" (Freud, 1919 [1918], pp. 167–168). Regarding the technique, he also admitted the possibility that "hypnotic influence, too, might find a place in it again, as it has in the treatment of war neuroses" (Freud, 1919 [1918], p. 168). Furthermore, he came to recognise that when taking patients under treatment "who are so helpless and incapable of ordinary life", as could have been common among severe war neurotics, it was necessary to "combine analytic with educative influence" (Freud, 1919 [1918], p. 165). However, the general orientation of his discourse diverged from that of the most common therapies in times of war: "the patient should be educated to liberate and fulfil his own nature, not to resemble ourselves" (Freud, 1919 [1918], p. 165), even if this meant going against the collective interests.

In short, in a context where the diversity of treatments was proportional to the urgency of obtaining high levels of effectiveness in a short time, Freud was willing to accept certain modifications that adapted the technique to the new conditions. Nevertheless, in a context where pragmatic criteria seemed to prevail, he attempted to preserve space for ethical reflection.

Next, as we had announced, we will continue onto the second part of this chapter.

4.2 Part II: The Effects of the War on Freud's Work: Towards a New Conception of Trauma

4.2.1 *Ethical Effects: Analysis of the Use of Electrotherapy*

Following the collapse of the Austro-Hungarian Empire, on December 19, 1918, the Austrian Parliament passed a law that created a "Commission of Inquiry into the Violation of Military Duty", which sought to investigate the actions of military officers, including their doctors (Brunner, 2000, p. 310; Ramirez Ortiz, 2007,

p. 164). As Ramirez Ortiz points out, one week prior to this, a social democratic newspaper called *Der Freie Soldat* published an article entitled "Electrical Torture", in which the medical corps were denounced for the mistreatment of soldiers. A few months later, a new article ("Doctors or Torturers") primarily accused Julius von Wagner-Jauregg, who was Titular Professor of Psychiatry and Neurology at the University of Vienna and Director of the Department of Psychiatry at the Vienne General Hospital (Ramirez Ortiz, 2007, pp. 164–165).

In this context, the commission of inquiry summoned Freud as a specialist so that he could express himself on the subject, which led him to write the "Memorandum on the Electrical Treatment of War Neurotics" (Freud, 1920b). This short text can be understood as a post-war reinterpretation of the respective positions of soldiers and doctors during the war.

As we have pointed out, the Central Powers' medical establishment did not consider there to be much difference between malingerers and soldiers whose symptoms did not quickly recede after receiving treatment. They assumed that in the latter, a desire was present that, even when described as unconscious, deserved to be morally criticised since it was opposed to the collective will and the interests of the Nation. Brunner argued that although Freud's statement "contained notions that were current in the mainstream medical discourse", it also presented "a significant difference in tone" (Brunner, 2000, p. 311). The founder of psychoanalysis argued that, during the war, it had been inferred that "the immediate cause of all war neuroses was an unconscious inclination in the soldier to withdraw from the demands (…) made upon him by active service" (Freud, 1920b, p. 210). Three years earlier, he himself had admitted in one of his lectures which we have already referenced, that in these war neuroses, it was possible to find "a self-interested motive on the part of the ego, seeking for protection and advantage" (Freud, 1916–1917d, p. 382).

However, at this point, where the moral criticisms would usually begin and the coercive treatment methods justified, Freud introduced a subtle but immense difference:

> Fear of losing his own life, opposition to the command to kill other people, *rebellion against the ruthless suppression of his own personality by his superiors* – these were the most important affective sources on which the inclination to escape from war was nourished.
>
> (Freud, 1920b, pp. 212–213; italics added)

The illness that prevented the fulfilment of military obligations thus ceased to be a sign of moral cowardice or of a state of selfishness opposed to the nation and became an act of resistance against the subjective flattening provoked by the war and by the soldiers' superiors. In the records of the judicial process, the following words are attributed to Freud. They were not included in the final version of the published article, but they point in the same direction:

> For many educated men, submitting to military service must have been a horrible thing, and both among us and in the German army, the mistreatment inflicted by superiors has been of a great influence (…) Anger towards superiors was often the main motive behind the illness, numerous cases of illness did not arise from the frontline; they did so from the rearguard in the hospitals which provide this explanation (…) (the national army) entrusted doctors to play in some way the role of a machine gun in the rearguard of the front, a role that consisted of pushing the fugitives.
>
> (Eissler, 1992, pp. 44–45; cited in Ramirez Ortiz, 2007, p. 168)

We agree with Brunner in his assertion that in the Freudian discourse, the "neuroses were no longer presented as a weakness of will, but as an assertion of individuality against oppressive, state-imposed conditions" (Brunner, 2000, p. 311). In this sense, the distinction between the conscious, selfish malingerer and the neurotic who resisted oppression was once again reaffirmed (Freud, 1920b, p. 213).

Freud's view was attentive to the attitude of the soldiers in regard to their illness and did not exclude the neurotic's subjective responsibility. As in his previous notions of trauma, the patient was not conceived as a completely passive victim of an external event. The patients, for Freud, took on a role of resistance, which saved them from putting their lives at risk, the obligation to kill and obedience to authority. However, at the same time, they were not the only ones to blame for the development of their symptoms. Their unconscious subjective position did not stem from an internal world (isolated from everything) nor did it arise from a completely individual egoistic desire. Rather, it was considered the result of the conditions of the experience they had gone through and a response to the actions of their superiors. In other words, for Freud, neither the illness nor the trauma depended solely on the objective/external pole of the experience nor on its subjective/internal pole, but rather on the *relationship* established between both poles.

In that memorandum, there was also a criticism of physicians' work during the war. If for the average physician, the illness served as a refuge for the neurotic to withdraw himself from his obligations, then the treatment should aspire to make "the illness (…) even more intolerable to him than active service (…) For this purpose, painful electrical treatment was employed, and with success" (Freud, 1920b, p. 213). If during the war, the choice of treatment often depended on the pragmatic criterion of effectiveness, when it was over, Freud chose to judge therapies despite their supposed achievements. He also stated that he was convinced that this painful treatment in the Vienna Clinics "was never intensified to a cruel pitch by the initiative of Professor Wagner-Jauregg", although "there were deaths at that time during treatment and suicides as a result of it" (Freud, 1920b, pp. 213–214). However, beyond the defence of his denounced colleague, he refused to "vouch" for other physicians, accusing them of having abandoned their duty of aiming for "the patient's recovery" in pursuit of another goal: that of "restoring his fitness for service" (Freud, 1920b, p. 214). In this way, he warned about the dangers that could arise from responding to demands that did not correspond with the primary purpose of medical activity. Nevertheless, he did not cease to comprehend his colleagues' attitudes:

> the physician himself was under military command and had his own personal dangers to fear – loss of seniority or a charge of neglecting his duty – if he allowed himself to be led by considerations other than those prescribed for him.
> (Freud, 1920b, p. 214)

The physician themself would have been faced with the "insoluble conflict between the claims of humanity, which normally carry decisive weight for a physician, and the demands of a national war", a conflict which "was bound to confuse his activity" (Freud, 1920b, p. 214).

According to Ramirez Ortiz, Freud was not summoned to respond in the second session of the Wagner-Jauregg case and psychoanalysis ended up accused of being "a long, costly, and fruitless treatment", and of being "too subtle when it comes to differentiating hysteria from simulation" (Ramirez Ortiz, 2007, p. 169). These accusations led Freud to complain about "the indignity and mendacity of local psychiatrists" (Falzeder, 2002, p. 455; Ramirez Ortiz, 2007, p. 170). Finally, Wagner was acquitted and reinstated in his position, while the discussion between a treatment's pragmatic and ethical criteria still continues today.

4.2.2 Conceptual Effects: An Economic Conception of Trauma

After the war and its urgencies were over, and although some of its consequences persisted (famine, ruins, unfinished mourning, etc.), Freud reorganised his theory. This conceptual twist could be understood as the effect of having worked through certain economic problems (that is, quantitative, libidinal issues, and issues of the drives) derived from the war and the introduction of narcissism into his theory.

As we saw in Chapter 1, since the end of the nineteenth century, the problem of psychical trauma was conceived around the interplay of two factors that made up the elementary cell of Freudian thought: ideas and affects. Whether the trauma depended to a greater extent on ideas or on certain types of affects was a problem lacking a sole answer. It could be said that with respect to trauma, in Freud's work, the emphasis progressively shifted from the interplay of ideas towards the affective components. To make ourselves clear, we are not affirming that the question of affect was not present in the first writings of the father of psychoanalysis, nor are we saying that ideas eventually ceased to have a role in shaping a traumatic experience. On the contrary, both elements were always present, although the relative importance given to each one in defining the trauma varied. We have pointed out that, in the times of catharsis, the fact that an affect could not be discharged was central to aetiology. However, the ideas also counted since, in many cases, the content of the experience determined the impossibility of reacting to it; furthermore, the splitting of groups of ideas was essential for the formation of symptoms. Later on, when Freud introduced the notions of conflict and defence, the unpleasure the subject sought to avoid was linked to an affect. However, its emergence depended on the relationship of incompatibility between an idea and the rest of the ideas that made up the ego. Finally, the trauma was circumscribed around childhood sexual experiences, which left memory-traces in the psyche. At times, Freud hesitated when determining what aroused the memory-trace and made it traumatic: was it the increase in tension due to the subject's entrance into puberty or was it the emergence of an idea associated with the trace? It would seem, rather, that he considered both factors indispensable. In addition, we have pointed out that the trace was linked with two elements. On the one hand, with the affects, since only the memory-trace could release the sum of excitation that would call for repression. On the other hand, with the ideas, because when the memory-trace became associated with these, a memory was awakened which operated unconsciously, since despite being repressed, it returned in the form of symptoms, thus generating another form of remembering.

However, although ideas and affects were present in those first Freudian texts, it is also true that in them, the trauma was *bound* to a scene. That is, bound to webs of representations which were the remnants of an experience and which seemed to structure the rest of the material of the neurosis.[14] Therefore, it was possible to construct a narrative based on the trauma; furthermore, the end of analysis seemed to coincide with the emergence and narration of the memory of that "traumatic" scene, which until then had remained repressed and whose recollection depended on overcoming the resistance to remembering this conflictive element. The fact that the distinction between the real or phantasised character of the narrated scenes was later considered a problem only confirms the close relationship between trauma and scenes, between trauma and ideas, and between trauma and narratives.

Subsequently, this way of thinking was modified as Freud increasingly established the idea that to conceive trauma, it was necessary to adopt an economic point of view that, obviously, considered the affective component to be more significant. In this way, the trauma ceased to be bound to a scene that could be narrated; rather, as we shall see, it was linked to the moment in which the narrative is interrupted by the emergence of something heterogeneous to it, something that the webs of representations cannot completely bind, something that seems to circumscribe what is processable in the framework of a scene.

This economic point of view was made explicit in 1917 in the framework of the XVIII Introductory Lecture on Psycho-Analysis, which we have analysed in the first part of this chapter. Let us remember that in this lecture, he proposed limiting the use of the expression "traumatic" to an

> experience which within a short period of time presents the mind with an increase of stimulus too powerful to be dealt with or worked off in the normal way, and this must result in permanent disturbances of the manner in which the energy operates.
> (Freud, 1916–1917a, p. 275)

We would like to summarise these ideas with the following formula: Trauma = Powerful increase of stimulus + Unprocessable + Permanent.

This turn was further developed in 1920 with the publication of *Beyond the Pleasure Principle* (Freud, 1920a). This paper was written between March and May of the previous year (Falzeder & Brabant, 2001, p. 197). We can find a first reference to it in a letter sent to Ferenczi on March 17, 1919 (Falzeder & Brabant, 2001, p. 196). However, Freud was probably already sketching out some of his ideas when he wrote one of the fragments that make up the letter addressed to Jones from February 18, 1919, to which we have already referred:

> Consider the case of the traumatic neurosis of peace. It is a narcissistic affection like dementia praecox, etc. The mechanism may be guessed. Anxiety is a protection against shock (*Shreck*). Now the condition of the traumatic neurosis seems to be that the soul had no time to recur to this protection and is (overrun) taken by the trauma unprepared. Its *Reizschuts* (protective shield against stimuli) is overrun, the principal and primary function of keeping off excessive quantities of *Reiz* (stimulus) frustrated. Then narcissistic libido is given out in shape of the signs of anxiety. This is the mechanism of every case of primary repression, a traumatic neurosis thus to be found at the bottom of every case of transference neurosis.
>
> (Paskauskas, 2001, p. 396; Ramirez Ortiz, 2007, p. 158)

Let us highlight two issues present in this excerpt. First, as in the introduction to the book on the war neuroses, the nosographic reference once again brought these neuroses closer to the narcissistic type. If one were consistent with what Freud proposed in the mid-1910s, it could be believed that he excluded the war neuroses from analytic treatment, since the latter was designed for the transference neuroses. However, both in this epistle and in that introduction, the father of psychoanalysis ended up admitting that (primary) repression lies at the base of every neurosis. This form of repression can be characterised as a "reaction to a trauma" (understood in economic terms) and "as an elementary traumatic neurosis" (Freud, 1919, p. 210). We, therefore, consider that Freud did not intend to state that it was impossible to treat traumatic neuroses through psychoanalysis; instead, we conjecture that he was seeking to affirm that in every neurosis, there is a trauma (which cannot be avoided and which insistently emits indicators of anxiety) whose treatment entails great difficulties, analogous to those that occur in the treatment of narcissistic neuroses.[15] Second, although some of the elements found in this excerpt were already present in previous writings (such as the relationship of traumatic neuroses with narcissistic neuroses, anxiety understood as a preparation for and protection against shock, and the role of narcissistic libido in these conditions), other elements (such as the idea of a protective shield against stimuli) were novel and anticipated certain developments which Freud only made public one year later.

The central thesis of the 1920 paper was based on questioning the pleasure principle. Until then, the Viennese psychoanalyst had maintained that the functioning of the psychical apparatus was organised around the attempt to avoid the unpleasure generated by the increase in tension within the system. In *Beyond the Pleasure*

Principle, certain features of traumatic and war neuroses constituted one of the primary sources that allowed him to address the problem of a tendency to repeat, which prevails despite generating unpleasure.

Furthermore, the text led to a new transformation in his theory of drive dualism (life drives/death drives). As Sulloway maintains, this transformation attempted to sustain itself on biological premises that referred to tendencies which exceed the psychical and even the human sphere (Sulloway, 1979, pp. 401–404). This can be observed in a quote such as the following: "*It seems, then, that an instinct is an urge inherent in organic life to restore an earlier state of things* which the living entity had been obliged to abandon" (Freud, 1920a, p. 36; italics in original). The conservative nature of the drives, which Freud believed could be found in the migratory flights of certain birds, or in specific hereditary phenomena and the facts of embryology (Freud, 1920a, p. 37), served as a conceptual foundation for understanding a compulsion to repeat that imposes itself beyond the pleasure principle. It also served to explain a drive that leads the organism towards the return to an inanimate state, towards the total cancellation of tension, towards death. However, as Freud himself admitted four years later (Freud, 1924), the fact that death is the final destination should not lead one to think that the compulsion to repeat is realised through a reduction of tension; on the contrary, it implies an excessive increase of unpleasurable tension.[16]

In *Beyond the Pleasure Principle*, Freud again differentiated between fright and anxiety: the first is a state that emphasises the factor of surprise and the lack of preparation in the face of an experience (Freud, 1920a, pp. 12–13). After this, he focused on a feature of dream life characteristic of traumatic neuroses. The dreams in these types of neuroses have the characteristic of "repeatedly bringing the patient back into the situation of his accident, a situation from which he wakes up in another fright" (Freud, 1920a, p. 13). "Another" fright which is not simply a past memory: it presents itself, at the same time, as a reiteration of the previous failed attempt at processing it and as a new production of an unpleasurable affect.[17]

To address the clinical problem of a repetition that imposes itself beyond the pleasure principle, Freud resorted to a model inspired by biology. It was a construct, which he himself described as "speculation" (Freud, 1920a, p. 24), based on the functioning of unicellular organisms concerning the treatment of quantities of external stimuli. According to this metaphor, in a simplified living being, as well as in the psychical apparatus, there exists a "protective shield against stimuli". It must "endeavour to preserve the special modes of transformation of energy operating in it against the effects threatened by the enormous energies at work in the external world"; effects which could disrupt the economical functioning of the system, thus generating enormous amounts of unpleasure (Freud, 1920a, p. 27). Making use of this fiction, he introduced a new definition of trauma:

> We describe as 'traumatic' any excitations from outside which are powerful enough to break through the protective shield (…). Such an event as an external trauma is bound to provoke a disturbance on a large scale in the functioning of

> the organism's energy (…) There is no longer any possibility of preventing the mental apparatus from being flooded with large amounts of stimulus.
>
> (Freud, 1920a, p. 29)

In this passage, the traumatic situation began to be conceived in relation to a *hole* (at the borders that circumscribe the interior of the system) and in relation to the *presence* of a heterogeneous element (the large amounts of stimulus outside the levels of normal functioning).

Henceforth, Freud made use of a conceptual opposition between "bound" and "unbound" elements, which, as Ruth Leys points out, played "a crucial role in his thought" (Leys, 2000, p. 23). The Viennese psychoanalyst derived these opposing notions from the difference that Breuer had established between the energy of the "psychical systems" (a quiescent – bound – cathexis) and the energy of the external world (a "freely flowing cathexis" [Freud, 1920a, pp. 26–31]). However, he added that certain "impulses arising from the instincts" and "the repressed memory-traces of his – the patients' – primaeval experiences" (Freud, 1920a, pp. 34–36) remain in a free (unbound) state. They are inside the body but outside a psychical apparatus which attempts to govern itself via the pleasure principle.

We now wish to highlight a few issues. On the one hand, as in the times of the papers that made up his *Neurotica*, here we once again find the memory-traces on the *edge* between the interior of the apparatus (because they are inscribed in it) and its exterior (because of its connection to unbound quantities of stimuli). This edge also signals the border between the set of ideas that makes up the apparatus and the hypertrophic quantitative elements. Alternatively, to use the terms highlighted by Sandra Berta, the traces constitute an *imprint* that could lead to something (quantitative) which is *not inscribed* in the web of representations (Berta, 2014, pp. 49–77).

On the other hand, the instinctual impulses that remain in a mobile or "unbound" state also occupy a strange space: even while belonging to the interior of the body, they are external to the psychical apparatus, even more so than certain experiences that seem to come from the external world.[18]

Let us review what we have developed thus far. Freud conceived the psychical apparatus as a web of representations and bound energy, which attempts to reduce the tension within it as much as possible. In turn, the *trauma* can be defined, in economic terms, as the presence of a quantitative excess unable to be bound to that web; and *traumatic* is the designation given to any element capable of producing that increase in quantity. In temporal terms, the trauma is a moment of discontinuity in the habitual functioning of the apparatus, which is usually governed by the pleasure principle. Finally, in logical terms, the trauma is conceived as an exclusive disjunction: either the apparatus is governed by the pleasure principle, thus capable of binding quantities of excitation to chains of representations, or a large amount of stimulus is introduced, which interrupts its functioning; *either web, or trauma.*[19]

The eruption of large amounts of stimulus presents the apparatus, at least in that instant, with an impossible task.

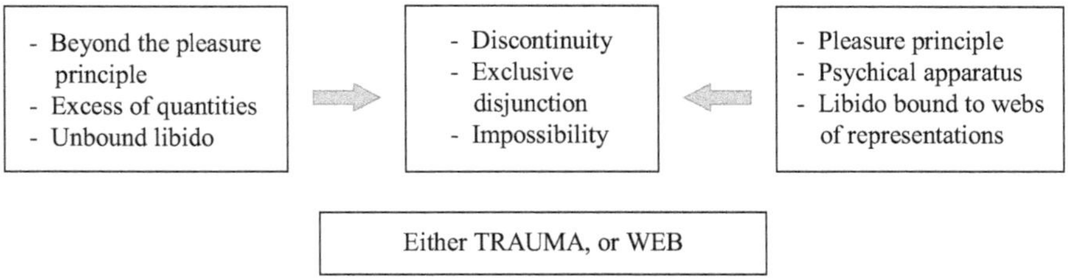

Until now, we have only used two elements of the formula we constructed from Freud's economic definition of trauma in 1917: trauma = powerful increase of stimulus + unprocessable. The third element is missing; it is evident that the trauma *endures* in time, is *repeated,* and, in each moment, seems to *resist being bound* to the webs of representations.

To address this question, let us consider that "the binding of the energy that streams into the mental apparatus" would be, according to Freud, a prior and more urgent task than avoiding unpleasure (Freud, 1920a, p. 31). For this reason, he argued that a part of the compulsion to repeat unpleasurable experiences responds to an attempt to dominate, to bind the heterogeneous element to the system, even when this could cause a momentary suspension of the pleasure principle.

For example, the reaction to bodily pain (produced by the rupture of the protective shield against stimuli in a certain area and the increase of free-flowing excitation in the apparatus), was explained by the displacement of bound energy to the affected area, in an attempt to produce an "anticathexis" or "hypercathexis" that would increase the chances of successful binding (Freud, 1920a, pp. 30–31). Here, we once again come across the model of the "open wound", which we had already found in relation to melancholia which, in turn, was defined by Freud as a painful process (Freud, 1917, p. 253). The same model also served to explain the "preparedness for anxiety" (Freud, 1920a, p. 31). Although it entails a small amount of suffering, the preparedness for anxiety implies the "hypercathexis of the systems that would be the first to receive the stimulus" and would therefore constitute "the last line of defence of the shield against stimuli" (Freud, 1920a, p. 31). In simpler terms, anxiety, thus understood, involves a preparation that protects the apparatus when faced with fright. In this sense, it would operate as a "screen" (not composed of matter, as in the unicellular organisms of the biological model he used) but of webs of representations bound with energy.

Nevertheless, the issue of bodily pain was not sufficient when trying to explain the trauma. Although he highlighted two issues linked to the latter (the increase in tension and the need for work to bind it), pain is a phenomenon that, unlike trauma, does not in itself entail subsequent repetition. In the paper from 1920, other examples appeared that were probably more apt for the proposed task. First, the example of particular repetitive play in children (the renowned "fort-da"). In one of his grandchildren's compulsion to throw objects, Freud found an indicator of the repetition of the unpleasurable situation brought about by the mother's departure. In his opinion, through this playful activity, children manage to "abreact the strength of the impression and, as one might put it, make themselves master of the situation" (Freud, 1920a, p. 17). The quantitative excess generated by the mother's departure would be bound to the scene outlined by the game, thus making the excess amount processable. In addition, the repetition would allow for a modification of the role that was taken up in the first situation: if "at the outset he was in a passive situation (…) by repeating it, unpleasurable though it was, as a game, he took on an active part" (Freud, 1920a, p. 16).

However, in this type of infantile game, another dimension of repetition compulsion also appeared, which differed from the supposed function of enabling dominance over a situation and from the objective of binding the quantitative excess. If in this phenomenon something was repeated beyond the pleasure principle, then the satisfaction of "an impulse of the child's" (a hostile impulse directed towards the mother) was also involved, which brought along with it "a yield of pleasure of another sort" (Freud, 1920a, p. 16). That is to say, this situation yielded a sort of pleasure that was not produced by the discharge of a quantity of excitation but by its increase.

In fact, all the clinical examples provided by Freud show this double facet of the compulsion to repeat: an (often unsuccessful) attempt at binding the excess energy and a paradoxical drive satisfaction, which imposes itself on the subject despite the unpleasure it generates. For example, the dreams which occur in traumatic neuroses also seek to bind the quantitative excess. If the fright that emerged during the traumatic situation was met with a lack of preparation for the reception of stimuli on behalf of the psychical apparatus, the dreams that repeated the trauma would be endeavouring to "master the stimulus retrospectively, by developing the anxiety whose omission was the cause of the traumatic neurosis" (Freud, 1920a, p. 32). Nevertheless, the reference (cited above) to patients waking up in "another fright" would prove the endeavour's failure.

Moreover, these types of dreams showed that it was not the scene of the accident in its entirety that is traumatic and produces fright, but more so the irruption within that scene of a surprising, inconceivable element that cannot be processed. Let us imagine, for example, the scene of a war trench: the dialogue with fellow soldiers, the complaints about fatigue and injuries, and the expectation of danger to come. These types of situations could be sad, painful or frightening. Nevertheless, they occurred (during the experience itself and in the memory of it) within a continuity that would only be interrupted by the unexpected explosion of a bomb, by the inconceivable subjection to torture, and so on. For this reason, according to the Freudian view, it is erroneous to conceive war (or a similar event) as a globally and unitarily traumatic experience. It would be necessary, rather, to consider that in said experience, certain elements could function in a traumatic way if they reach the limit of what can be processed by the webs of representations with which each human being faces the experience.

Something analogous to the oneiric life of traumatic neuroses occurs, according to Freud, in "the dreams during psycho-analyses which bring to memory the psychical traumas of childhood" (Freud, 1920a, p. 32). In relation to these dreams, the author gave an indication that we consider essential in order to define certain characteristics of memory and repetition in relation to the trauma. For the Viennese psychoanalyst, these dreams obey "the compulsion to repeat, though it is true that in analysis that compulsion is supported by the wish (which is encouraged by 'suggestion') to conjure up what has been forgotten and repressed" (Freud, 1920a, p. 32). The analytic treatment would attempt to recover the memory of the past that has been repressed. However, by following the tracks that lead to it, the recovery process runs into a *hole* through which an *unbound* drive element *repeatedly* emerges. Once again, attempting to remember would not be enough to process a trauma; rather, it could lead to an encounter with something that is far too alive, far too present, something that refuses to become a memory or a fragment of the past. Indeed, the repetitions (in dreams, in transference or in certain actions) are not only evidence of the presence of an excess of unbound quantities but also of the attempt to realise the binding. In other words, the repetitions are an attempt to escape from the state of "helplessness" (Freud, 1926, p. 142), to which the subject succumbed when the traumatic disturbance shook his psychical economy. However, if no transformation were to take place in the mode of articulating the webs of representations, the binding would remain impossible.

Having reached this point, we wish to return to and recapitulate the main argument of this part of the chapter, which aimed at analysing the economic view of trauma. According to this perspective, a trauma is produced at the moment in which excessive amounts of excitation that cannot be bound invade the psychical apparatus. Presented in this way, it is clear that the traumatic character of a situation like this lies in the quantitative, affective, non-representational excess. However, these quantities are hypertrophic, and the impossibility of their binding is *only related to* two variables: on the one hand, in relation to the time it takes the quantities to enter the apparatus – lesser time, more difficulty (Freud, 1917, p. 255); on the other hand, in relation to the particularities of each specific psychical apparatus, that is, in relation to the structuring of the elements within the system, structuring that will leave it better or worse prepared to process those excessive quantities. In this sense, the representational domain ends up being just as important as the affects, since a different structure in that domain could entail that a situation, once traumatic for the subject or traumatic for others, ceases to be so.

We can glimpse the relative nature of the trauma in several passages of the Freudian work. It can be found at the end of the nineteenth century, when the trauma was defined based on a *relationship* of incompatibility between one or several ideas and the ego's set of ideas. It can be found after 1920 in *Inhibitions, Symptoms and*

Anxiety (Freud, 1926). Here Freud addressed the individual variations regarding a possible trauma: "Each individual has in all probability a limit beyond which his mental apparatus fails in its function of mastering the quantities of excitation which require to be disposed of" (Freud, 1926, p. 148). These limits, specific to each person and different when compared between people, would explain why the same situations do not acquire a traumatic character in all cases. In Lecture XXXII (Freud, 1933a), Freud made a remark along those same lines. When faced with an experience that needs to be processed, there would be two possibilities: either that said processing is carried out according to the pleasure principle or that it leads to the emergence of a state of high tension experienced as unpleasure. The outcome is a question of "relative quantities. It is only the magnitude of the sum of excitation that turns an impression into a traumatic moment (…) and gives the situation of danger its significance" (Freud, 1933a, p. 94).

Finally, if the trauma has been produced due to the entry of a sum of unbound excitation, the repetition would then be unleashed if a contingent encounter awakens the memory of the trace that functions as a hole in the web of representations. Said repetition would be motivated by an attempt at binding and the compulsion to reiterate the same paths and modalities of satisfaction despite the unpleasure generated. In repetition, the trauma resists being bound to the webs of representations. Paraphrasing the famous book compiled by Friedlander, the trauma, as Freud outlined it after the experience of the Great War, would "probe the limits of representation" (Friedlander, 1992).

Notes

1 In Lecture XXIII Freud introduces the aetiological schematic picture known as "complemental series" (see Figure 4.1). Note that the word "traumatic" is used here in relation to adult experiences and as an apposition or a synonym for "accidental", contingent.

2 Robert Gaupp was a famous German psychiatrist and neurologist, who trained with Wernicke and Kraeplin, and obtained the title of professor of psychiatry at the University of Tübingen in 1908, where he worked until 1936. At that university, another important figure in German psychiatry, Ernst Kretschmer, served as Gaupp's assistant.

3 The idea of an "open wound" was not mentioned at that congress, but Freud used it in that same year, 1917, although in relation to an apparently different problem: melancholia. His approach to this illness was also carried out from an economic point of view. Freud maintained that "the complex of melancholia behaves like an open wound, drawing to itself cathectic energies – which in the transference neuroses we have called 'anticathexes' – from all directions, and emptying the ego until it is totally impoverished" (Freud, 1917, p. 253). This melancholic wound seemed to generate a fixation comparable to that of the traumatic accident, at least because it impelled the psychical apparatus to attempt to solve a task which it experienced as being current and unavoidable and because both implied an alteration of the libidinal economy.

4 This book was the first of those published by the International Psychoanalytic Publishing House, founded in 1919.

5 A similar legitimisation process regarding war-related nervous diseases occurred in the United States (Cox, 2001).

6 F.J Robinson is the author of a website entirely dedicated to disseminating the career and ideas of William Halse Rivers Rivers, who -according to Robinson- is "still a largely

forgotten figure, only recently re-discovered due to Pat Barker's trilogy of 'Regeneration' novels" (Robinson, 2005). In this case, literature seems to have contributed to modifying the collective memory of war experiences independently of official historiography. We thank the psychologist and historian of psychology Marcela Borinksy for giving us the information about Robinson's site. We also refer readers to the book "Tierra de nadie (poesía inglesa de la Gran Guerra)", by Rolando Costa Picazo (2015), in which a sketch of the life of Siegfried Sassoon (and several other English poets) is developed, with the transcription and translation from English of several of his poems written on the battlefront.

7 According to Rivers, the instinct of self-preservation is concerned with "the welfare of the individual", while the sexual instinct subserves "the continuance of the race" (Rivers, 1920, p. 52). To these two kinds of drives, Rivers added a third: the "gregarious instinct" which "maintain the cohesion of the group" (Rivers, 1920, pp. 52–53). Freud, on the other hand, was opposed to admitting the existence of a specific gregarious instinct. From his view, a group is held together by its libidinal ties (Freud, 1921).

8 Freud had made a similar comment one year earlier. In Lecture XXV of his "Introductory Lectures on Psycho-Analysis", he dealt with distinguishing and linking "realistic" anxiety, which constitutes the reaction to an external danger, and "neurotic" anxiety, which occurs because the ego considers "the demand by its libido" as dangerous (Freud, 1916–1917e,f, p. 405). In the following lecture, he went a step further and even affirmed that the libido also participates in the state of anxiety triggered in the face of an external danger. The only "realistic" response to such a danger would be action, be it flight or defence. If instead of action, anxiety appeared (which, in many cases, leads to paralysis, to "inaction"), then Freud believed it pertinent not to attribute this affect to the self-preservation drives (which would push one to action) but to the ego-libido (Freud, 1916–1917f, p. 430).

9 Or rather, the decisive factor is the relationship between that magnitude and the *particular* capacity of each psychical apparatus to process it.

10 With this allusion to the avoidance of danger, Freud recognised the benefit that refuge in the illness could bring; but his conception made it impossible to conceive this manoeuvre as a conscious objective, typical of a simulator who refuses collective demands since, for him, it was the ego who found itself traversed by a conflict to which it could only give a neurotic resolution.

11 See Chapter 3.

12 For this book, the International Psychoanalytic Association awarded Simmel the prize for the best clinical work of the year, following a proposal by Freud (Falzeder & Brabant, 2001, p. 177)

13 For example: "The neurotic, in my opinion, succumbs in the first instance to auto-suggestion, that is to say, to over-strong emotionally toned ideas which have arisen in him at a time when the ego-complex is weakened in power or completely suspended" (Simmel, 1919, p. 34).

14 The choice of the word "bound" to define the link between trauma and scene is not random. The question of quantitative components which are "bound" or "unbound" to the set of representations that make up the psychical apparatus will be crucial to Freud's final conceptions of trauma.

15 In the text from 1920, he also brought traumatic neurosis nosographically closer to transference and narcissistic neuroses: "The symptomatic picture presented by traumatic neurosis approaches that of hysteria in the wealth of its similar motor symptoms, but it surpasses it as a rule in its strongly marked signs of subjective ailment (in which it resembles hypochondria or melancholia) as well as in the evidence it gives of a far more comprehensive general enfeeblement and disturbance of the mental capacities" (Freud, 1920a, p. 12).

16 In the paper of 1920, the notion of the death drive was associated with the reduction of tension: "The dominating tendency of mental life (…) is the effort to reduce, to keep constant or to remove internal tension due to stimuli (the 'Nirvana principle'…) – a tendency which finds expression in the pleasure principle; and our recognition of that fact is one of our strongest reasons for believing in the existence of death instincts" (Freud, 1920a, pp. 55–56). In "The Economic Problem of Masochism", Freud argued that a view which sees the pleasure principle as being identical to the Nirvana principle and that puts the former at the service of the death drive (instead of conceiving it as "the watchman over our life" (Freud, 1924, p. 161)) "cannot be correct" (Freud, 1924, p. 167). In any case, death could indeed be the final destination of repetition compulsion which imposes itself beyond the pleasure principle, or beyond healing, or beyond the preservation of life. However, that destination is reached by the increase of tension and not by its reduction, as exemplified by masochism and a subject's fixation to the trauma. Or, even melancholia, which in 1917 was already characterised by the libidinal cathexes that were not given up but instead drawn back to the ego (Freud, 1917, p. 257), thus generating "the self-tormenting (…), which is without doubt enjoyable" (Freud, 1917, p. 251). Perhaps he found in these clinical situations an argument to establish the plausibility of the death drives more firmly than with the biological model of the return to an inanimate state.

17 Strictly speaking, if an affect such as fright can be "remembered" it implies that a distancing from it has been produced; thus, it would not re-emerge in the present situation and can be registered as having occurred in the past. It would merely be the colour, the quality that stains a past memory. However, if the affect arises again, there is no memory or quality: rather, it would signal the new production of a quantitative process. In a lengthy discussion, Ruth Leys, supporting her arguments on Borch-Jacobsen's, seems to confuse these two aspects, both contained in the word "affect", but which must be differentiated in Freud's work (Leys, 2000, pp. 93–100). From an economic point of view, only a quantitative increase can produce the irruption of (a sum of) affect. If this quantitative disturbance does not occur, then no affect emerges: at most, one could remember ("point out") that this once took place and one could act to avoid its re-production. The distinction between these two situations and between both uses of the word "affect" is at the base of the differentiation between "the signal of anxiety" and the "automatic" development of anxiety in the text *Inhibitions, Symptoms and Anxiety* (Freud, 1926). It also justifies the difference established by Freud between remembering and the compulsion to repeat.

18 As many authors have pointed out, Lacan invented a neologism that refers to this type of topographical problem, a notion that alludes to something that is external and intimate at the same time: the category of "*extimacy*" (Lacan, 1959–1960; Miller, 1985)

19 See *translator's note* in the Introduction.

References

Abraham, K. (1907). La experimentación de traumas sexuales como una forma de actividad sexual. In K. Abraham (Ed.), *Psicoanálisis clínico* (pp. 35–47). Buenos Aires: Hormé. 1980.

Abraham, K. (1919). II. Symposium held at the Fifth International Psycho-Analytical Congress at Budapest, September 1918. 2. Dr. K. Abraham. In VVAA. *Psycho-Analysis and the War Neuroses* (pp. 22–29). London, Viena, New York: The International Psycho-Analytical Press.

Babinski, J. (1901). Définition de l'hystérie. *Revue neurologique, organe officiel de neurologie*, 1074–1080.

Baños Orellana, J. (2013). *La novela de Lacan. De neuropsiquiatra a psicoanalista.* Buenos Aires: El cuenco de plata.

Bernheim, H. (1903). *Hypnotisme, Suggestion, Psychothérapie, études nouvelles avec considérations nouvelles sur l'hysterie.* Paris: Doin.

Berta, S. (2014). *Escribir el Trauma, de Freud a Lacan.* Buenos Aires: Letra Viva.

Brunner, J. (2000). Will, desire and experience: Etiology and ideology in the German and Austrian medical discourse on war neurosis. *Transcultural Psychiatry, 37* (3), 295–320.

Cox, C. (2001). Invisible wounds: The American legion, shell-shocked veterans, and American Society, 1919–1924. In M. Micale & P. Lerner (Eds.), *Traumatic Pasts. History, Psychiatry, and Trauma in the Modern Age, 1870–1930* (pp. 280–305). Cambridge: Cambridge University Press.

Dejerine, J. (1904). *Le traitemente des hystériques à l'hôpital.* Paris: Le Bulletin médical.

Dejerine, J. & Gauckler, E. (1911). *Les manifestations fonctionnelles des psychonévroses. Leur traitement par la psychothérapie.* Paris: Masson.

Edelman, N. (2003). *Les métamorphoses de l'histérique. Du debut du XIX siècle à la Grande Guerre.* Paris: La Découverte.

Eder, M.D. (1917). *War-Schock: The Psycho-Neuroses in War Psychology and Treatment.* London: William Heinemann.

Eissler, K.R. (1992). *Freud sur le front des névroses de guerre.* Paris: Presses Universitaires de France.

Falzeder, E. (2002). *The Complete Correspondence of Sigmund Freud and Karl Abraham. 1907–1925.* London and New York: Karnac.

Falzeder, E. & Brabant, E. (2001). *Sigmund Freud, Sandor Ferenczi. Correspondencia complete, 1917–1919: Vol. II.* Madrid: Síntesis.

Ferenczi, S. ([1916/1917] 1927). Two types of war neurosis. In S. Ferenczi (Ed.), *Further Contributions to the Theory and Technique of Psycho-Analysis* (pp. 124–141). New York: Boni and Liveright Publishers.

Ferenczi, S. (1919). II. Symposium held at the fifth international psycho-analytical congress at Budapest, September 1918. 1. Dr. S. Ferenczi. In VVAA. *Psycho-Analysis and the War Neuroses* (pp. 5–21). London, Viena, and New York: The International Psycho-Analytical Press.

Freud, S. ([1894] 1962). The neuro-psychoses of defence. In S. Freud (Ed.), *The Standard Edition of the Complete Psychological Works of Sigmund Freud, Vol. III: Early Psycho-Analytic Publications* (pp. 41–68). London: The Hogarth Press and the Institute of Psycho-Analysis.

Freud, S. ([1905] 1953). On psychotherapy. In S. Freud (Ed.), *The Standard Edition of the Complete Psychological Works of Sigmund Freud, Vol. VII: A Case of Hysteria, Three Essays on Sexuality and Other Works* (pp. 255–268). London: The Hogarth Press and the Institute of Psycho-Analysis.

Freud, S. ([1906] 1953). My views on the part played by sexuality in the aetiology of the neuroses. In S. Freud (Ed.), *The Standard Edition of the Complete Psychological Works of Sigmund Freud, Vol. VII: A Case of Hysteria, Three Essays on Sexuality and Other Works* (pp. 269–279). London: The Hogarth Press and the Institute of Psycho-Analysis.

Freud, S. ([1911] 1958). Psycho-analytic notes on an autobiographical account of a case of paranoia (Dementia paranoides). In S. Freud (Ed.), *The Standard Edition of the Complete Psychological Works of Sigmund Freud Vol. XII: The Case of Schreber Papers on Technique and Other Works* (pp. 1–79). London: The Hogarth Press and the Institute of Psycho- Analysis.

Freud, S. ([1914] 1957). On narcissism: And introduction. In S. Freud (Ed.), *The Standard Edition of the Complete Psychological Works of Sigmund Freud Vol. XIV: On the History of the Psycho- Analytic Movement, Papers on Metapsychology and Other Works* (pp. 67–102). London: The Hogarth Press and the Institute of Psycho-Analysis.

Freud, S. ([1916–1917a] 1963). Lecture XVIII. Fixation to traumas, the unconscious. In S. Freud (Ed.), *The Standard Edition of the Complete Psychological Works of Sigmund Freud Vol. XVI: Introductory Lectures on Psycho- Analysis (Part III)* (pp. 273–285). London: The Hogarth Press and the Institute of Psycho-Analysis.

Freud, S. ([1916–1917d] 1963). Lecture XXIV. The common neurotic state. In S. Freud (Ed.), *The Standard Edition of the Complete Psychological Works of Sigmund Freud Vol. XVI: Introductory Lectures on Psycho-Analysis (Part III)* (pp. 378–391). London: The Hogarth Press and the Institute of Psycho-Analysis.

Freud, S. ([1916–1917e] 1963). Lecture XXV. Anxiety. In S. Freud (Ed.), *The Standard Edition of the Complete Psychological Works of Sigmund Freud Vol. XVI: Introductory Lectures on Psycho-Analysis (Part III)* (pp. 392–411). London: The Hogarth Press and the Institute of Psycho-Analysis.

Freud, S. ([1916–1917f] 1963). Lecture XXVI. The libido theory and narcissism. In S. Freud (Ed.), *The Standard Edition of the Complete Psychological Works of Sigmund Freud Vol. XVI: Introductory Lectures on Psycho-Analysis (Part III)* (pp. 412–430). London: The Hogarth Press and the Institute of Psycho-Analysis.

Freud, S. ([1917] 1957). Mourning and melancholia. In S. Freud (Ed.), *The Standard Edition of the Complete Psychological Works of Sigmund Freud, Vol. XIV: On the History of the Psycho-Analytic Movement, Papers on Metapsychology and Other Works* (pp. 237–260). London: The Hogarth Press and the Institute of Psycho-Analysis.

Freud, S. ([1918] 1955). From the history of an infantile neurosis. In S. Freud (Ed.), *The Standard Edition of the Complete Psychological Works of Sigmund Freud, Vol. XVII: An Infantile Neurosis and Other Works* (pp. 1–123). London: The Hogarth Press and the Institute of Psycho-Analysis.

Freud, S. ([1919 (1918)] 1955). Lines of advance in psycho- analytic therapy. In S. Freud (Ed.), *The Standard Edition of the Complete Psychological Works of Sigmund Freud, Vol. XVII: An Infantile Neurosis and Other Works* (pp. 157–168). London: The Hogarth Press and the Institute of Psycho-Analysis.

Freud, S. ([1919] 1955). Introduction to psycho-analysis and the war neuroses. In S. Freud (Ed.), *The Standard Edition of the Complete Psychological Works of Sigmund Freud, Vol. XVII: An Infantile Neurosis and Other Works* (pp. 201–215). London: The Hogarth Press and the Institute of Psycho-Analysis.

Freud, S. ([1920a] 1955). Beyond the pleasure principle. In S. Freud (Ed.), *The Standard Edition of the Complete Psychological Works of Sigmund Freud, Vol. XVIII: Beyond the Pleasure Principle, Group Psychology and Other Works* (pp. 1–64). London: The Hogarth Press and the Institute of Psycho-Analysis.

Freud, S. ([1920b] 1955). Introduction to psycho- analysis and the war neuroses. In S. Freud (Ed.), *The Standard Edition of the Complete Psychological Works of Sigmund Freud, Vol. XVII: An Infantile Neurosis and Other Works* (pp. 207–215). London: The Hogarth Press and the Institute of Psycho-Analysis.

Freud, S. ([1924] 1961). The economic problem of masochism. In S. Freud (Ed.), *The Standard Edition of the Complete Psychological Works of Sigmund Freud, Vol. XIX: The Ego and the Id and Other Works* (pp. 157–170). London: The Hogarth Press and the Institute of Psycho-Analysis.

Freud, S. ([1926] 1959). Inhibitions, symptoms and anxiety. In S. Freud (Ed.), *The Standard Edition of the Complete Psychological Works of Sigmund Freud, Vol. XX: An Autobiographical Study. Inhibitions, Symptoms and Anxiety. The Question of Lay Analysis and Other Works* (pp. 75–175). London: The Hogarth Press and the Institute of Psycho-Analysis.

Freud, S. ([1933a] 1964). Lecture XXXII. Anxiety and instinctual life. In S. Freud (Ed.), *The Standard Edition of the Complete Psychological Works of Sigmund Freud, Vol. XXII: New Introductory Lectures on Psycho- Analysis and Other Works* (pp. 81–111). London: The Hogarth Press and the Institute of Psycho-Analysis.

Friedlander, S. (Ed.). (1992). *Probing the Limits of Representation: Nazism and the 'Final Solution'*. Cambridge and London: Harvard University Press.

Gilles, A. (1917). L'Hystérie et la guerre, Troubles fonctionnels par commotion, Leur traitement par le torpillage. *Annales médico-psychologiques*, *8*, Abril 1917, 207–227.

Jones, E. (1919). War shock and Freud's theory of the neuroses. In VVAA (Ed.), *Psycho-Analysis and the War Neuroses* (pp. 44–59). London, Viena, New York: The International Psycho-Analytical Press.

Jones, E. (1953–1957). *The Life and Work of Sigmund Freud: Volume I, II and III.* New York: Basic Books.

Kaufmann, F. (1916). Die planmässige Heilung komplizierter psychogener Bewegunsstörungen bei Soldaten in einer Sitzung. *Münchner medizinische Wochenschrift, Feldärztliche Beilage, 22*, 802–804.

Lacan, J. (1959–1960). *The Seminar of Jacques Lacan. The Ethics of Psychoanalysis. Book VII.* New York and London: W.W. Norton & Company, 1992.

Laignel-Lavastine, M. & Carbon, P. (1919). *Les Accidentés de la guerre: leurs éspirit, leurs réactions, leur traitement.* Paris: Baillière et fills.

Leese, P. (2001). "Why are they not cured". British shellshock treatment during the Great War. In M. Micale & P. Lerner (Eds.), *Traumatic Pasts. History, Psychiatry, and Trauma in the Modern Age, 1870–1930* (pp. 205–221). Cambridge: Cambridge University Press.

Lerner, P. (2001). From traumatic neurosis to male hysteria: The decline and fall of Hermann Oppenheim, 1889–1919. In M. Micale & P. Lerner (Eds.), *Traumatic Pasts. History, Psychiatry, and Trauma in the Modern Age, 1870–1930* (pp. 140–171). Cambridge: Cambridge University Press.

Leys, R. (2000). *Trauma. A Genealogy*. Chicago, IL: The University of Chicago Press.

Loughran, T. (2008). Hysteria and neurasthenia in pre-1914 British medical discourse and in histories of shell-shock. *History of Psychiatry, 19* (1), 25–46.

Micale, M. & Lerner, P. (2001). Trauma, psychiatry, and history: A conceptual and historiographical introduction. In M. Micale & P. Lerner (Eds.), *Traumatic Pasts. History, Psychiatry, and Trauma in the Modern Age, 1870–1930* (pp. 1–27). Cambridge: Cambridge University Press.

Miller, J.A. ([1985] 2010). *Extimidad. Los cursos psicoanalíticos de J. A. Miller.* Buenos Aires: Paidós.

Nonne, M. (1915). Soll man wieder 'traumatische Neurose" bei Kriegsverletzten diagnostizieren? *Medizinische Klinik, 11*, 849–854.

Oppenheim, H. (1916). *Die Neurosen infloge von Kriegsverletzungen.* Berlin: Karger.

Paskauskas, R.A. (2001). *Sigmund Freud, Ernest Jones. Correspondencia complete, 1908–1939.* Madrid: Editorial Síntesis.
Ramirez Ortiz, M.E. (2007). *Psicoanalistas en el frente de batalla. Las neurosis de guerra en la Primera Guerra Mundial.* Antioquía: Editorial Universidad de Antioquía.
Rivers, W.H.R. (1920). *Instinct and the Unconscious: A Contribution to a Biological Theory of the Psycho-Neuroses.* Cambridge: Cambridge University Press.
Robinson, F.J. (2005). *Rivers. The Forgotten Healer.* See https://whrrivers.com/
Rose, N. (1999). 1. The psychology of war. In N. Rose (Ed.), *Governing the Soul. The Shaping of the Private Self* (pp. 15–21). London and New York: Free Association Books.
Roudebush, M. (2001). A battle of nerves: Hysteria and its treatments in France during World War I. In M. Micale & P. Lerner (Eds.), *Traumatic Pasts. History, Psychiatry, and Trauma in the Modern Age, 1870–1930* (pp. 253–279). Cambridge: Cambridge University Press.
Simmel, E. (1918). *Kriegsneurosen und psychisches Trauma. Ibre gegensseitigen Beziehungen, dargestellt auf Grund psychoanalytischer, hypnotischer Studien.* Munich and Leipzig: Editorial Otto Nemnich.
Simmel, E. (1919). II. Symposium held at the fifth international psycho-analytical congress at Budapest, September 1918. 3. Dr. E. Simmel. In *Psycho-Analysis and the War Neuroses* (pp. 30–43). London, Vienna, and New York: The International Psycho-Analytical Press, 1921.
Sollier, P. (1901). *L'Hystérie et son traitement.* Paris: Alcan.
Sulloway, F. (1979). *Freud Biologist of the Mind. Beyond the Psychoanalytic Legend.* New York: Basic Books.
Swain, G. (1994). Du traitment moral aux psychothérapies. Remarques sur la formation de l'idêe contemporaine de psychothérapie. In G. Swain (Ed.), *Dialogue avec l'insensé* (pp. 237–262). Paris: Gallimard.
Tausk, V. (1916). Diagnostic consideratiosn concerning the symptomatology of the so-called war psychoses. *The Psychoanalytic Quarterly, 37*, 382–405.
VVAA (1919). *Psycho-Analysis and the War Neuroses.* London, Vienna, and New York: The International Psycho-Analytical Press.

Chapter 5

On Collective Traumas

The Persistence and Transmission of Past Experiences (1913 and 1939)

Throughout the various chapters of this book, we have attempted to defend the idea that, in Freud's work, trauma *persists*. First, it persists because, despite its variations and apparent abandonments, the notion never ceased to allude to problems central to psychoanalytic practice and theory: unconscious and psychical conflict, aetiology and sexuality, memory and repetition, non-linear temporalities, etc. Second, trauma persists because, when it was linked to memory (Chapter 1) and to a *nachträglich* temporality (Chapter 3), it became a notion that implies the idea of its permanence and its return. Trauma *insists*: it seeps in, in a distorted form, between the representations of the present. Third, trauma persists because, from an economic point of view (Chapter 4), it indicates an aspect of psychical life that cannot be wholly bound to the field of representations that make up the psychical apparatus and with which we approach experience. In other words, trauma refers to that which *resists* symbolisation.

Could these notions of trauma, which persist in different ways, be applied to human groups? Freud was the first to conceive this possibility; until the 1980s, he was probably the only one to do so. In *Totem and Taboo* (Freud, 1913) and, more so, in *Moses and Monotheism* (Freud, 1939), he defended the idea that certain past experiences (which occurred at some distant moment in the history of humanity and which could be termed "traumas") remained present in the collective memory and conserved their ability to produce effects in subsequent generations, despite not being explicitly rememberable. We will attempt to demonstrate that this thesis, far from being a marginal excursion into the field of anthropology and social memory, was central to Freudian thought. We have come across certain aspects of this thesis in Chapter 3, in the context of the discussion about the real or phantasised nature of certain scenes recounted repeatedly in Freud's analyses: scenes of castration and seduction and primal scenes. Towards the middle of the 1910s, in the context of his disputes with Jung, Freud allowed himself to leave it unclear whether a scene had occurred or not in the "Wolf Man's" childhood. In opposition to the Swiss doctor, he maintained with certainty the actual and historical nature of this event and similar ones, whether they took place in the person's life or in that of their ancestors. Even though the three "primal phantasies" (Freud, 1916–1917d, p. 371) can *also* occur during a person's life, he considered them "an inherited endowment, a

DOI: 10.4324/9781003380016-6

phylogenetic heritage" that allows an individual to fill in "the gaps in individual truth with prehistoric truth", to replace "occurrences in his own life by occurrences in the life of his ancestors" (Freud, 1918, p. 97). The scene of parental intercourse described in the case history of the "Wolf Man" exemplified well the Freudian approach. It also delimitated a zone of overlap between collective and individual experience, between group psychology and the analysis of a neurotic subject. In this text, Freud conjectures the existence of a process of *transmission* carried out over many generations, which ties the evolution of an individual's life to what was experienced by the individual's ancestors. How was this "inherited endowment" preserved if it did not seem to exist in explicit traditions? By what means was this "phylogenetic heritage" produced? Or, in more general terms: what is *preserved* from the experience of the humans who preceded us and how would it be *transmitted* throughout the generations? Could a *trauma* experienced by ancestors *persist* in social memory? Could it *insist* and eventually return many years later? Could it have effects in the present despite *resisting* its full inclusion in collective representations? These questions, linked to the Freudian texts that dealt with collective traumas, remain valid in many of the contemporary approaches to these problems in the field of historiography and studies on social memory.

In this chapter, we will first attempt to analyse the historical reasons why Freud was confronted with these questions. Undoubtedly, certain internal aspects of the development of the doctrine and of the psychoanalytic movement (in particular, Jung's interest in religious phenomena and his criticism of the role of sexuality in the neuroses) pushed the Viennese psychoanalyst to study certain collective processes with the use of psychoanalytic categories. Later, after the First World War and the increasingly notorious rise of Nazism, the articulation between collective and individual psychology became more and more notorious, finally giving rise to the last great book published by Freud (1939). In this book, the category of trauma was intimately tied to the origins of Jewish monotheism, the development of the neuroses and the context in which the text was written. The latter found the psychoanalyst going through his last days in exile due to the beginning of the Jewish genocide perpetrated by the Nazis.

Second, we seek to study the responses given by Freud to the questions regarding the existence, persistence and transmission of collective traumas. We are interested in investigating the arguments that he offered to justify the comparison and the articulation of individual and collective psychology regarding a problem of difficult resolution: the permanence and transmission of the traces from past traumatic experiences within a community, despite these not having been preserved in its explicit traditions. Finally, for Freud, the effects of the marks of past experiences in a human group were not permanent. They depended on processes of forgetting and compulsive returns analogous to those found in the development of a neurosis. In this way, the issue of trauma constituted one of the privileged ways that Freud found to question the traditional division between individual psychology and collective psychology.

5.1 The Historical Bond between Savages and Neurotics

There are several works by Freud in which he intended to shorten the divide between the individual and collective dimensions of psychology and attempted to apply psychoanalysis to areas other than the clinic of the neuroses: "Obsessive Actions and Religious Practices" (1907), "'Civilized' Sexual Morality and Modern Nervous Illness" (1908), *Group Psychology and the Analysis of the Ego* (1921), *The Future of an Illusion* (1927), *Civilization and its Discontents* (1930) and *Moses and Monotheism* (1939), among others. Of these, *Totem and Taboo* was most likely one of the most ambitious attempts (1913). This book had a subtitle that narrowed down the domain of his interest and foreshadowed some elements of the thesis he intended to defend: "Some Points of Agreement between the Mental Lives of Savages and Neurotics". In the introduction, James Strachey clarified that "the major elements of Freud's contribution to social anthropology made their first appearance in this work" (Freud, 1913, p. xi). If it was possible to find "points of agreement" between savages and neurotics, then the bridging of psychoanalysis and anthropological knowledge would be justified. However, this subtitle did not explain the nature of the similarities between the two objects of analysis or how the link between the two disciplines could be established.

In Freud's preface, we find a second reference that aimed to define the terms in which he understood that relationship. At the same time, he made explicit an important aspect of the context in which the book was written: the growing differences with his favourite disciple, Carl Jung. In those years, the latter had been studying the relationships between prehistory, myths, religion and psychoanalysis. His book *Psychology of the Unconscious. A Study of the Transformations and Symbolisms of the Libido* (Jung, 1911–1912) appeared as one of the references from which Freud's work sought to differentiate itself.[1] As stated in the preface, the contrast between the two books was a "methodological" one. While the Swiss doctor endeavoured "to solve the problems of individual psychology with the help of material derived from social psychology" (Freud, 1913, p. xiii), the Viennese physician intended to do the opposite, that is, to apply "the point of view and the findings of psycho-analysis to some unsolved problems of social psychology" (Freud, 1913, p. xiii). It was a question of "extending", of "applying" the psychoanalytic method to a new field: the psychology of primitive peoples.[2]

However, this reference concealed more than it exposed the situation. We say this because, initially, it did not make any mention of the conflict regarding the importance that each one of the authors intended to attribute to sexuality, a conflict that was very noticeable in the epistolary exchange between them.[3] Furthermore, it is not possible to ignore the fact that what Freud elucidated regarding the mental life of primitive people by using the categories and the method of psychoanalysis ended up having an impact on the latter. Most importantly, Freud required the hypothesis of a phylogenetic heritage that would be transmitted to future generations in order to explain certain occurrences that took place in his analyses, such as the recurrence of narratives about seduction, castration threats and parental intercourse (Freud, 1916–1917d, 1918). If these events did not always actually occur in a patient's childhood, what would be the source of these scenes or other common features in the different types of neuroses? The answer to this question was not long in coming; rather, it was already present in the 1913 book. According to Freud, the source of these common features in the neuroses, which were not a part of the individual's history, was found in certain experiences that the person's ancestors actually lived; these experiences were preserved in the memory of peoples and transmitted throughout successive generations, despite not appearing in official education.

In other words, for Freud, the "points of agreement between savages and neurotics" were not mere analogies nor different historical expressions of certain universal and immutable symbols but rather the consequence of the transmission of events that occurred at the very origin of culture. A historical bond would thus unite the savages of yesteryear with those investigated by the anthropologists of the nineteenth century and with the neurotics who presented themselves in Freud's consulting room. Although there was no empirical proof for some of his conjectures, he never gave up on considering that his constructions referred to historical events, even though the latter could be manifested in a distorted way.

Before investigating the Freudian hypotheses about a key historical experience which he believed to have been transmitted from prehistory, we consider it necessary to clarify the "points of agreement" and the anthropological problems that the psychoanalyst intended to make explicit. The book's first chapter aimed to explain the origins and the main characteristics of "the horror of incest" (Freud, 1913, pp. 1–17). On this issue lay one of Freud's main differences with Jung. While the latter rejected the existence of incestuous desires in the age of matriarchal law (because he assumed that there were no recognised fathers to compete with and that promiscuity was allowed), the former sought to demonstrate the universal nature of those desires and of their prohibition since the origins of culture.[4] The first "point of agreement" between savages, children and neurotics would thus reside in the fact that they were all considered to be caught up in a conflict between incestuous desires and interdictions that, initially (that is, before being internalised), originated in an external agency.

To justify this assertion, Freud presented ethnographic material on certain Australian tribes which were known for not building houses, not having kings, not worshipping superior beings, not knowing of agriculture, not using clothes, and nevertheless "avoiding incestuous sexual relations" between members of the same clan (that is, between people who shared the same totem) (Freud, 1913, p. 2). Thus, totemism and exogamy seemed to co-belong.[5] The savage's horror of incest was then conceived under the psychoanalytic lens, as "an infantile feature (…) that (…) reveals a striking agreement with the mental life of neurotic patients" since "a boy's earliest choice of objects for his love is incestuous and (…) those objects are forbidden ones – his mother and his sister", a choice which ends up constituting "the nuclear complex of neurosis" (Freud, 1913, p. 17).

The second point of agreement between savages and neurotics appeared in the second chapter, where he discussed the prohibitions of taboo, a term that condenses two opposing meanings: "to us it means, on the one hand, 'sacred', 'consecrated', and on the other 'uncanny' 'dangerous', 'forbidden', 'unclean'" (Freud, 1913, p. 18). The violation of taboo infected the violator with the attributes (sacred/unclean) of the violated object: no one may come into contact with them. The *ambivalent* question of *contact* (its prohibition, but also the attraction generated by that which is prohibited), as well as the "acts of atonement and purification" (Freud, 1913, p. 20), made it possible to point out the similarities between the savage's behaviour towards the prohibited object and that of the obsessional neurotic, who responds to seemingly senseless prohibitions and limitations and performs innumerable expiatory actions (Freud, 1913, pp. 26–27).

Freud was not satisfied with the possibility that this resemblance was limited to a formal analogy (Freud, 1913, pp. 26–27). Just like the prohibitions of obsessional neurosis, which would imply the internalisation and distortion of an originally external interdiction of incestuous desires,

> taboos, we must suppose, are prohibitions of primaeval antiquity which were at some time externally imposed upon a generation of primitive men (...) These prohibitions must have concerned activities towards which there was a strong inclination. They must then have persisted from generation to generation.

until becoming "an inherited psychical endowment" (Freud, 1913, p. 31). This point of agreement was not a mere analogy: neurotics, who in the present behave like prisoners of a taboo, "may be said to have inherited an archaic constitution as an atavistic vestige" (Freud, 1913, p. 66).

This inheritance of a particular psychical endowment was not limited to neurotics. In the third chapter of *Totem and Taboo*, Freud established another point of agreement between the stages of libidinal development common to every individual (narcissism, incestuous object-choice, exogamic object-choice) and certain phases of the "evolution of human views of the universe" (animistic, religious, scientific) (Freud, 1913, p. 88). With this simple gesture, the founder of psychoanalysis was not only establishing points of agreement between these stages but also applying Haeckel's *fundamental law of biogeny* to the field of psychology (Acha, 2007, pp. 40–41; Sulloway, 1979, p. 259). According to this law

> every organism (...) reproduces in its individual development, in virtue of certain hereditary processes, a part of its ancestral history. The very word 'recapitulation' implies a partial and abbreviated repetition of the course of the original phyletic development, determined by the 'laws of heredity and adaptation'.
>
> (Haeckel, 1904, p. 139, cited in Acha, 2007, p. 41)

Freud, in this way, reinforced the idea of a historical bond and a heritage that would tie not only ancient people with contemporaries but also the history of humanity with the development of the individual.

The fourth and final chapter of the book was called "The Return of Totemism in Childhood" (Freud, 1913, pp. 100–161). Its main objective was to elucidate the origin of the institution of totemic organisation and to explain the relationship between the totem and the taboo upon incest, of which exogamy is the expression (Freud, 1913, p. 108). In addition, the title alluded to one of the most important theses of the book: that which occurred in those origins *returns* in childhood.

At this point, Freud began to construct an explanatory edifice supported by three pillars, with which he intended to resolve these questions and demonstrate the historical bond between savages and neurotics. The first pillar was a Darwinian hypothesis (McGuire, 1974, p. 504). According to this deduction that "might be described as 'historical'" (Freud, 1913, p. 125), before the totemic organisation was established, human beings would have lived in small hordes under the command of a male whose jealousy prevented, in fact, the sexual promiscuity that Jung supposed to be in the origins of humanity (Freud, 1913, p. 125).

The second pillar stemmed from psychoanalytic research and made it possible to establish a new "point of agreement": "There is a great deal of resemblance between the relations of children and of primitive men towards animals" (Freud, 1913, p. 126). Neither of the two believes to have any essential difference with respect to animals, and both feel related to them. However, the child's relationship with animals is disturbed by the emergence of zoophobia, which is common in childhood. Therefore, psychoanalysis is in charge of shedding "one single ray of light"[6] into the obscure enigma of the origins of totemism: the anxiety produced when in the presence of the animal originated in the relationship with the father (Freud, 1913, pp. 126–131). Consequently, in Freud's opinion, "these observations justify (…) substituting the father for the totem animal in the formula for totemism" (Freud, 1913, p. 131).

In short, in the phase prior to totemism, a primal father would have effectively barred access to the women of the horde; in the stage of totemic organisation (which implied exogamy), the totem was a substitute for the father. And so:

> "the two taboo prohibitions (…) – not to kill the totem and not to have sexual relations with a woman of the same totem – coincide in their content with the two crimes of Oedipus (…) as well as with the two primal wishes of children, the insufficient repression or the re-awakening of which forms the nucleus of perhaps every psychoneurosis.
>
> (Freud, 1913, p. 132)

As can be seen, the points of agreement appeared to become deeper and deeper. Only one piece was missing to account for the origin of the totem: the explanation of the transition from the horde to a totemic organisation, that is, from exogamy sustained in fact, by force, to a law that prohibited incest, erected around the totem. At this point, Freud made use of the third leg of his explanatory edifice: William Robertson Smith's hypothesis about the "totem meal", in which all the clan members had to eat the totemic animal in a ceremony full of ambivalent attitudes (Freud, 1913, pp. 132–133).

Having installed the three pillars of his explanatory edifice (the Darwinian hypothesis, the equivalence between the totem and the father and the totem meal), Freud found himself in a position to go a step further and present a construction with which he sought to explain the unresolved enigmas of totemism and exogamy. Said construction was based on a scene in which the act committed in it was thought to have had lasting consequences in the forms of human organisation. No explicit or conscious memory of that scene is preserved; however, for Freud, it *persists* in collective memory, thanks to a process of transgenerational transmission, and *insists* on appearing in distorted forms. With this construction, Freud hoped to solve some anthropological problems and to give a historical and material foundation to the points of agreement between savages and neurotics. To justify the historical and material nature of the concordances, the psychoanalyst conceived a process of hereditary transmission analogous to Lamarck's proposals.

In other words, for Freud, all these enigmas would find a solution if it were true that…

> One day the brothers who had been driven out came together, killed and devoured their father and so made an end of the patriarchal horde. United, they had the courage to do and succeeded in doing what would have been impossible for them individually. (…) The violent primal father had doubtless been the feared and envied model of each one of the company of brothers: and in the act of devouring him they accomplished their identification with him, and each one of them acquired a portion of his strength. The totem meal, which is perhaps mankind's earliest festival, would thus be a repetition and a commemoration of this memorable and criminal deed, which was the beginning of so many things – of social organization, of moral restrictions and of religion.
>
> (Freud, 1913, pp. 141–142)

Freud knew that there was no conventional empirical evidence of that act; nevertheless, he firmly believed that the crime had left *traces* that, from time to time, *returned.* These traces are repeated and expressed in a *distorted* manner that, thanks to psychoanalysis, can be interpreted. The totem meal, observed by anthropologists in certain communities which maintained ancient customs at the end of the nineteenth century, is one of these distorted repetitions. The child's ambivalent relationship with their father in the context of the Oedipus Complex is another distorted testimony of that founding murder. If the "points of agreement" between children, neurotics and savages are so abundant, and if the psychoanalytic method is able to interpret the present remnants of those primal times correctly, then it would be possible to assume that these brothers also had *ambivalent* feelings regarding that primal father. Thus:

> After they had got rid of him, had satisfied their hatred and had put into effect their wish to identify themselves with him, the affection which had all this time been pushed under was bound to make itself felt. (…) The dead father became

> stronger than the living one had been (...). What had up to then been prevented by his actual existence was thenceforward prohibited by the sons themselves, in accordance with the psychological procedure so familiar to us in psychoanalyses under the name of 'deferred obedience'. They revoked their deed by forbidding the killing of the totem, the substitute for their father; and they renounced its fruits by resigning their claim to the women who had now been set free. They thus created out of their filial sense of guilt the two fundamental taboos of totemism, which for that very reason inevitably corresponded to the two repressed wishes of the Oedipus complex.
>
> (Freud, 1913, p. 143)

What Freud was trying to explain with this sort of "theoretical fiction" (De Certeau, 1988, p. 294) is nothing more and nothing less than the origin of culture. In the transition from the horde to the clan via the murder of the father, an impediment in fact became specific prohibitions in law (the two main taboos of totemism), which were established as the minimum norms for the organisation of a truly human collective to be possible. Without the prohibition of incest (which falls on sexual and hostile desires), the divisions between the brothers would have grown until one of them returned to occupy the father's place. With this narrative about the origins, conflict and death were exposed as the original background of the law and life in society (Acha, 2007; Braunstein, Fuks & Basualdo, 2013).

At the same time, Freud converted ambivalence into a fundamental category to expand his construction about the primal murder. According to his hypothesis, the displaced brothers not only hated their father but also loved and admired him. Only under the assumption of ambivalent feelings is it possible to explain why the young brothers felt guilt after the act. Thus, they did not continue fighting for a place as the horde's leader; instead, after killing him, they turned that terrible father's will into the law of the brothers: clan women are forbidden for all men. The "deferred" nature of their love hidden behind hostility allowed for a new meaning to be given to the deceased's actions and to begin obeying his desire, which had become law. As can be seen, ambivalence is not, for Freud, a contingent and minor detail but rather a central element to understanding the transition from the primal horde to culture (Le Gaufey, 1995).

Jacques Lacan, who made an extensive commentary on *Totem and Taboo* in his seventeenth Seminar, has rightly pointed out a fundamental difference between the Oedipus myth and the narrative about the murder of the primal father. While in the former, killing the father granted access to the mother, in the Freudian conjecture, that act of murder converted the impediment into law: no one else could have access to the prohibited object (Lacan, 1969–1970, pp. 113–114). However, this comment could generate in non-attentive readers a shift concerning the point that interested Freud. The father of psychoanalysis did not intend to compare both narratives as myths. He was not looking for matches between Oedipus, a character from Sophocles, and the band of brothers, protagonists of another narrative of a purely phantasist nature; rather, what he intended to compare in order to point out their concordance is the situation in which savages, children and neurotics *actually* find themselves in: they are affected by the same *conflict* between their incestuous desires and a repressive agency. Although his conjecture could lack empirical evidence and have a mythical structure, he was trying to give an account of something real.

At the same time, Lacan refused to refer to the leader of the horde as a "father": "We have seen orangutans. But not the slightest trace has ever been seen of the father of the human horde" (Lacan, 1969–1970, p. 113). In this way, he turned the distance between one time and another into a gap between nature and culture. From the outset, in Lacan's view, to be human implies the law and the symbolic; about the earlier time, we can only a posteriori construct myths. This standpoint ignores a problem dear to Freud: that of the origin, that is, of the transition from the impediment de facto to the prohibition in law. The Viennese psychoanalyst could acknowledge that laws were only erected during clan organisation, and he could recognise the distance between the time of the horde and that of the totem. However, his way of thinking was much more historicist than that of the French psychoanalyst. He needed to construct a link, a bridge, a series of continuities (not just ruptures) between the supposed primal stage and the observable totemic phase. If the conflict with Jung is taken into account, we can find some reasons for this need. For sexuality and the Oedipus complex to not be displaced from the core of the theory (a shift that the Swiss psychoanalyst was carrying out), both had to be present in that primal period. The "Darwinian hypothesis" allowed him to conceive that the struggle between the incestuous desires of a generation and a repressive agency (which Freud insisted on calling "father") had existed since before the latter's symbolic interdiction. From his view, prohibition does not engender desire, as Jung suggested; instead, desire exists before prohibition, even when its satisfaction can not be effectively realised due to the violence exerted by that strange father.

After considering that the transition from nature to culture was already explained by the murder and by the conflict of ambivalence, Freud dedicated himself to tracking the traces of that act, which he believed appeared in distorted forms throughout humanity's history. The successive transformations in the modes of social organisation, religious practices, the myths and legends of different cultures and so on also account for the *persistence* of a type of ambivalent relationship with the father (Freud, 1913, pp. 144–156). A tragic act seems to *insist* on returning in a distorted manner and produces *deferred effects*, despite the fact that its trace *resists being* fully bound to shared representations.

Here we come across many of the elements mentioned throughout the analysis of the Freudian notions of trauma. Freud thought that this scene, like certain traumatic experiences, persists in the history of humanity, produces deferred effects and contains elements that resist symbolisation. And yet, he *did not once mention the notion of trauma* throughout the 164 pages of his book. One year before the start of the First World War, this category seemed doomed to be forgotten, both in Freud's work and in the entire field of psychopathology. However, the scene of the murder of the primal father, the hypothesis of its preservation in collective memory through a process of transgenerational transmission and the equivalence between certain processes of individual and collective psychology constitute a set of ideas that continued to be valid in Freud's work and that returned insistently in several of his writings. These ideas can be found in writings such as the unpublished manuscript entitled "Overview of the Transference Neurosis (1915c)"; the unfinished project of writing with Ferenczi a work on Lamarck[7]; Chapter 10 of *Group Psychology and the Analysis of the Ego* (1921) entitled "The Group and the Primal Horde"; and in *Civilization and its Discontents* (1930).

It was not until the book on Moses (1939), which was published in the year of his death and the beginning of the Second World War (whose horrors had already determined Freud's final exile), that this scene and other events that occurred in the history of humanity were explicitly conceived as *collective traumas*. We will address this topic below.

5.2 The Writing of History and Its Marks

The book about Moses is divided into three essays that vary significantly in structure and length. The first, entitled "Moses an Egyptian" (Freud, 1939, pp. 7–16), was published in the first issue of the journal *Imago* in 1937. The second, "If Moses was an Egyptian…" (Freud, 1939, pp. 17–53), was included in the fourth issue of that journal in the same year. A small part of the third essay was read by Anna Freud at the International Psychoanalytical Congress of 1938 which was held in Paris. During that year, the first essay and a fragment of the second were published together in the journal *Almanach*. Finally, in 1939, while Freud was already in London during his forced exile due to the Nazi occupation of Vienna, the complete book was published in Holland and then in England. This book included the longest chapter, "Moses, his People and Monotheist Religion" (Freud, 1939, pp. 54–137), which was divided into two parts and had two different prefatory notes and a recapitulatory summary before the beginning of its second part.

This long editorial journey, which was well explained by Strachey in his introduction to the version included in the *Standard Edition* (Freud, 1939, pp. 3–5), paired with the complexity of the internal organisation of the text, are elements which do not conceal (but rather, expose) the traces of the writing process that culminated in this book. *Totem and Taboo*, despite containing a hypothesis that (even for Freud himself) might seem phantasist in nature, respected the canons of scientific and academic writing: it presented the methodology used, a state of the art, the great enigmas that were still valid in the field and the hypothesis that might solve them. The book about Moses, even though it addressed a subject that belonged to the same territory, was characterised by a much more convoluted writing style. The four years needed to produce the final draft, the fears, the need for explanations, the censorship imposed by the fear of reprisals, the repetitions, the doubts, the detours and the political situation: all these elements appear in the book almost without veils throughout its pages. In this strange way, towards the end of his existence, a Jew, father of psychoanalysis, approached, during his own exodus, the most important figure in Judaism. He did so through the lens of the instrument that he himself had designed and transformed throughout 45 years of his life. In this way, he was once again faced with a problem dear to the Hebrew tradition and his own work: how is an intergenerational transmission possible? How is the memory of a people constructed?[8]

The reasons behind this peculiar form of writing remain locked away in the author's tomb. However, two things are certain. First, as Strachey points out (Freud, 1939, pp. 4–5), the particular way in which the text was presented cannot be attributed to the effects of old age in Freud since his "Outline of Psycho-Analysis" (Freud, 1940) was just as organised and neat as most of his works. Second, this text full of amendments, contradictions, vacillations, censorship, recapitulations and so on, was in many respects homologous to the form of the Holy Scriptures, which were the primary source of the analytical work undertaken by the elderly psychoanalyst. Freud was attempting to demonstrate that in the Bible and his book, it was possible to find a nucleus of "historical truth" (Freud, 1939, p. 58) hidden behind the guise of "phantasy", "legend" or "novel". Michel de Certeau understood the book as "interplay between religious 'legend' (Sage) and Freudian 'construction' (Konstruktion), between the object under study and the discourse performing the analysis (…), -in which- its elucidation does not escape what it is elucidating" (De Certeau, 1988, p. 308). This is why he described it with the *ambivalent* term of "theoretical fiction": a text that "in the fashion of a fantasy, (…) *narrates* a story about what *is produced* in a tradition" (De Certeau, 1988, pp. 308–309; italics in original).

What, then, in this case, is the hidden historical truth? Which were the experiences that were imprinted and expressed in a distorted fashion in the biblical narrative? First, something that would be irreconcilable with what the tradition intended to be remembered: that Moses was an Egyptian. The conflict between two peoples (Jews and Egyptians) appeared internalised in Moses, the Jewish leader, whom Freud considered to have been Egyptian. Second, an even more *traumatic* experience can be read in certain marks present in the Holy Scriptures. For Freud, Moses was assassinated by members of the people he founded, who also tried to bury the traces of that act. On what was the Viennese psychoanalyst basing this almost sacrilegious gesture, which forced a reconsideration of the entire tradition he himself was a part of?

In the book's first essay, the hypothesis of the Jewish Moses was based on an etymological investigation of his name and, above all, on an interpretation, through the lens of psychoanalysis, of the Biblical narrative about his birth. According to the point raised by Freud, many authors had already suggested that "Moses" would likely derive from the Egyptian word "*mose*", which means child. However, they had not reached the conclusion that the person who bore that name was Egyptian (Freud, 1939, p. 8). The psychoanalytical interpretation of the myths about the origins of heroes reinforced this idea.[9] The story of Moses was unlike most legends, which try to embellish their narratives. In traditional myths, the hero is born noble but is separated from his family and raised by a humble family. Instead, the Biblical narrative claims that Moses was Jewish but was raised by an

Egyptian royal family. This particularity, for Freud, far from constituting an error to be ruled out, was the mark, within the texts on Moses, of a "special feature of his history" (Freud, 1939, p. 15).

This reference illuminates a central aspect of the Freudian procedure when faced with obscurities in a text referring to a remote past. Whether dealing with a patient's narrative or a text on the origins of a human group, the truth emerges not from the accurate affirmations but from *the text's missteps* and from everything that is considered disposable or contradictory from the point of view of the conscious representations that constitute the identity. In Freud's words:

> "Thus almost everywhere noticeable gaps, disturbing repetitions and obvious contradictions have come about – *indications which reveal things to us which it was not intended to communicate*. In its implications the distortion of a text resembles a murder: the difficulty is not in perpetrating the deed, but in getting rid of its traces. (…) '*Entstellung* (distortion)'" means "not only 'to change the appearance of something' but also 'to put something in another place, to displace'. Accordingly, in many instances of textual distortion, *we may nevertheless count upon finding what has been suppressed and disavowed hidden away somewhere else*, though changed and torn from its context.
>
> (Freud, 1939, p. 43; italics added)

For Freud, the attempts to erase and distort the traces of the past, far from achieving their goal, allow these marks to be archived (that is, hidden but preserved) (Derrida, 1996). When faced with narratives which cannot be verified empirically, which refer to a remote past, which remit to experiences marked by a conflict or which involve memories that the subject once tried to forget, the psychoanalyst believed he could find a fragment of truth in those places where a misstep had altered a text's coherence.

After presenting his thesis and two routes that attempted to substantiate it, Freud halted the essay, fearing that his arguments were insufficient to justify his conjecture's historical veracity. *And yet...* as a mark of one of the many contradictions that appeared in the text, a few months later, he published a second essay in which he returned to his endeavour by communicating the inferences derived from the initial hypothesis. "If Moses was an Egyptian and if he communicated his own religion to the Jews", it would not have been the traditional polytheistic religion, but "Akhenaten's, the Aten religion" (Freud, 1939, p. 24). According to historical investigations known by Freud, around 1375 BC, the pharaoh Amenhotep IV changed his name to Akhenaten and attempted to impose a rigorous form of monotheism throughout the kingdom, in which Aten, the sun, was considered a universal and sole god. However, following his death, his religion was thought to have been prohibited, and his memory was proscribed (Freud, 1939, pp. 20–24). Many of the characteristics of this creed were very similar to those of Judaism: the strictness of monotheism, the denial of a kingdom of the dead and circumcision as a mark of belonging. Moses, therefore, would have been a supporter of Akhenaten who, in the light of the new political situation "chose -certain Semitic tribes- to be his new people" (Freud, 1939, p. 28). Freud also believed he could calculate the date of the Exodus to be between 1358 and 1350 BC, during an anarchic period, where the chances of its realisation would have been easier.

However, other historical investigations provided information that contradicted this conjecture: according to these, the Jewish lineages adopted a new religion, not in Egypt or Sinai, but in an oasis known as Meribah-Kadesh. Their new god, Yahweh, was in fact a volcano god, "an uncanny, bloodthirsty demon" who was adored by the neighbouring Arabian tribe of Midianites (Freud, 1939, p. 34). The mediator between God and the people was a shepherd, Moses, the son-in-law of the Midianite priest Jethro. How would it be possible to reconcile this story (studied by E. Meyer) with that of the Exodus, to reconcile the noble and Egyptian Moses with the Midianite shepherd Moses? Just like we saw with the two meanings of taboo, with the relationship that the child has with respect to the father within the framework of the Oedipus complex, with the bond that tied the brothers to the primal father, we find here two distinguishable elements occupying the same space. This "two in one" structure, is that which Guy Le Gauffey highlighted when analysing the same texts we are addressing here (Le Gaufey, 1995, pp. 95, 109–110).

Finally, Freud added another piece of information. In 1922, Ernst Sellin put forward a hypothesis according to which in the Prophet Hosea's book there were "unmistakable signs of a tradition to the effect that Moses, the founder of their religion, met with a violent end" (Freud, 1939, p. 36). According to Freud, this tradition was at the core of what "reappears in most of the later Prophets" (Freud, 1939, p. 36). Once again, an act of murder was central to a Freudian development on a key aspect of culture and religion; and once again, that fact, which was apparently forgotten, insisted until finding distorted ways of returning.

The threads of his analysis converged towards the contradiction between two Moses and two different origins of the Jewish people and their religion. As is to be expected, this contradiction, far from becoming an insurmountable obstacle, was transformed into the spearhead of a new interpretation. According to the latter, the Jewish people were effectively made up of two different Semitic tribes that had come together in Meribah-Kadesh: one that lived through the Exodus and another that inhabited a stretch of country between Egypt and Canaan (Freud, 1939, pp. 37–38).[10] The first murdered Moses before uniting with the other tribe. However, among them were the Levites, who probably had the closest ties to the Egyptian nobleman and who "remained loyal to their master, preserved his memory and carried out the tradition of his doctrines", even after the fusion with the rest of the people had taken place (Freud, 1939, p. 39). Two generations later, in Kadesh, a "compromise" had been reached (Freud, 1939, p. 40). Freud understood the new religion as a kind of symptom that attempted to condense certain elements from both tribes.

> Yahweh, who lived on a mountain in Midian, was allowed to extend over into Egypt, and, in exchange for this, the existence and the activity of Moses -the murdered Egyptian- were extended to Kadesh and as far as the country east of the Jordan. Thus, he was fused with the figure of the later religious founder, the son-in-law of the Midianite Jethro, and lent him his name of Moses.
>
> (Freud, 1939, p. 41)

So far, we have outlined the central aspects of this Freudian construction, which he likened to a "dancer"[11] balancing its entire body on the tip of one toe, supported by the "analytic interpretation of the exposure myth" and "Sellin's suspicion about the end of Moses" (Freud, 1939, p. 58). This brief history was full of dualities: two tribes, two kingdoms, two gods' names and two religious founders. According to Freud, all of these dualities were "the necessary consequences of the first one: the fact that one portion of the people had an experience which must be regarded as *traumatic* and which the other portion escaped" (Freud, 1939, p. 50; italics added). In this way, towards the end of the second essay and seemingly not having much conceptual importance, the adjective *traumatic* reappeared in a Freudian text.

Its inclusion, however, should not be considered random or irrelevant. The third essay in *Moses and Monotheism* was plagued with detours, repetitions and contradictions. However, it stood out because it allowed two central concerns in Freud's work to return in full force: *the problem of trauma* (its temporality, its mechanism and its lasting marks on mental life) and *the problem of transgenerational transmission* (which had been developed in depth for the first time in "Totem and Taboo"). Furthermore, both problems were closely linked because, according to Freud, *only traumatic experiences are capable of being transmitted unconsciously throughout the generations.* We will address these issues below.

5.3 The History of Jewish Monotheism and the Trauma

At the beginning of the third essay, after summarising his hypotheses about the origin of Moses and monotheism, Freud began using the notion of trauma to address the enigma behind the temporal gap between the Mosaic teaching and the moment in which his ideas were finally imposed. This gap was compared to the so-called "'incubation period'" of symptoms following a serious accident, such as a railway collision (Freud, 1939, p. 67). "In spite of the fundamental difference between the two cases – the problem of traumatic neurosis and that of Jewish monotheism – there is nevertheless one point of agreement: namely, in the characteristic that might be described as 'latency'" (Freud, 1939, p. 68). This Freudian text was written almost 75 years after Erichsen's book, which we examined in the first chapter. However, the clinical evidence regarding the late development of symptoms seemed to remain valid. As we shall see, many of the ideas about trauma which he had developed in the days of his *Neurotica* also persisted in his thinking.

In the case of the Jewish religion, Freud considered that the solution to the problem of *latency*, that is, of the delay in the emergence of the characteristics that related it to the faith of Aten, should be looked for "in a particular psychological situation" of the alliance formed in Kadesh (Freud, 1939, p. 68). On the one hand, those who came from Egypt had vivid memories of their leader and his religion but also strong motives to repress what they had done to him. On the other hand, those already residing there sought to deny Yahweh's foreignness. Therefore, both portions of the people

> had the same interest in disavowing the fact of their having had an earlier religion and the nature of its content. So it was -Freud stated- that the first compromise came about, and it was probably soon recorded in writing.
>
> (Freud, 1939, p. 68)

As of then, "a discrepancy was able to grow up between the written record and the oral transmission of the same material – *tradition*" (Freud, 1939, p. 68; italics in original). In other words, the Jewish tradition, like so many others, became *split* between a *written, fixed, official* version and an *oral, changing, alternative* version that refuted the other. The first version was more greatly subject to distortions, which tended to embellish it and (unsuccessfully) attempt to eliminate its conflictive features; the second was more veracious but also imprecise and prone to change. Freud considered that, in general, oral traditions tended to either deviate and end up being forgotten or to remain fixed to the written text. Nevertheless, the Mosaic tradition, which was intended to be forgotten, ended up prevailing. "These traditions, instead of becoming weaker with time, became more and more powerful in the course of the centuries" (Freud, 1939, p. 69).

We will attempt to place Freud's outline of the history of Jewish monotheism on a timeline:

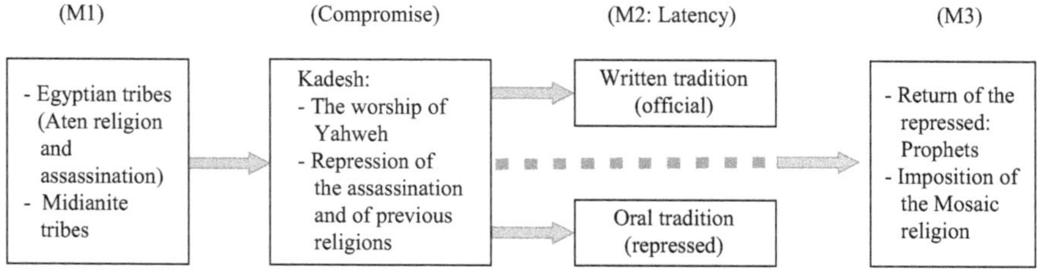

Before delving into the analogy between this historical development and the development of the neuroses, Freud summarised his theory of *trauma* by utilising a conceptual schema that repeated, in condensed form, many of the elements that he had linked to that notion in the past. "We give the name of *traumas* to those impressions, experienced early and later forgotten, to which we attach such great importance in the aetiology of the neuroses" (Freud, 1939, p. 72; italics in original).

Just as if we were revisiting the texts that constituted his *Neurotica*, here we once again find that these phenomena were "experienced early" and left "impressions", that is, traces. Only through the influence of the latter (and the elements that could later be associated with them) could the trauma occur. At the same time, the issue of aetiology came up again: "We may leave on one side the question of whether the aetiology of the neuroses in general may be regarded as traumatic" (Freud, 1939, p. 72). He was then quick to admit what was already known: not all neurotics seem to have gone through a "manifest trauma", while others manifest an excessive and "abnormal reaction to experiences and demands which affect everyone" (Freud, 1939, p. 72). These two dissimilar situations, which impede the classification of all neuroses as being "traumatic", do, however, have a common feature: in both, "the experience acquires its traumatic character only as a result of a quantitative factor" whose excessive character is always relative to each person (Freud, 1939, p. 73). In other words, if the subject's predisposition is greater, an apparently banal experience can be impossible to process (and, therefore, becomes traumatic).

Thus, in just a few pages, we are able to rediscover several of the components that make up the various notions of trauma that we have analysed throughout this book: the traces left by experiences and the relationships between trauma, memory and forgetting (Chapter 2); the early character of traumatic experiences and their role in aetiology (Chapter 3); the quantitative and relative nature of trauma (Chapter 4).

Furthermore, Freud highlighted two traits of neurotic symptoms: they all indicate a fixation to the trauma and are of a compulsive nature. The first trait, however, manifests itself in two different ways. The first modality refers to a *positive* influence of trauma on the symptoms:

> -characterised by- attempts to bring the trauma into operation once again – that is, to remember the forgotten experience or, better still, to make it real, to experience a repetition of it anew (…) We summarize these efforts under the name of 'fixations' to the trauma and as a 'compulsion to repeat'.
>
> (Freud, 1939, p. 75)

The second and *negative* modality pursues the opposite aim:

> that nothing of the forgotten traumas shall be remembered and nothing repeated. We can summarize them as 'defensive reactions'. Their principal expression are what are called 'avoidances', which may be intensified into 'inhibitions' and 'phobias' (…) Fundamentally they are just as much fixations to the trauma as their opposites.
>
> (Freud, 1939, p. 76)

Once again, we find two opposing tendencies (repetition and avoidance, the vivid memory and complete amnesia) united by the same element (fixation to the trauma). This apparent contradiction, far from invalidating the reasoning, seems to explain the disturbing effects of trauma better. Seemingly opposed symptoms, such as hallucinations and forgotten memories, share the same trait of being fixated to the trauma. Both differ from the objective of psychoanalysis: to promote a form of remembering that allows for the separation of the subject from the compulsive nature of the consequences of trauma. The compulsive quality of these phenomena denotes their capacity to impose themselves to the detriment of "other mental processes, which are adjusted to the demands of the real external world and obey the laws of logical thinking" (Freud, 1939, p. 76).

Finally, Freud summarised "the formula" that he lay down to account for "the development of a neurosis": "Early trauma – defence – latency – outbreak of neurotic illness – partial return of the repressed" (Freud, 1939, p. 80). If we add to this schema the idea that traumas and constitutional factors complement each other in producing the predisposition and that they require a second element to "awaken them", thus triggering the pathological effect, we can then outline the following diagram.

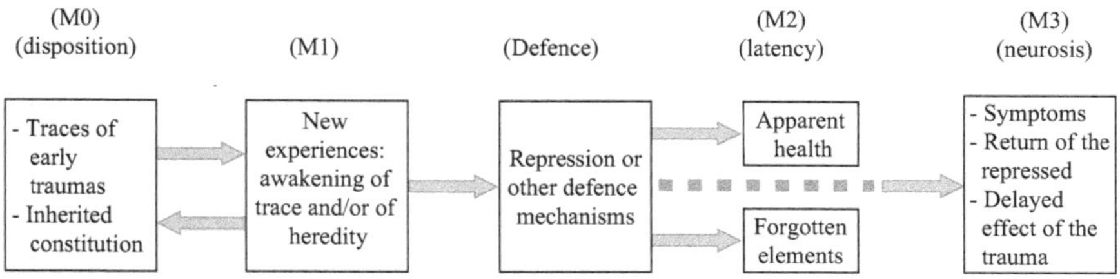

After having concluded this recapitulation of his ideas on trauma and the development of the neuroses, Freud addressed the promised concordance:

> something occurred in the life of the human species similar to what occurs in the life of individuals: of supposing, that is, that here too events occurred of a sexually aggressive nature, which left behind them permanent consequences but were for the most part fended off and forgotten, and which after a long latency came into effect and created phenomena similar to symptoms.
>
> (Freud, 1939, p. 80)

Freud strengthened the analogy by adding that "the human race has a prehistory (…) that is, forgotten (…) When we learn that in both cases – in the origins of humanity and the individual's prehistory – the operative and forgotten traumas relate to life in the human family" (Freud, 1939, p. 80). In this late book, that element transmitted from prehistory through the generations was given the name of *trauma*. The content of this traumatic inheritance was that which Freud conjectured in "Totem and Taboo": the sons' bond to the primal father (who killed, castrated or expelled his male offspring)[12] and the act of parricide (Freud, 1939, pp. 80–82). Freud considered this *transgenerationally transmitted collective trauma* to be at work both in the *history of humanity* (because it affects the psychology of the peoples by contributing to the production of religious phenomena) and in each *individual's history* (since it constitutes part of what every subject is endowed with in the form of inheritance, and its effects can be triggered by the new experiences of personal life).

Furthermore, it is worth noting that this scene, with its events "of a sexually aggressive nature", in which the brothers united to murder the being who prevented their access to the women, did not leave the survivors in a passive position: they were the ones who, with their act, killed the father. However, that act did not cease to be incompatible with the bond that, despite everything, tied them to their father. Perhaps the most horrific aspect resided precisely in the fact that they themselves (and not strangers) killed the being they simultaneously loved and hated.

Something analogous occurred in the story of Moses: its traumatic nature was not due to the murder itself but because it was committed by those the leader had chosen as his people. The traumatic nature of the situation, therefore, resided in the proximity of the bond, in its familiar character, in the fact that it was an act of parricide. And also, that this homicidal act was a *repetition* of the murder of the primal father. "It was a case of 'acting out' instead of remembering, as happens so often with neurotics during the work of analysis" (Freud, 1939, p. 89). The new experience awoke the trace of the ancient trauma and doomed both to be forgotten. However, this, far from eliminating its potential effects, laid the foundations for its return and its repetition.

As in the neuroses, the traces of past collective traumas *insist* on coming to light in the history of humanity and *resist* all attempts to fully bind them to a narrative that definitively makes them a thing of the past. The following diagram attempts to synthesise the complete development of monotheism as it was reconstructed by Freud, by also establishing the zero point that predisposes the murder of Moses, its repression and the compulsive return of his teaching. In this way, the analogy to the development of a neurosis is complete:

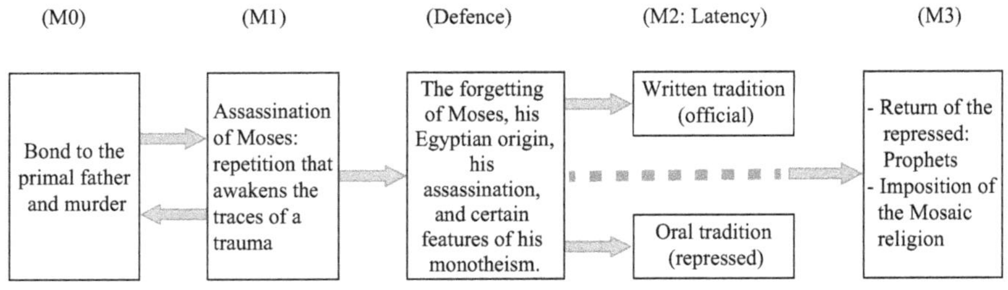

5.4 The Traces of Collective Traumas

To conclude this chapter, we would like to analyse the hypotheses that Freud utilised to justify the permanence of past traumas in human groups. From his perspective, these experiences are preserved and transmitted in two ways: through the traces of the experiences left behind in the biblical text and other religious, folkloric and traditional writings (Freud, 1939, p. 84) and through the inheritance of acquired characters (Freud, 1939, p. 100). The "impressions" (Freud, 1939, p. 72) that make up these traumas are "imprinted" onto two different substrates but are nevertheless capable of being marked and inscribed (Derrida, 1996, p. 30).

Regarding the first of these ways of transmission, Freud thought that, despite the efforts of the tradition to forget those traumatic experiences, some marks, *scars*, remain in the texts, which account for what took place and the attempts to censor it. Almost without announcing it explicitly, or at least without drawing all the possible consequences from his statements, Freud was putting forward another substrate that allows for the past to endure and traces to be transmitted, different from the one he conjectured in *Totem and Taboo*. Thus, alongside the old *body of phylogenetic endowment*, a *literary corpus* was added as a means of supporting the hypothesis about the transgenerational transmission of the impressions left by traumas.

An apparently similar interpretation was put forward by Jan Assmann, in an article published in the journal *Annales*, entitled "Monothéisme et mémoire. Le Moïse de Freud et la tradition biblique" (Assmann, 1999). The author agreed with Freud on the need to "place the notions of memory, trauma and guilt at the centre of the history of religion" and "to interpret this history in the light of forgetting and remembering" (Assmann, 1999, p. 1011). However, he criticised the psychoanalyst for resorting to a phylogenetic explanation and for assuming the existence of acts of violence that actually occurred (Assmann, 1999, p. 1012). According to Assmann,

> the archaic heritage and the hypothesis of a repressed death are not necessary (…) It is not necessary to search in collective psychology to discover the semantics of memory and forgetting, of repression and latency, of traumatism and guilt: all this is clearly specified in the texts, that is what they speak of.
>
> (Assmann, 1999, p. 1014)

In others words, from his view, the conflicts linked to the collective memory of Judaism only have a literary, intratextual reality.

This idea, of course, differs greatly from the Freudian theses. From our point of view, the founder of psychoanalysis began to envision the possibility that texts and customs can *also* preserve the traces of the past and contribute, unconsciously and in a distorted manner, to their transmission. However, he never allowed himself to consider that the conjectured scenes were *only* fiction, nor did he resign to his faith in a certain version of Lamarckism. This is why he admitted that "for a long time" he had behaved:

> "…as though the inheritance of memory-traces of the experience of our ancestors, independently of direct communication (…) were established beyond question. (…) When I spoke of the survival of a tradition among a people or of the formation of a people's character, I had mostly in mind an inherited tradition of this kind and not one transmitted by communication.
>
> (Freud, 1939, pp. 99–100)

Freud recognised that "biological science (...) refuses to hear of the inheritance of acquired characters by succeeding generations"; but he nevertheless confessed that he "cannot do without this factor in biological evolution" (Freud, 1939, p. 100).

Far from abandoning this pre-Darwinian theory, Freud broadened and made the scope of Lamarck's theses more complex. He broadened them because he supposed that not only trends but also past scenes and forms of bonds with others can be transmitted and can develop a compulsive character, which leads to the same types of relationships being repeated. In Freud's words: "the archaic heritage of human beings comprises not only dispositions but also subject-matter – memory-traces of the experience of earlier generations" (Freud, 1939, p. 99).

He made them more complex because he differentiated the "acquired characters" of the Lamarckian theory, which were "hard to grasp", from his own views on the "memory-traces of external events -which are- something tangible, as it were" (Derrida, 1996, p. 35; Freud, 1939, p. 100). As Derrida argues, by making this distinction, Freud seemed to admit the criticism of Lamarck's ideas while at the same time affirming the "survival of these memory-traces in the archaic heritage" (Freud, 1939, p. 100).

In addition, Freud made Lamarck's theses more complex by introducing his own ideas on repression and the return of the repressed into the field of heritage:

> A tradition that was based only on communication could not lead to the compulsive character that attaches to religious phenomena. It would be listened to, judged, and perhaps dismissed (...) It must have undergone the fate of being repressed, the condition of lingering in the unconscious, before it is able to display such powerful effects on its return, to bring the masses under its spell, as we have seen with astonishment and hitherto without comprehension in the case of religious tradition.
>
> (Freud, 1939, p. 101)

In Freud's view, the experiences of the past can be listened to, judged and finally accepted or rejected by logical thought if, and only if, their memory was not previously repressed and therefore forgotten. If, instead, they underwent a process of repression, then they will return in a distorted manner that will be imposed on the masses, thus making the task of properly judging them more difficult. Repression, as we anticipated, far from eliminating the trauma and burying it in the past, generates the conditions for its perpetuation and its compulsive form of return.

In other words, the Freudian hypothesis that states that the same laws that structure the neuroses also govern collective psychology leads us to think that if a people seek to leave behind a conflict arising from an experience without first trying to resolve it, or if any of the elements of that experience are impossible to signify and process within the framework of shared representations, then the conditions are in place for a *fixation to the trauma* to be produced. This fixation is expressed by attempts to *avoid* everything related to that collective trauma ('pathological' amnesias, inability to address any aspect associated with the memory of the past experience, etc.) or by a *compulsion to repeat* what happened (without knowing, of course, that they are repeating it) (Freud, 1939, p. 75).

Failed attempts at forgetting and reliving the trauma seem to be the most common "symptoms" of those peoples who sought to cover up and leave behind their most painful past processes without having faced and dealt with them sufficiently or without having taken the time to grieve for the irreparable things that occurred. In these groups, the past trauma continues to make itself present; it behaves like "an excess of life which resists annihilation" (Derrida, 1996, p. 60); it remains an *open wound* that, without healing, affects the generations to come.

Notes

1 The other source with which Freud argued was Wundt's body of work on Folk Psychology.

2 "Applied" or "in extension" psychoanalysis did not suppose, for Freud, a new object of analysis (for example, a collective subject that would be radically different from the individual subject) but simply a new domain. At the beginning of *Group Psychology and the Analysis of the Ego*, he questioned the opposition between individual and social psychology: he considered it impossible to address an individual without regarding their relations to others. Thus the phenomena analysed by psychoanalysis "may claim to be considered as social phenomena" (Freud, 1921, p. 69). As Michel De Certeau stated, psychoanalytic investigations are only distinguished "from the phenomena treated by collective psychology by a 'numerical factor' (…)"; therefore, "the social life that postulates from the beginning the constitution of the subject through a reference to others (parents, etc.) and to language" would present "only broader social units" but which "obey the same laws" (De Certeau, 1998, p. 82). In this sense, the border between individual and collective phenomena (on which the specificity of different disciplines for each field is intended to be erected) is revealed as arbitrary, at least from Freud's point of view. The ideas of libidinal bonds and identification, fundamental in psychoanalytic theory and practice, are located from the outset in the terrain of the bonds with others and became Freud's key for attempting to elucidate not only the relationship between the individual and society but also the organisation of culture itself. In this direction, we agree with Omar Acha when he maintained that "it was not a simple application of psychoanalytic theory to the 'empirical' material offered by anthropological and historiographical research, but rather the integration of these into a *network of readings of culture, whose key was given by the libidinal bonds* that underlay the formation of (social, political and economic) institutions and the cultural achievements of the civilisation of his time" (Acha, 2007, p. 35; italics added).

3 For example, on March 31, 1907, Jung asked Freud the following question: "Is it not conceivable, in view of the limited conception of sexuality that prevails nowadays, that the sexual terminology should be reserved only for the most extreme forms of your 'libido', and that a less offensive collective term should be established for all the libidinal manifestations?" (McGuire, 1974, p. 25). Freud's response took place on April 7 of the same year and was conclusive: "even if we do not call the driving force in the broadened conception of sexuality 'libido', it will still be libido, and in every inference we draw from it we shall come back to the very thing from which we were trying to divert attention with our nomenclature (…) Perhaps you are underestimating the intensity of these resistances if you hope to disarm them with small concessions. We are being asked neither more nor less than to abjure our belief in the sexual drive. The only answer is to profess it openly" (McGuire, 1974, p. 28). Despite Freud's suggestion, the Swiss analyst insisted on questioning libido. At the beginning of the following decade, he wrote to his master that in his new book he had tried to "replace the descriptive concept of libido by

a genetic one. Such a concept covers not only the recent sexual libido but all those forms of it which have long since split off into organized activities" (McGuire, 1974, p. 471). The conflict culminated in 1913, coinciding with the publication of "Totem and Taboo".

4 Jung's position was reflected in the letter of May 8, 1912 (McGuire, 1974, pp. 502–503). Two days later, Freud sent him a response in which he tried to impugn his viewpoint. First, because he considered that "there have been father's sons at all times" since the former would not necessarily coincide with the progenitor: "a father is one who possesses a mother sexually (and the children as property)" (McGuire, 1974, p. 504). But fundamentally, Freud did not agree with his disciple because he favoured a "different hypothesis in regard to the primordial period – Darwin's", for which a "primordial state of promiscuity" was highly unlikely (McGuire, 1974, p. 504). We will return to this hypothesis later.

5 "Totemism and Exogamy" was the title of one of the works most cited by Freud in his book: the enormous four volumes published by J.G. Frazer in 1910.

6 As Le Gaufey points out, this metaphor is falsely modest.

7 In a letter sent to Ferenczi on December 22, 1916, the Vienesse psychoanalyst proposed to his Hungarian disciple to carry out a joint work on Lamarck and psychoanalysis (Falzeder & Brabant, 2001, V.II.2, p. 10).

8 Yosef Yerushalmi, in his work entitled: *Freud's Moses: Judaism Terminable and Interminable* (1991), carried out an excellent analysis of the Jewish question in Freud's book.

9 On this point, Freud referred to Otto Rank's book *The Myth of the Birth of the Hero* (Rank, 1909).

10 According to what is recorded in the Bible, these two tribes would later be separated again, thus constituting the kingdom of Israel and the kingdom of Judah (Freud, 1939, p. 38).

11 This is how Freud described his own work (Freud, 1939, p. 58).

12 Note that in *Totem and Taboo* the fate conjectured by Freud for the sons of the primal father was limited to a single possibility: to be driven out of the horde. Here, instead, he conceived two other options: castration or death (as in his "Overview of the Transference Neuroses", Freud, 1915).

References

Acha, O. (2007). *Freud y el problema de la historia.* Buenos Aires: Prometeo.

Assmann, J. (1999). Monothéisme et mémoire: Le Moïse de Freud et la tradition biblique. *Annales Histoire, Sciences Sociales, 54* Année, 5 (September–October), 1011–1026.

Braunstein, N., Fuks, B. & Basualdo, C. (Ed.). (2013). *Freud: A cien años de Tótem y tabú (1913–2013).* México, DF: Siglo XXI.

De Certeau, M. (1988). *The Writing of History.* New York: Columbia University Press.

De Certeau, M. (1998). *Historia y psicoanálisis. Entre ciencia y ficción.* México, DF: Universidad Iberoamericana.

Derrida, J. (1996). *Archive Fever. A Freudian Impression.* Chicago, IL and London: The University of Chicago Press.

Falzeder, E. & Brabant, E. (2001). *Sigmund Freud, Sandor Ferenczi. Correspondencia complete, 1917–1919, Vol. II.* Madrid: Síntesis.

Freud, S. ([1907] 1959). Obsessive actions and religious practices. In S. Freud (Ed.), *The Standard Edition of the Complete Psychological Works of Sigmund Freud, Vol. IX: Jensen's 'Gradiva' and Other Works* (pp. 115–127). London: The Hogarth Press and the Institute of Psycho-Analysis.

Freud, S. ([1908] 1959). 'Civilized' sexual morality and modern nervous illness. In S. Freud (Ed.), *The Standard Edition of the Complete Psychological Works of Sigmund Freud, Vol.*

IX: Jensen's 'Gradiva' and Other Works (pp. 177–204). London: The Hogarth Press and the Institute of Psycho-Analysis.

Freud, S. ([1913] 1955). Totem and taboo. In S. Freud (Ed.), *The Standard Edition of the Complete Psychological Works of Sigmund Freud, Vol. XIII: Totem and Taboo and Other Works* (pp. 1–164). London: The Hogarth Press and the Institute of Psycho-Analysis.

Freud, S. ([1915] 2018). Sinopsis de las neurosis de transferencia. In S. Freud (Ed.), *Textos Inéditos y Documentos Recobrados* (pp. 173–191). Buenos Aires: Miño y Dávila.

Freud, S. ([1916–1917d] 1963). Lecture XXIII. The paths to the formation of symptoms. In S. Freud (Ed.), *The Standard Edition of the Complete Psychological Works of Sigmund Freud, Vol. XVI: Introductory Lectures on Psycho- Analysis (Part III)* (pp. 358–377). London: The Hogarth Press and the Institute of Psycho-Analysis.

Freud, S. ([1918] 1955). From the history of an infantile neurosis. In S. Freud (Ed.), *The Standard Edition of the Complete Psychological Works of Sigmund Freud, Vol. XVII: An Infantile Neurosis and Other Works* (pp. 1–123). London: The Hogarth Press and the Institute of Psycho-Analysis.

Freud, S. ([1921] 1955). Group psychology and the analysis of the ego. In S. Freud (Ed.), *The Standard Edition of the Complete Psychological Works of Sigmund Freud, Vol. XVIII: Beyond the Pleasure Principle, Group Psychology and Other Works* (pp. 65–143). London: The Hogarth Press and the Institute of Psycho- Analysis.

Freud, S. ([1927] 1961). The future of an illusion. In S. Freud (Ed.), *The Standard Edition of the Complete Psychological Works of Sigmund Freud, Vol. XXI: The Future of an Ilussion, Civilization and Its Discontents and Other Works* (pp. 1–56). London: The Hogarth Press and the Institute of Psycho-Analysis.

Freud, S. ([1930] 1961). Civilization and its discontents. In S. Freud (Ed.), *The Standard Edition of the Complete Psychological Works of Sigmund Freud, Vol. XXI: The Future of an Ilussion, Civilization and Its Discontents and Other Works* (pp. 57–145). London: The Hogarth Press and the Institute of Psycho-Analysis.

Freud, S. ([1939] 1964). Moses and monotheism: three essays. In S. Freud (Ed.), *The Standard Edition of the Complete Psychological Works of Sigmund Freud, Vol. XXIII: Moses and Monotheism, an Outline of Psycho-Analysis and Other Works* (pp. 1–137). London: The Hogarth Press and the Institute of Psycho-Analysis.

Freud, S. ([1940] 1964). An outline of psycho- analysis. In S. Freud (Ed.), *The Standard Edition of the Complete Psychological Works of Sigmund Freud, Vol. XXIII: Moses and Monotheism- An Outline of Psycho-Analysis & Other Works* (pp. 141–207). London: The Hogarth Press and the Institute of Psycho-Analysis.

Haeckel, E. (1904). *The Wonders of Life*. London: Watts & Co.

Jung, C. ([1911–1912] 1952). *Transformaciones y símbolos de la libido*. Buenos Aires: Paidós.

Lacan, J. (1969–1970). *The Seminar of Jacques Lacan: The Other Side of Psychoanalysis. Book XVII*. New York and London: W.W. Norton & Company, 2007.

Le Gaufey, G. (1995). *La evicción del origen*. Buenos Aires: Edelp.

McGuire, W. (1974). *The Freud/Jung Letters*. Princeton, NJ: Princeton University Press.

Rank, O. (1909). *Der Mythos von der Geburt des Helden*. Leipzig and Wien: Deuticke.

Sulloway, F. (1979). *Freud Biologist of the Mind. Beyond the Psychoanalytic Legend*. New York: Basic Books.

Yerushalmi, Y. (1991). *Freud's Moses: Judaism Terminable and Interminable*. New Haven, CT and London: Yale University Press.

Conclusions

Luis Sanfelippo

We have reached the end of this journey where we sought to study the processes through which the notion of trauma transformed its meaning (from the old surgical meaning of damage to different forms of psychical disturbance); extended its field of application to cover a large number of dissimilar experiences; reached a high degree of recognition and of institutionalisation; was associated with various problems, different conceptual configurations and diverse images; and, lastly, entered new domains (psychopathological, legal, among others) until managing to establish itself in certain sectors of collective psychology and historiography. Thus, *the history of trauma* was faced with the problem of the *trauma in history*.

The historical panorama that we have described justifies our decision to consider trauma to be an open notion characterised by its multiplicity and diffuse limits instead of conceiving it as a closed, single, well-defined concept. When this is taken into consideration, it becomes clear that *this* history of trauma cannot be *the* history of trauma. It also cannot be considered *a story*, if we understand the latter as the unfolding of a unified totality within a linear and continuous temporality; rather, each chapter was organised in a relatively independent way around certain problems that conditioned the territory from which new conceptions and new practices related to trauma emerged. These transformations in the conceptualisation and use of the notion then gave rise to new questions that, in many cases, transcended the specific domain from which they emerged.

Chapter 1 covered the area of clinical and legal problems that arose at the intersection of railway accident expertise and the clinic of neuroses. Within this context, the notion of trauma underwent changes that conferred certain psychological features to these conceptions originally constructed from anatomical and physiological matrices. Finally, a new problem arose, which remains valid to this day: the complex relationship between the event and its representation, between the objective conditions and the subjective particularities of an experience. Chapter 2 focused on the early works of Janet and Freud to investigate the way in which the notion of trauma was linked to the problems of memory in a context where this function was beginning to be established as a scientific object (while the arts of memory and the weight of tradition began to lose importance). In this context, the trauma itself was not only associated with mnemic processes but also

DOI: 10.4324/9781003380016-7

was its treatment. These therapeutic practices inspired new questions on the role that memory, forgetting and the individual's current subjective position had with respect to the traumatic nature of a past experience. Chapter 3 began with Freud's search for a sexual, specific and acquired aetiology of the neuroses that displaces heredity from the causal role it had been given in the French clinical tradition. However, other problems soon unfolded: on the one hand, that of temporalities that articulate past and present in a non-linear way and determine reciprocal effects between both temporal moments; on the other hand, the tension between reality and phantasy in the narratives and testimonies about traumatic experiences. Chapter 4 sought to briefly address the great debates on the war neuroses in Great Britain, France, Germany and the Austro-Hungarian Empire. Within this context, different problems emerged around the question of limits: on the one hand, the ethical limits in the treatment of traumatised individuals; on the other hand, the limits of the webs of representations in approaching and processing certain elements of traumatic experiences. Lastly, in Chapter 5, we addressed Freud's attempts to apply psychoanalysis to certain problems of collective psychology, such as the origin of totemism and Jewish monotheism. We were then led to question the problem of the existence, persistence and transgenerational transmission of collective traumas, as well as the influence of these traumas in individual and collective history.

In other words, when studying the different processes of transformation of the notion of trauma, we found ourselves facing a series of problems that remain valid today and whose scope cannot be reduced to the field of psychopathology. These problems can be summarised as follows: the tension between event and representation; the relationship between trauma and memory; the articulation between memories, forgetting and repetitions; the reciprocal influence between the past and the present; the difficulties that come up when receiving and interpreting testimonies of trauma; the ethical questions regarding "treatments" (in a broad sense) which seek to overcome the consequences of trauma; the limits of representations when addressing certain aspects of traumatic experiences; and the transmission of the latter to subsequent generations. From the 1980s onward, when the problem of memory became crucial in Western culture and the notion of trauma was implanted into certain sectors of historiography and studies on collective memory, many of these issues came to the fore. These issues continue to be interrogated by scholars who seek to study and overcome the consequences of experiences such as the Shoah and other genocides, certain aspects of the Latin American dictatorships, the apartheid, terrorist attacks with great symbolic impact (such as the attack on the Twin Towers) and so on.

Furthermore, since each chapter was structured around different problems, we were led to slightly modify our historiographical approach in each of them. Thus, Chapters 1 and 4 required a broadened scope in order to cover different national contexts, as well as the technological, cultural and political processes that exceed strictly psychological developments. On the other hand, Chapters 2, 3 and 5 required more focused attention on the works of Freud and certain key debates in the field of psychoanalysis and the clinic of the neuroses. However, our analyses always included broader epistemic and cultural transformations than those demarcated by each author, work or disciplinary domain. At all times, we found ourselves facing the porous and contingent borders between the different disciplines, as well as the diffuse line that marks the limits between the academic, clinical or scientific territory and the "extra-disciplinary" space. Therefore, the changes in our approach only implied differences in emphasis. By positioning our investigation in the field of intellectual history, we aimed to avoid the biases characteristic of internal histories (which ignore contextual references) and external histories (which call into question the importance and relative autonomy of the conceptual debates of the time). We thus sought to construct the web of interlocutors, knowledges, practices and events that determined the transformations of the notion of trauma and tied this category to multiple issues.

In this sense, we believe to have demonstrated that the trauma in Freud was not developed solely by the work and grace of the author, but that the notion's modifications and, even, the entire "work" and the "author" were subject to a heterogeneous series of historical factors, of which we can mention: the vicissitudes of his personal and professional development (such as the scholarship that allowed him to meet Charcot); the internal obstacles tied to the psychoanalytic theory and practice (such as the limits of catharsis; the developments made by other authors in the field of the treatment of the neuroses (Janet, Jung, Ferenczi, etc.); certain advances and changes in other adjacent disciplines (physiology, infectology, biology, etc.); certain epistemic turns that impacted in different fields of knowledge (such as the rise of evolutionism or of energeticism); certain cultural transformations that affected various areas of Western thought (such as various technological developments and alterations in the importance of tradition and memory); and, finally, certain historical and political processes (such as the wars).

At the same time, this way of historically approaching our object of study, which seeks to question the limits between the exterior and the interior of the disciplines and the epistemic domain, seemed adequate to study a notion that, *in different ways*, brings into question the supposed limits that separate *the external world from the internal world.* In the anatomical conceptions of trauma, the mechanical action of the accident was considered to be a completely external factor to the person who suffered it passively. However, in a strict sense, the trauma also encompassed the lesion produced within the organism, which was considered the material and immediate cause of the symptoms. Without this interior and organic element, which mediated between the accident and the symptoms, there was no traumatic experience. Thereafter, the first physiological conceptions of trauma relativised, even more, its supposed exteriority. From this physiological point of view, the accident was still a condition for a traumatic experience; however, it did not act directly, but through the emotion it generated and the ideas it suggested since these were the elements that altered nervous functioning. Furthermore, on occasions, the symptoms seemed to depend on the way in which the subject had represented the accident and not on how it had actually occurred. Subsequently, the different Freudian conceptions of trauma made the relationships between exterior and interior even more complex. For example, the notion of the psychical conflict tied the trauma to an event which introduces an idea contradictory to the representations of the self. This idea is not external to the psychical domain, but nevertheless it is alien to the ego's territory. When Freud associated the trauma to the posthumous effect of a childhood sexual experience, he introduced the category of memory-traces. These mark the edge between the external world and the internal world, since they are inscribed in the psychical apparatus but as the remnant of an event that, from the external world, had affected the body. In many passages of his later work, Freud refused to consider phantasies as a completely internal phenomenon; rather, he affirmed that they always originate from an episode that has effectively occurred and that they make it possible to express, address and process something real that has taken place beyond psychical interiority. Finally, by explicitly adopting an economic point of view in the context of the First World War, Freud defined trauma based on a quantitative excess, which cannot be bound to the webs of representations that make up the psyche and through which the experience is processed. The sum of excitation is aroused by a current event or by the activation of the memory-traces and the unbound drives. This quantity is internal and is perceived by the subject; however, at the same time, it remains unbound, external to the psychical apparatus that seeks to be governed by the pleasure principle. In summary, the different conceptions of trauma, far from consecrating the idea that an event external to a subject could single-handedly generate pathological phenomena, questioned the limits between the exterior and the interior.

The notion which is the object of our research also questioned the usual modes of conceiving the relationship between *the past and the present* in our culture (in general) and in historiography (in particular). In modernity, time was conceived linearly. According to this conception, the past is dead and closed off. In turn, the present is well distinguished from the past, and this difference allows the latter to be studied objectively (De Certeau, 1988; Hartog, 2003; Koselleck, 1993). However, trauma implies specific features that force us to rethink modern temporality: its persistence despite the distance from the facts, its insistence on making itself present in symptomatic forms and its resistance to fully becoming something of the past and something wholly representable.

In Janet's view, for example, automatic association and fixed ideas accounted for a *total imposition of the past on the present*, given the weakness in synthesis, which prevents the articulation of the current experience with past experiences. On the other hand, Freud never believed that the past could completely determine the present. Despite the fact that the fixations to the trauma seem to suggest this idea, the articulation between both temporal categories was more complex and took on two main forms in the writings of the founder of psychoanalysis. On the one hand, the notion of *nachträglich* temporality implies a double directionality: *prospective* and *retrospective*. According to Freud, certain past experiences leave marks that condition the present and predispose the emergence of malaise in the subject. However, they cannot determine the latter by themselves: in order to become traumatic, these past experiences need to be resignified in the present, thus giving way to a pathological effect that had not emerged on the first occasion. However, this effect is not automatic: the activation of the past trace via its association with a present idea leads to repression. After this defence has operated, the past can compulsively return as a symptom. But not even then does it fully impose itself; instead, the past returns in a distorted manner and expresses a compromise between the repressed past and the repressive agencies in the present. On the other hand, the economic conception locates trauma at the moment (the "short period of time", as Freud called it) in which there occurs a discontinuity in the normal functioning of the psychical apparatus. In that moment, the webs of representations run into a hole through which, as we have said, an unbindable quantity appears. In other words, the association between ideas stops, making it impossible to incorporate, process and signify whatever emerged in the experience. And, to the extent that the articulation between past, present and future depends on this symbolic articulation, *time is suspended* until the chains of representations can be once again set in motion. Only then is it possible for the subject to affirm: "I am the one who, *now*, can say that I suffered such and such *in the past*". However, at the very moment of trauma, the *temporal categories remain undifferentiated.* This experience leaves a mark, more like a hole than an inscription, more like an open wound than a scar. This trace acts as a fixation point and impulses repetition. In each repetition, there is a reiteration of the past and a current development of malaise, an attempt to realise the missing bond and the production of a new trauma.

In Freud's works, the notion of trauma also contributes to questioning the traditional division between *individual* and *collective* psychology. If the difference between them is only a question of numbers and if the same principles govern both domains, then certain collective experiences can become traumatic not only for the individuals who are directly affected by the events but also for the community as a whole and future generations. Just as a trauma leaves an indelible impression on the psychical apparatus, the traces of the traumas experienced collectively are preserved in a people. However, as in neurosis, these marks are not part of the set of conscious memories; rather, they are usually forgotten (repressed) and return later in a distorted and compulsive way. As we have seen, on the question of the preservation and transmission of the traces of collective traumas, Freud conceived two possibilities: either a certain process of hereditary transmission more or less comparable to Lamarckian ideas is in force, or the impressions are preserved and distorted in a literary *corpus* made up of traditional and religious texts. In any case, the posthumous consequences of those traumatic experiences are felt both in the history of each individual that belonged to that group of people and in certain collective processes.

From the developments we have laid out in this book, we can extract a fourth problematisation. The trauma also questions the objective and subjective dichotomy.

Some of the conceptions we have studied considered that the traumatic consequences solely depend on the objective conditions of the situation, regardless of the characteristics of the person who is going through it or the responses that they can give to what they experience. In this way, the event is understood as the absolute determining factor, and the person is left in the position of a victim in a way that does not contribute to their active participation in the subsequent processing of the malaise. In short, according to these types of conceptions, in the face of an objective trauma, there can only be passive victims who, at most, can be compensated. In general, this way of understanding the phenomena is common in those who held somatic conceptions of trauma in relation, for example, to railway accidents or war experiences. In those same contexts, other authors held the opposite view. For them, the pathological effects of an experience depend exclusively on subjective particularities independent of the event's characteristics. When taken to an extreme, this reasoning considers that there is no such thing as trauma, only people susceptible to falling ill. The subjective particularities can be rooted in the past (hereditary traits or previous experiences that predisposed the illness) or current circumstances (most often, expectations or desires of obtaining a benefit from being ill). In the most extreme cases, the subject is considered guilty of what is happening… and is treated as such. However, a good part of the conceptions we analysed throughout this book distanced themselves from these two extreme views. Thus, someone can be the victim of a traumatic experience (which entitles them to some sort of reparation and which will require some kind of treatment) and, at the same time, can assume the responsibility, if not for the events that occurred, at least for the response given to what they had to live through. In these types of views, the trauma depends on a combination or relationship between the objective conditions of the situation and the particularities of the person who experienced it (as well as previous factors, the current experience and the *individual* and *collective* responses given after the facts). The Freudian idea of "complemental series" falls under these types of conceptions.

Having reached this point, we wish to focus again on Sigmund Freud's work and recap some of the hypotheses we used in our investigation. First, we sought to establish that the notion of trauma accompanied Freudian thought from his first works in the field of the clinic of the neuroses until his last great book published during his lifetime (we are referring, of course, to the work on Moses and monotheism). The presence of trauma in his work does not consist in the mere persistence of a habitual term from the medical and psychopathological thought of that time. Rather, this category was linked to many of the great problems that Freud set out to address: the development of a possible therapy, pathological defence, the aetiology of neuroses, necessity and contingency, the unconscious and sexuality, the role of events and phantasies, the problem of memory (of remembering, forgetting and repetitions), the limits of representations and quantitative excesses and the transgenerational transmission of lived experiences.

Second, we verified that Freud did not adopt a single conception but constructed several varying notions of trauma, which can be organised into at least four different conceptual configurations. The first of these, presented in the Preliminary Communication in 1893, established that a trauma is produced when an idea that arouses affect is combined with a lack of reaction. This combination leads to the idea being separated from the ego along with the undischarged affect. The second posits that a trauma occurs when a psychical conflict takes place, that is, a contradiction between an idea and the rest of the ideas of the ego, leading to the defence and the splitting of the incompatible idea via repression. The third combines the idea of conflict with *nachträglich* temporality. In this way, certain childhood sexual experiences have a delayed effect and become traumatic if a current situation awakens their memory, thus resignifying what had happened and generating an unpleasurable quantitative increase which had been absent in the original situation. The final configuration of the trauma states that it occurs at the instant in which a certain aspect of the experience arouses such a large amount of stimulus in the mental apparatus that the webs of representations cannot bind and process it.

Third, despite the differences between these conceptions, a common factor remained constant throughout the transformations. For the Viennese psychoanalyst, no experience is intrinsically traumatic, nor are there subjects especially predisposed to suffer the pathological consequences of a trauma. The latter's production does not entirely depend on the objective conditions of the situation nor wholly on the particularities of the subject; neither is it produced solely by present circumstances or by predisposition rooted in the past; it is never completely external or fully internal. In other words, no single factor can define trauma in absolute terms since it can only be defined in *relative* terms. From the works of the founder of psychoanalysis, it can be deduced that a trauma occurs when there is a *relationship of incompatibility between an element and an organisation*. This relationship was understood in different ways throughout the different configurations that we have indicated. In the first of these, the relationship is fundamentally stated in topical terms: an element is *left out* of the ego's organisation. In the second configuration, this split is considered the consequence of a relationship of *incompatibility* or *contradiction* between an idea and the ideas that constitute the ego. In the third, the association of a current circumstance with the memory-trace of a childhood sexual experience comes into conflict with the ego and also produces the same type of relationship of incompatibility that we have indicated for the second conception; but to this, the increase of excitation due to the arrival of puberty is added, which leads to a sum of affect being released from the memory-trace that had not been originally produced during the experience in the past. This last point is accentuated in the final configuration: a sum of excitation that enters the mental apparatus becomes *unprocessable* for it. The affect aroused by certain aspects of an experience *cannot be bound* to the webs of representations, not because it is intrinsically unrepresentable or ineffable, but because, in *relative* terms, it entails too much affect in too little time for that particular psychical organisation.

In short, whether defined in terms of *exteriority*, *incompatibility* or *impossibility*, in all the conceptual configurations outlined by Freud we can find a *relationship of incompatibility* between a certain *element* and *an entity* which intends to function as an *organised totality*. In this way, the organisation is called into question by the presence of the element. This relationship, therefore, generally leads to some form of defensive action that, far from succeeding in overcoming the trauma, produces symptoms. In turn, these symptoms account for a fixation to the trauma. Finally, once a trauma has occurred, an indelible mark lives on: something from the experience remains "uncurable", which does not exclude the possibility of treating the malaise generated by it if some aspect of the *traumatic relationship* can be modified (or, in others words, if the subjective position held at that moment in respect to the past experience is transformed).

Fourth, in this history of trauma, which came up against (and attempted to initiate dialogue with) the problem of trauma in history, it is possible to outline two different ways of articulating *trauma* and *history*. In Chapters 3 and 4, we pointed out a shift in the relative importance given by Freud to the webs of representations and the sum of affect. At the time of the construction of his *Neurotica*, the trauma was situated in a *scene* that the representations could organise and narrate. In this way, trauma *and* history (and story) seem to *be conjugated*: a story can become traumatic and be structured as a unified and cohesive narrative that revolves around a scene lived in the past. In the most extreme examples, the entire identity would seem to be defined by the identification to a certain element of that scene: "I am like this because I lived through a trauma that has marked my history" (the same could be applied to a group). Later, in the context of the First World War, the trauma was situated at the *limits* of what the webs of representations can process from an experience and in the *holes* that are produced in the narration of a scene from the past. Thus, here it is not a matter of conjunction but of *exclusive disjunction*: *either* history (that is, story, narrative, scene, plot, cohesion, identity) *or* trauma (that is, something that introduces a discontinuity or a rupture in the plot, the cohesion, the coherence, the identifications, etc.) Without a doubt, the first of these versions of the trauma is more compatible with history and with "story".[1] The second version, on the other hand, poses more difficulties with regard to its narration and historicisation. This forces us to develop a way of narrating the past that includes in the story the elements left out of the plots of past experiences within the confines of representation. Undoubtedly, this way of conceiving the relationship between trauma and history is at the centre of certain historiographical debates regarding the representation of borderline events and the writing of historical traumas. Here we can find questions that are very difficult to resolve: Is it possible to write a history of past traumas that does not imply their denial or trivialisation nor their sacralisation or perpetuation? Is it possible to inscribe in a narrative the things that remain alive from those experiences without either erasing its traumatic specificity or provoking the repeated encounter with a hole?

These questions evoke, in the field of history, problems that are not only of a cognoscitive nature, since they refer to a practical dimension that englobes both the debates on the ways of constructing historical narratives about traumatic experiences and the concerns about finding strategies to mitigate the collective consequences of historical traumas. The interest of historians and researchers concerned with the recent past in notions from the field of psychopathology is probably due to the expectation of finding in this field not only doctrinal developments but also conceptions about practices that seek to transform the experiences they address and not just understand them.

In turn, the transformations in the ways of approaching the treatment of trauma in the clinical domain not only expressed different conceptual configurations that were prior to the practices but also contributed to defining and modifying what was understood by trauma at each time and place. At the time of the Preliminary Communication, the cathartic method was presented as a technique designed as a counterpart to the pathological mechanism and to the conception of trauma. If the latter was considered to occur due to a lack of reaction to an event that generated unpleasure, the therapy sought to recover the forgotten memory in order to produce the reaction which had been absent in the original experience, and, in this way, discharge the affect and reintegrate the idea to the ego. However, when Breuer and Freud explained the technique in more detail, two features came to light. First, according to how the authors conceived their own practice, its efficacy seemed to depend more on the discharge of affect than on the possibility of remembering the event by overcoming the split. In fact, if the association of the idea to the ego was not achieved, it would still be possible to eliminate its effects via suggestion; in contrast, eliminating the strangled quantitative element seemed essential to achieve success (Breuer & Freud, 1893). In other words, "abreacting" and discharging seemed to matter more than remembering. This way of presenting the technique leads us to affirm that the conception of trauma held by the authors at that time gave affect a much more important role than the one we can derive solely from their conceptual developments. Second, the act of remembering was not central to this practice for an even more important reason: the therapy sought the repetition of the trauma, not its recollection.

Would reliving the trauma make it possible to overcome it? Or would it reinforce and perpetuate its effects? Both Janet and Freud seem to have favoured this second option. For both authors, the repetition of the past could be as automatic, compulsive or symptomatic as any other pathological phenomenon based on the forgetting of a past experience. Indeed, remembering a forgotten trauma was not considered enough to mitigate its consequences. If the therapy was limited to promoting the retrieval of the memory from the past, if it established the idea that it was enough to talk about the trauma to overcome it, then paradoxical effects could be generated. In the hypothetical case that the act of remembering made possible the elimination of the symptoms, the risk remained for the latter to be replaced by a narrative that structures the subject's entire life around a traumatic experience. Thus, whoever suffered that event would become a *traumatised* person whose being is defined entirely by the trauma they had experienced. These types of identity narratives, which consolidate fixations to a point in the past, are usually the – more or less desired – consequence of certain treatments that are limited to the search for and the expression of the forgotten trauma.

For these kinds of reasons, Janet and Freud considered that therapy should aim at something other than just remembering. For the French doctor, that "something" implied different variants of *forgetting*. In his first texts, he stated that, after the recovery of the memory split from the personality, it was necessary to implement processes of *decomposition* of the memory and the *suppression* or *substitution* of the elements that still generated malaise. Towards the beginning of the 1920s, he maintained that therapy should set in motion processes of *assimilation* of the past experience into the subject's personality through recounting that experience. However, it should also promote the simultaneous *liquidation* of certain past aspects that are still present. In particular, what must be liquidated is, according to this doctor and philosopher, the motor and affective attitude that the subject had adopted in the past. Because if it remained unchanged, they would be led to the hallucinatory repetition of the past and not to an exercise of memory (which Janet sought to distinguish from repetition).

The founder of psychoanalysis also stated that remembering on its own was not enough to overcome trauma and its pathological consequences. If the neuroses depend on the response given in the face of a conflict, a defensive response that has doomed a contradictory element with respect to the ego organisation to be forgotten, then the cure should seek not only to remember what was forgotten but also to *modify the contradictory relationship between that element and the organisation.* As we have seen, Freud tried to resolve this point in different ways throughout his texts: via thought-*activity* that *resolves* the contradiction, through *melting the resistances* to remembering, by allowing the patient to *work-through the resistances* once they had been discerned, etc. These resistances are expressed not only by the impossibility of consciously accessing what is forgotten but also by the compulsion to repeat it. He recognised that in both modalities of resistance, the same forces which at the time had generated the process of repression continue to be currently in force. Therefore, retrieving the forgotten past is useless if the subject does not want to know anything about it. In short, Freud assumed that in order to overcome the consequences of a trauma it is necessary to modify the subjective position that, in the present, is adopted with respect to the conflictive element from the past.

As can be seen, Janet's ideas regarding therapy seem to emphasise the modification of the past: it aims for some part of the past experience to be lost (forgotten, suppressed, substituted, liquidated, etc.) to avoid it being automatically imposed in the present. Freud's ideas seem to stress the importance of transforming the present subjective position in order to remember what in the past was repressed and doomed to be forgotten. However, in this author, the reference to the necessity of some type of loss is not absent either. At the end of Chapter 2, we had already referred to the fact that working with the contradictions and the resistances could be compared to the work of mourning, a process that not only involves a change of subjective position with respect to a fragment of the past but also the production, inscription and acceptance of a loss. We now wish to make a final development that allows us to understand the type of work required to mitigate the effects of trauma from an economic point of view.

When, in 1926, Freud performed a detailed analysis of anxiety, his first impression was that it is a reaction to a loss (of the mother, of the penis, of parental love, etc.). When any of these losses occur, or simply threaten to occur, the anxiety functions as a signal that initiates the defence mechanisms, given the danger that these losses imply for the psyche. However, here Freud introduced another question: what does the danger consist of? He approached this question from an economic perspective, and the issue of loss was subordinated to it:

> The reason why the infant in arms wants to perceive the presence of its mother is only because it already knows by experience that she satisfies all its needs without delay. The situation, then, which it regards as a 'danger' and against which it wants to be safeguarded is that of non-satisfaction, (…) the economic disturbance caused by an accumulation of amounts of stimulation which require to be disposed of. It is this factor, then, which is the real essence of the 'danger'.
> (Freud, 1926, p. 137)

This economic disturbance, caused not by a loss but by a greater presence of stimulation, is what Freud calls, strictly speaking, "trauma". It generally does not occur since it is usually limited to being an expectation: the anxiety signals the imminence of danger, and it calls upon "actions of defence which amount to the psychical binding of the repressed (impulse)" (Freud, 1933, p. 90), thus avoiding the helplessness that would be felt if large amounts of excitation were to invade the psychical apparatus without being bound. That is why a loss does not often become traumatic. There are ways of responding to it that avoid the degree of discomfort, paralysis and discontinuity that are typical in a traumatic situation. The signal of anxiety is one of these ways; mourning seems to be another.

However, mourning could also be thought of, from an economic point of view, as an excess that resists being lost. Already in 1917, Freud pointed out that once reality testing has shown that the loved object no longer exists, the work of mourning implies that "all libido shall be withdrawn from its attachments to that object" (Freud, 1917, p. 244). This task runs into resistance, which Freud considered universal: "people never willingly abandon a libidinal position" (Freud, 1917, p. 244). For this reason, the demand proceeding from reality testing is: "carried out bit by bit (…) Each single one of the memories and expectations in which the libido is bound to the object is brought up and hypercathected, and detachment of the libido is accomplished in respect of it" (Freud, 1917, p. 245). As long as this detachment is not fully consummated, while the work of mourning lasts "the existence of the lost object is psychically prolonged" (Freud, 1917, p. 245) and the quantitative excess continues to be *present* because the psychical apparatus responds to the object's presence by means of a hypercathexis.

Note that at that time, Freud was already invoking a schema similar to the one used in 1920. When faced with the entry of a sum of excitation, the psychical apparatus summons energy from all sides and moves it towards the ruptured zone in which the excess is found. It does so in order to create an anticathexis that allows for the intruding quantity of stimulus to be bound (Freud, 1920, pp. 29–30). Freud believed that if a system is "in itself highly cathected", that is, if it strengthens the bonds between its components, it will be better prepared to receive and bind inflowing energy (Freud, 1920, p. 30). This conception explains well why in such circumstances, the person does not only feel unpleasure due to the increase in quantity but also experiences the impoverishment of "all the other psychical systems", which provided the energy for the anticathexis. Thus, "the remaining psychical functions are extensively paralysed or reduced" (Freud, 1920, p. 30). During the traumatic moment and the response given to it, the person seems absorbed in a task comparable to the one of someone who is going through mourning. In both cases, the subject seems fixated on an activity in which all the energy is used to respond to the quantitative excess. While these processes last, the person who undergoes them seems to find themselves in the state described by the epigraph from the start of this book: "he abandons all interest in the present and future and remains permanently absorbed in mental concentration upon the past" (Freud, 1916–1917, p. 276). To this description, we can add the comparison with melancholia, whose complex behaves like an "open wound, drawing to itself cathectic energies (...) from all directions" (Freud, 1917, p. 253). As can be seen, the economic perspective and the fixation to the past make it possible to bridge trauma, melancholia and mourning in Freudian thought.[2]

However, the treatment given to the trauma cannot be content with this state of affairs. Reinforcing the components of a system in an attempt to accommodate a component that is heterogeneous to it seems to be a common response, but it runs the risk of perpetuating the fixation to the trauma and the loss of all interest outside of it. If the relationship of impossibility established between an element and an organisation is not modified; and if the latter does not transform its internal structure in pursuit of cancelling the element's inconceivability and incompatibility, then it could repeatedly find itself with the same failure in each attempt to assimilate and process the traumatic elements.

Perhaps the resolution of the work of mourning could serve as a model for a possible treatment of the consequences of trauma. While it lasts, mourning involves an economic disturbance comparable to that of melancholia and trauma. However, its possible outcome is different: a change in the subjective position regarding the past and a loss of the (libidinal) ties that continue to bind the subject to an object that is no longer there. If the subject maintains the ties that bind him to the object, the former may lose himself along with the latter. For Freud, mourning (understood as psychical work and as a collective ritual) does not lead to forgetting or trivialising what has happened. It does not deny the undeniable, irretrievable and irreplaceable nature of what is lost, but neither does it perpetuate the fixation to the past.

Rather, it makes it possible for something experienced as being all too present to be inscribed as a part of the past. Thus, a (surely indelible) scar remains, but the wound is no longer open.

With these ideas, we can conclude this history of trauma. All that is left for us to do is present some possible lines of inquiry that, in our opinion, the work in this book give rise to. At the beginning of our endeavour we had proposed to study not only the transformations of the notion of trauma in the psychopathological field but also the processes that had led to its implantation in the fields of historiography and the studies on social memory and history of the recent past. We obviously do not intend to judge the precision with which historians and social scientists utilise psychoanalytic categories nor do we intend to denounce alleged deviations from an orthodoxy that should supposedly be defended. Doing so would constitute an error equivalent to criticising the inaccurate way in which Freud or other psychoanalysts utilised categories from the natural sciences without taking into account that this type of use allows for the resolution of specific problems in psychoanalysis. Even though the way in which historiography utilises *conceptual configurations* and *images* (that is, as *models* or *theoretical fictions*) arising from the "psy" field is imprecise, what is interesting to evaluate are the possibilities and limits that these uses have produced when addressing specific issues in the field of history or issues in common with the field of psychopathology. Below we point out some of the problems that, in our opinion, merit further research.

First, the topic of memory: that is, the forgetting, the repetitions and the remembering of past collective experiences considered traumatic. This problem is central to LaCapra's work on the Holocaust (LaCapra, 2008, 2009, 2014) and Rousso's on the Vichy regime (Conan & Rousso, 1994; Rousso, 1990). These authors made use of the Freudian ideas of repression and the return of the repressed to address the way in which these historical processes affect the present. Cathy Caruth, on the other hand, preferred to utilise the hypothesis of a literal reiteration of the trauma, which she drew from the readings about Janet made by contemporary authors such as Van der Hart and Van der Kolk (Caruth, 1995a,b, 1996). The question of the memory of past experiences is also present in Hugo Vezzetti's books about collective representations of the last Argentine dictatorship and revolutionary violence (Vezzetti, 2002, 2009).

Second, the problem of the limits of representation. This issue was explicitly raised in a series of conferences held in 1990 entitled "Probing the Limits of Representation: Nazism and the 'Final Solution'" which Saul Friedlander (1992) was in charge of publishing in a book that contains most of these expositions. The idea of "Limits of Representation" condensed at least two meanings. On the one hand, it referred to the debate on the pertinence of the imposition of limits in the ways of representing events such as the Shoah. Would it be possible to represent it as a comedy? Do all possible approaches have the same value? Would certain representations be truer than others? Would there be "external" or "objective" criteria to limit the representation of that kind of experience and determine its truthfulness, or would there only be internal, linguistic criteria? Should a certain form of relativism be accepted such that it would not be possible to determine a stable criterion of truth about the facts of the matter?, etc. (Friedlander, 1992). The meaning given to the "limits of representation", understood as the determination of the validity or invalidity of certain historical narratives, became more urgent around 1980 when a revisionist movement arose in Germany that denied the existence of the gas chambers. On the other hand, the "limits of representation" refer to another problem, closer to certain Freudian topics. We are referring to the question (mentioned in Chapter 4 of this book) of whether it is possible or not to wholly inscribe certain experiences into representations or if there are certain elements still unable to be bound to a plot, to a story.

Both meanings are connected, in turn, with two other central problems that largely correlate with one another: the writing of history and the transgenerational transmission of collective traumas. The works mentioned above by LaCapra and Caruth and several of the papers compiled in Friedlander's book dealt with the ties between writing, limits of representation and transmission. One of the risks when creating a historical narration about traumatic experiences seems to be that of constructing "fetishised" narratives (LaCapra, 2009; Santner, 1992) which seek to deny the horror and loss in order to build homogeneous and conflict-free identities, as if the conflictive past can be left behind without attempting to face and work-through certain aspects that are still very much alive. At the opposite extreme, are the "sacralised" narratives, which, in order to avoid trivialising the trauma, end up consecrating and eternalising it to the point of excluding it from a possible rational approach. This seems to be the case of Caruth, who strongly questioned the possibility of historicising trauma and raised the question of whether its integration into memory and the consciousness of history is not "a *sacrilege of the traumatic experience*" (Caruth, 1995b, p. 154; italics added).

Another important problem is the reception and interpretation of the testimonies about traumatic experiences. Events such as the Shoah and some Latin American dictatorships have a common feature: the attempt of the perpetrators to erase the trace of their crimes. The lack of written documents on many of these crimes – above all, of the extermination camps – grants capital importance to the testimonies of the survivors, which have become the almost exclusive source of evidence when carrying out the judicial processes and the historical investigations. To the list of traditional difficulties associated with any type of witness testimony (contradictions, memory flaws, more or less deliberate distortions, among others), two other issues are added. On the one hand, if the witness is not only a spectator but also a victim of the traumatic experience, to what extent would it be expected (and fair) to demand from their account the (illusory) objectivity sought by the jurist? On the other hand, regarding the extermination camps, the most important testimony is considered that of the person who reached the end and, therefore, can no longer testify. Many revisionist histories that tried to deny the facts were based on this paradox. Nevertheless, works have also emerged, such as those by Carlo Ginzburg

(1992) or Giorgio Agamben (2002), which highlight the importance of these accounts even when they come from a single witness, are unverifiable or contain inconsistencies or are incomplete. These testimonies are situated in a zone, common in Freudian practice, in which it is difficult to fully distinguish between reality and phantasy or determine the accuracy of the facts, despite which it is possible to extract a particular truth from those experiences.

The last topic that we want to mention in this brief description of the historiographical problems that open up for future research is the analysis of the attitudes, strategies and policies that were implemented or proposed to alleviate the subjective and collective consequences of historical traumas. Authors such as Ricoeur (2008), LaCapra (2005) and Todorov (2008) did not content themselves with studying the historical experiences considered traumatic or the problems that they pose to collective memory and historiography. They also conceived concrete alternatives for their overcoming, discussed the treatments (in a broad sense) given to traumas in communities, warned about the dangers of memories that seek to preserve everything or that are permanently looking to the past and pointed out the need to mourn, assume losses and generate processes of forgetting.

In summary, the problems of memory, the limits of representation, the writing of the past, transgenerational transmission, testimony and the treatments of trauma constitute a series that we have come across in our journey which revolved around Freud's works and that have tangible consequences in the field of history of the recent past. In particular, it becomes necessary to study the intersections between psychoanalysis, memory and history in order to approach our dictatorial past and its consequences, which make themselves felt even today. In the book *Historia reciente. Perspectivas y desafíos para un campo en construcción* (Franco & Levín, 2007), which well illustrates the main features of the disciplinary field that deals with the recent past, the compilers maintain that in this domain, there is a

> … strong predominance of issues and problems linked to the social processes considered *traumatic*: wars, massacres, genocide, dictatorships, social crises and other extreme situations that threaten the maintenance of social bonds and are experienced by their contemporaries as moments of profound ruptures and discontinuities, both at the level of individual and collective experience.
>
> (Franco & Levín, 2007, p. 34)

In Argentina, this description is applicable to, above all, the enormous amount of historical works that, in recent years, dealt with the experience of the last military dictatorship and utilised, in many cases, the notion of trauma and other categories from the "psy" terrain, without an exhaustive study of these uses having been carried out up to now.[3]

Lastly, we also consider it important to study the intersection between history and psychoanalysis from another point of view. So far, we have mentioned the works inscribed in the historical discipline that made use of psychoanalytic instruments.

It is also possible to address the specific practices that certain groups of "psy" practitioners (psychiatrists, psychologists, psychoanalysts) carried out to alleviate the consequences of traumatic historical experiences, such as State Terrorism or Shoah. These practices, of which we often only have the account of the protagonists, were carried out by different groups in various state institutions, human rights organisations and non-governmental organisations and, to date, have not been exhaustively studied in their entirety. At the same time, it would also be interesting to address the way in which these professionals conceptualised their tasks and the categories they used or constructed to think about the subjective and collective effects of these events. Thus, not only could the existence of new conceptual configurations or new images (or the recovery of some of those we have already studied throughout this book) be explored, but also the particularities of that historical experience, read in the light of its subjective consequences and its treatments.

In summary, we believe that many of the ideas and problems addressed throughout this book that deals with the history of trauma can be used to study in greater depth some of the topics related to the presence of traumas in recent history. Much remains to be investigated in the problematic area framed by the intersection of psychoanalysis and history. We hope this book constitutes a useful contribution to developing further in that direction.

Notes

1 That is, as a narration and as a discipline, as *story* and as *history*. In Spanish, the term "*historia*" contains both meanings: history and story.
2 Let us remember that in *Beyond the Pleasure Principle,* Freud once again compared traumatic neuroses with melancholia (Freud, 1920a, p. 12).
3 The works that began to problematise the uses of psychoanalytic notions in approaching the recent past in our country are those of Hugo Vezzetti (2002, 2009, 2010) and María Inés Mudrovcic (2005, 2009).

References

Agamben, G. (2002). *Homo Sacer III. Lo que queda de Auschwitz. El archivo y el testigo.* Madrid: Editora Nacional.

Breuer, J. & Freud, S. ([1893] 1955). On the physical mechanism of hysterical phenomena: Preliminary communication. In S. Freud (Ed.), *The Standard Edition of the Complete Psychological Works of Sigmund Freud Vol. II: Studies on Hysteria* (pp. 3–47). London: The Hogarth Press and the Institute of Psycho-Analysis.

Caruth, C. (1995a). Part 1: Trauma and experience. Introduction. In C. Caruth (Ed.), *Trauma: Explorations in Memory* (pp. 3–12). Baltimore, MD: The Johns Hopkins University Press.

Caruth, C. (1995b). Part 2: Recapturing the past. Introduction. In C. Caruth (Ed.), *Trauma: Explorations in Memory* (pp. 151–157). Baltimore, MD: The Johns Hopkins University Press.

Caruth, C. (1996). *Unclaimed Experience: Trauma, Narrative and History.* Baltimore, MD: The Johns Hopkins University Press.

Conan, E. & Rousso, H. (1994). *Vichy, un passé qui ne passe pas.* Paris: Fayard.

De Certeau, M. (1988). *The Writing of History*. New York: Columbia University Press.
Franco, M. & Levín, M. (2007). El pasado cercano en clave historiográfica. In M. Franco & M. Levín (Ed.), *Historia reciente. Perspectivas y desafíos para un campo en construcción* (pp. 31–66). Buenos Aires: Paidós.
Freud, S. ([1916–1917] 1963). Lecture XVIII. Fixation to traumas, the unconscious. In S. Freud (Ed.), *The Standard Edition of the Complete Psychological Works of Sigmund Freud, Vol. XVI: Introductory Lectures on Psycho-analysis (Part III)* (pp. 273–285). London: The Hogarth Press and the Institute of Psycho-Analysis.
Freud, S. ([1917] 1957). Mourning and melancholia. In S. Freud (Ed.), *The Standard Edition of the Complete Psychological Works of Sigmund Freud, Vol. XIV: On the History of the Psycho-analytic Movement, Papers on Metapsychology and Other Works* (pp. 237–260). London: The Hogarth Press and the Institute of Psycho-Analysis.
Freud, S. ([1920] 1955). Beyond the pleasure principle. In S. Freud (Ed.), *The Standard Edition of the Complete Psychological Works of Sigmund Freud, Vol. XVIII: Beyond the Pleasure Principle, Group Psychology and Other Works* (pp. 1–64). London: The Hogarth Press and the Institute of Psycho-Analysis.
Freud, S. ([1926] 1959). Inhibitions, symptoms and anxiety. In S. Freud (Ed.), *The Standard Edition of the Complete Psychological Works of Sigmund Freud, Vol. XX: An Autobiographical Study. Inhibitions, Symptoms and Anxiety. The Question of Lay Analysis and Other Works* (pp. 75–175). London: The Hogarth Press and the Institute of Psycho-Analysis.
Freud, S. ([1933] 1964). Lecture XXXII. Anxiety and instinctual life. In S. Freud (Ed.), *The Standard Edition of the Complete Psychological Works of Sigmund Freud, Vol. XXII: New Introductory Lectures on Psycho-analysis and Other Works* (pp. 81–111). London: The Hogarth Press and the Institute of Psycho-Analysis.
Friedlander, S. (1992). Introduction. In S. Friedlander (Ed.), *Probing the Limits of Representation. Nazism and the 'Final Solution'* (pp. 1–21). Cambridge and London: Harvard University Press.
Ginzburg, C. (1992). Just one witness. In S. Friedlander (Ed.), *Probing the Limits of Representation. Nazism and the 'Final Solution'* (pp. 82–96). Cambridge and London: Harvard University Press.
Hartog, F. (2003). *Régimes d'Historicité. Présentisme et expériences du temps*. Paris: Seuil.
Koselleck, R. (1993). *Futuro pasado. Para una semántica de los tiempos históricos.* Barcelona: Paidós.
LaCapra, D. (2008). *Representando el Holocausto. Historia, teoría y trauma.* Buenos Aires: Prometeo.
LaCapra, D. (2009). *Historia y memoria después de Auschwitz*. Buenos Aires: Prometeo.
LaCapra, D. (2014). *Writing History, Writing Trauma*. Baltimore.MD: John Hopkins University Press.
Mudrovcic, M. I. (2005). Alcances y límites de perspectivas psicoanalíticas en historia. In M. I. Mudrovcic, *Historia, narración y memoria. Los debates actuales en filosofía de la historia* (pp. 139–154). Madrid: Akal.
Mudrovcic, M. I. (2009). Trauma, memoria e historia. In D. Brauer (Ed.), *La historia desde la teoría, Vol. 2. Una guía de campo por el pensamiento filosófico acerca del sentido de la historia y del conocimiento del pasado* (pp. 105–126). Buenos Aires: Prometeo.
Ricoeur, P. (2008). *La memoria, la historia, el olvido.* Buenos Aires: Fondo de Cultura Económica.

Rousso, H. (1990). *Le syndrome de Vichy. De 1944 a nos jours.* Paris: Éditions du Seuil.
Santner, E. (1992). History beyond the pleasure principle: Some thoughts on the representation of trauma. In S. Friedlander (Ed.), *Probing the Limits of Representation. Nazism and the 'Final Solution'* (pp. 143–155). Cambridge and London: Harvard University Press.
Todorov, T. (2008). *Los abusos de la memoria.* Barcelona: Paidós.
Vezzetti, H. (2002). *Pasado y presente.* Buenos Aires: Siglo XXI.
Vezzetti, H. (2009). *Sobre la violencia revolucionaria.* Buenos Aires: Siglo XXI.
Vezzetti, H. (2010). La figura del trauma histórico en la formación de la memoria pública. *Jornadas Internacionales. Historia, memoria y patrimonio. Las conmemoraciones y el Bicentenario entre reflexión y experiencias.* Buenos Aires. Noviembre de 2010.

Index

Note: *Italic* page numbers refer to figures.

Abraham, K. 7, 147, 171, 174–175, 182–183, 188–189, 195–196
abreaction 82, 175
accident: as cause of illness (or symptoms) 1, 28, 30–36, 44, 50, 52–53, 57–61, 161, 183, *185,* 240; and emotion 41–43, 50, 55, 79; factors 81; as minor event 29–30, 33; as opposite of stigmata 84, 87, 95, 162; patient or subject or victims 25, 44, 54, 56; as a synonym for contingencies 88, 104, 117, 151, 162, 172, 173, 187, 203; *see also* railway
aetiology 4, 16, 31, 60, 73, 75–77, 88, 118, 121–122, 125, 127, 200; hereditary 59, 164; of hysteria or neuroses 5, 112, 116, 117, 119, 124, 130–131, 135, 137, 145–146, 149–150, 229–230; and sexuality 13, 119, 120, 123, 135, 167, 178, 215; specific 16, 124, 133; and trauma 117, 147, 239
affect: as opposite of physical shock 41; as a quantitative factor and in contrast to ideas or representations 4, 15, 23, 80–85, 88–91, 96, 100, 116, 139–140, 152, 171–172, 194, 200–201, 207, 244–246; sexual 120, 124, 128; as synonymous of emotion 77, 80–81, 94, 120, 127–129, 173, 198, 203
anatomy: framework or model 25, 35, 37, 39, 46–48, 52, 58, 60, 66, 78–79, 116, 238; pathological 8, 31–32, 35, 37, 39, 46–47; *see also* lesion
antecedents *see* predisposition
benefit for illness 33, 44–45, 162, 169–170, 183, 186, 190, 192, 243

catharsis 16, 98, 102, 191, 193–195, 200, 240; effect 80; method or therapy 82, 93, 96, 103, 119, 194
cathexis: with affect 152; anty- 205, 249; freely flowing 204; hiper- 205, 248; libidinal 179–180, *182*–183; quiescent 204; side- 129
cause: causality 17, 31, 36, 116, 126, 138, 184–185; of damage or lesion 2, 32–33, 35–36; and effect relationship 32, 80; emotional 41, 43, 51, 60, 171; heredity 131–132, 162, 167, 239; of illness 35, 43, 47, 66, 96, 112, 135, 137, 146, 150, 161; of neuroses 14, 74, 77, 92, 117, 119–126, 131–133, 142, 148, 164, 184, 191, 198, 206; organic 28, 168, 171; sexual 16, 112, 120, 122–125, 130–135; specific 116, 125–127, 132–133, 136; of symptoms 32, 77, 80, 87, 89, 95, 100, 104, 118, 151, 240; traumatic 24, 68–69, 80, 97, 101, 112, 165, 174; *see also* aetiology and accident
Charcot, J.M. 7, 9–10, 15, 24, 25, 29, 31, 33, 41–42, 45–60, 66, 70, 74–80, 84, 88, 92, 117, 120–122, 131, 142, 148, 162–163, 168, 171, 195, 240
compensation 36, 44–46, 53, 59, 169, 174, *185*, 190

conceptual configuration (or framework or schema) 6, 13–15, 17, 31, 34, 39–42, 44, 51, 54–55, 57, 60, 68, 73, 78, 82, 116, 135, 151, 195, 229, 238, 244, 246, 250, 253
concussion of the spine 28, 32–33, 35–39, 45
contingency/contingent 12, 16, 36, 116, 131, 164

defence: hysteria or neurosis (or neuro-psychoses) 88, 96, 112, 113, 118, 120, 123–124, 126, 130, 131, 133, 137, 145; as mechanism 68, 69, 73, 84–86, 89–91, 96, 112, 116, 126–129, 131, 137, 178, 180, 183, 200, 230–232, 242–245, 247–248
drives 13, 16, 69, 143, 154, 173, 176–177, 179, 200, 203, 206–207, 241
dynamic point of view (or conception) 66, 76, 89, 102, 134, 167, 184

economic: dimension 134, 172, 203; disturbance 117; point of view (or conception) 6, 10, 16, 76, 89, 156, 161, 173–174, 180, 183–184, 200–202, 204–205, 207, 215, 241–242, 248–249
electro-shock 192
element: current 4, 44; as opposite of entity or organization 13, 15, 17, 72, 85–87, 104, 196, 201–202, 204–207, 223, *231*, 234, 244–247, 249, 251; past 44; psychical or psychological 23–24, 40–41, 49–52, 55, 61, 69, 76, 163, 169, 194; sexual 122, 123, 147, 178; traumatic 91, 148, 155, 164, 173, 249
emotion (emotional): in contrast to ideas or representations 194; as opposite of physical shock 35, 37, 51; as part of pathological mechanism 15, 25, 27, 36, 40–44, 54–58, 66, 68, 70, 74, 76–77, 162–163, 168; as a synonym of feeling 33, 37, 40, 42, 43, 52, 73, 79, 87, 88, 125, 149, 240; *see also* affect
energy: as a model 8, 89, 240; as a quantitative factor 13, 53, 76, 173, 188, 196, 201, 203–206, 249; sexual 77, 184
epistemic framework (or matrix) 37; *see also* conceptual configuration
Erichsen, J.E. 7, 15, 25, 27–38, 40–41, 44–45, 47–48, 53, 55, 60, 66, 95, 164, 185, 228
evolutionism 8, 42, 240
external: conditions or factors 4, 32, 36, 38, 118, 121, 131, 138, 140, 142, 164, 177–178, 182–183, 185, 189, 196, 199, 203–204, 218–219, 231, 234, 241, 244, 250; history 6, 11, 240

fear 26, 35, 37, 41, 43, 44, 47, 60, 73, 92, 176, 178, 198
Ferenczi, S. 7, 171–176, 181–182, 189–190, 195–196, 202, 224, 240
forgetting 5, 15, 91, 98, 102, 162, 216, 230, *232*, 233, 235, 239, 243, 246–247, 249–250, 252
Freud, S. 4–17, 23–24, 31, 42, 57–58, 61, 66–67, 69, 74–85, 87–93, 96–104, 112–156, 164–168, 171–184, 189–191, 193–208, 215–235, 238–252; Freudism 68
fright 27, 34, 37, 40–41, 50–51, 76–77, 80, 125, 129, 173, 183–184, 190, 203, 205–206
functional alteration (or disturbance) 30, 32, 34, 37, 39, 40, 43, 47, 51, 53–55, 58–59, 66, 68, 95, 132, 140, 240, 242; *see also* lesion

group psychology 12, 13, 17, 51, 215–217, 224, 226, 232, 245

helplessness 29, 37, 40, 207, 248
heredity (or hereditary): factors 1, 68–69, 81, 88, 191; as a class of disease 30; as opposed to accident or trauma 16, 57, 61, 81, 84, 96, 113, 131, 133, 186–187; as predisposition or cause of illness 45, 50–51, 55, 57, 59, 77, 88, 91, 95, 97, 101, 104, 112, 117–126, 129–135, 137, 144, 149, 151–152, 161–162, 164, 167, 168, 239; as a process of transmission 203, 219, 221, 231, 242–243; as a psychiatric tradition or a theory 5, 16, 66, 92, 98, 117
history: external history 4, 6; historiography 7; of hysteria or illness 58; intellectual history 4,

6–7, 14, 240; internal history 4, 6; of the patient or his family 43–44, 50, 56, 59, 75–76, 92, 97–98, 141, 148, 150, 152, 155, 216, 218, 232, 239, 242; of a people or humanity 155, 169, 215, 217–219, 223–224, 226, 228–229, 231–233, 239; of practices 5; of present or recent past 2, 12, 17, 250, 252–253; and psychoanalysis 252–253; of psychoanalysis 6 – 8, 17, 69, 114, 121, 145–146, 153, 164; of psychiatry 31; traditional history 3; and trauma 80, 238, 245; of trauma 8–10, 12, 14–15, 28–29, 238, 245, 250, 253; as writing 224, 251
hypnosis: as a model 42, 53, 54, 66; as a nervous or mental state 15, 42–43, 49, 54, 76; as a technique 5, 10, 16, 23, 25, 48–50, 54–55, 66, 69–70, 73–74
hysteria: anxiety (hysteria) 171–172, 176; conversion (hysteria) 171–172, 176; as disease or nosographic category 5, 9, 10, 14, 23, 25, 29, 33, 42, 45, 47, 58, 61, 68–70, 76–90, 95–98, 101–102, 112–113, 117–120, 129–134, 136–137, 141, 147, 149, 152, 161–164, 168–170, 174, 181, 185, 192, 200, ; male 41, 50, 52, 74–75; mechanism of 48, 53, 76; medicalisation of 10, 43, 46, 50, 56; psychologisation of 162; traumatic (hysteria) 24, 45, 48, 51, 59–60, 97, 146; *see also* defence

ideas: of ego 55, 57, 79, 82, 90–91, 100, 139–140, 207, 246; fixed (ideas) 56, 84, 92–95, 201, 207, 241; incompatible (idea) 88–91, 96–99, 104, 120, 137–140, 201, 207, 244; as a psychological factor and in contrast to affect or emotion 4, 15, 25, 50–51, 53, 55–59, 66, 72, 74–83, 86–91, 127–128, 130, 138, 162, 168, 192, 200–202, 204, 240, 242; split off from the ego 54, 79, 81, 83, 87, 89, 90, 194; suggest (ideas) 54; unconscious (ideas) 76, 93
images: linked to trauma or its victims 6, 10, 15, 44, 57, 95, 98, 138, 141, 164, 185, 187–188, 238, 250, 253
incubation 57, 228
injury: as physical damage 1, 2, 5, 23, 27–28, 30–40, 46–48, 51, 58–59, 165, 171–172, 174, 189–190; as psychic damage 52, 61, 98; *see also* lesion
insidious (or progressive) development 30, 33, 34, 38, 42; *see also* latency
insurance 5, 23, 25–26, 58, 61
interlocutors 4, 7, 11, 13, 14, 240

Janet, P. 5, 7, 9, 10, 15, 23, 24, 42, 57–58, 61, 66–74, 76, 78–81, 84–88, 92–98, 100–101, 104, 112, 117–118, 142, 162, 168–169, 176, 193, 238, 240, 241, 246–247, 250
Jones, E. 7, 114, 171, 174–175, 177–179, 183, 191, 202
Jung, C. 7, 121, 146–147, 153, 176, 179, 215–218, 220, 223, 240

lesion: anatomical or mechanical 24–25, 28, 30–39, 43, 46–48, 53–54, 59–60, 66, 167, 185, 240; dynamic or functional 27, 48, 52–53, 73, 78–79, 95
limits of representation 4, 14, 16–17, 117, 156, 208, 239

mechanical action (or impact or accident) 1, 15, 25, 34–37, 40–41, 46, 51, 54–55, 57, 59–60, 68, 78, 82, 161, 165, 181, *185,* 187, 240
mechanism of symptoms (or pathological mechanism) 5, 35, 41–43, 46–49, 51–57, 66, 73–90, 98, 104, 116–118, 123–124, 129, 136, 162, 164, 172, 178, 182–183, 202, 228, *231,* 241, 248
memory: biological 5, 67; collective or social 2, 6, 12, 17, 67, 216, 218, 221, 223, 225, 250, 252; forgotten 58, 66, 73, 80, 82–84, 90, 94, 99–101, 104, 141, 150, 172, 194, 230–231, 234, 242, 246–247; as a function, in the sense of recall 1, 5, 9, 27, 33, 58, 66–67, 69, 78, 81, 85–86, 94–95, 99, 102, 127, 194, 215, 230, 233, 238–240, 243–244, 251–252; literal 68; narrative 68, 93; phylogenetic 155; as a psychic element, synonymous with recollection 3, 71–73, 80, 86, 92, 94, 96, 102–104, 113, 115–116,

128–129, 131, 136, 139, 141, 143, 145, 148–150, 154, 176, 193–194, 203, 206–208, 226–227, 229, 242, 248; (memory)-trace 90, 113, 116, 138–140, 201, 204, 234, 241; trauma and 4, 14–15, 17, 61, 69, 77, 112; traumatic (memories) 93–94, 97–101
model 6, 10, 14–15, 35, 40, 44, 47–48, 50, 53, 66, 70, 76, 78, 80, 89, 94, 97, 120, 122, 125, 127, 134, 203, 205, 249–250
moral 5, 10, 45, 59, 88, 97, 163, 168, 177, 185–187, 191, 221

nachträglich 11, 16, 116–117, 138–139, 141–142, 151, 215, 244
Nancy (school of) 49, 73, 77–78, 162
nervous: functioning 55, 59, 240; illness 27, 30, 50, 59, 112, 121, 132, 162, 172, 187, 217; predisposition 131; schema 44; shock 31, 37–41, 48, 53–54, 66, 162; system 15, 25, 28–29, 32–33, 37, 40, 42–43, 46–49, 51–52, 60, 70, 74–79, 88, 122, 127–128, 163, 167; tissue 34, 165, 168
neurology 24, 43, 76, 78, 131, 156, 198
neuroses/neurosis: actual (neuroses) 120–122, 125, 133; aetiology (or causes) of 5–6, 14, 77, 112, 117–127, 129–130, 134–135, 142, 145, 147–149, 164, 187, 229–230, 239, 243; clinic of 5, 12, 67, 217, 238, 240, 243; as illness or nosographic category 24, 30, 47–48, 50, 58, 69–70, 75, 89–92, 95, 100–102, 113, 116, 119, 131–133, 137–138, 140–141, 144, 150–156, 165, 176, 193, 199, 201, 216, 218, 220, 224, 229–234, 242, 247; obsessional 90, 119, 126, 129, 131, 133, 219; traumatic (neurosis) 25, 31, 45, 58, 60–61, 173, 190, 202–203, 228; treatment of 16, 96, 99, 104, 176, 240; war (neuroses) 10, 14, 16, 117, 161, 166–172, 174–175, 177–185, 190–191, 194–198, 203, 206–207, 239; works on 15, 74; *see also* pension
Neurotica 16, 112–113, 116–117, 119, 125, 127–128, 130–131, 133–138, 140–147, 150–153, 155–156, 164, 204, 228, 230, 245

objective: conditions 4, 13, 14, 16, 41, 59, 61, 142, 165, 185, 189, 191, 199, 238, 242–244, 250; (objective) event, experience or fact 17, 36, 57, 187
Oppenheim, H. 7, 15, 25, 29, 31, 58–61, 66, 75, 161–162, 167–171, 174, 176, 185–186

Page, H. 7, 15, 25, 29, 31, 32, 34, 37–45, 47–48, 51, 53–54, 60, 66, 76, 142, 171
pension 23, 59, 61, 161–162, 167, 169–170, 183, 190
persuasion therapy 16, 163–164, 168, 191–192
phantasy 4, 8, 16, 57, 114, 116–117, 142–147, 149–150, 152–155, 225, 239, 252
phylogenetic 155, 164, 216, 217, 233
physiology: in contrast to anatomy 4, 15, 25, 39–40, 42–43, 48, 53, 66, 76–78, 88, 116, 239–240; in contrast to psychology 44, 51, 56–57, 70, 74, 126–127, 129, 148, 185; (physiological) mechanism 34, *41*, 43, 49, 57, 66, 124, 168; neurophysiology 8, 43, 78, 89, 162
predisposition (or disposition): hereditary 46, 50, *55*, *77*, 87, 88, 92, 97, 118, 121, 125–126, 131, 161, 178, *187*; non-hereditary 91, 112–113, 130–131, 133, 136–142, 151; as a past factor, in contrast to current element 4, 41, 43–46, 55, 61, 74, 81, 117, 120, 122, 132, 142, *165*, 169, 175, 177, 183, 188–190, 195, 230–231, 234, 244
psychical (or psychological) conflict 13, 24, 85, 89, 90, 96, 98–100, 104, 112, 118, 120, 137–141, 164–165, 177–179, 183–184, 190–191, 196, 200–201, 215, 217–218, 223, 226, 241, 244, 247
psychoanalysis: (psychoanalytic) concepts or theory 2, 6, 10, 143, 153, 155, 170, 175, 178–181, 184, 215, 250; as a discipline or field of knowledge 1, 4, 6–12, 16, 17, 25, 58, 67–69, 100–101, 116, 121, 129, 135, 145, 149, 152, 164, 167, 174, 176, 188, 193, 195, 202, 217, 220, 222, 224, 231, 239–241,

247, 252–253; (psychoanalityc) movement 7, 11, 14, 100, 114, 121, 145, 146, 153, 166, 175, 186, 216; (psychoanalytic) practices 6, 8, 69, 103, 155, 194, 200, 215; psychoanalyst 16–17, 24, 98–99, 113, 117, 129, 131, 133, 137, 139, 144, 149, 154, 164, 168, 171–175, 177–180, 182, 184, 187–189, 196, 202, 204, 218, 221, 223, 225–226, 233, 244
psychology: in contrast to biological or organic approaches or dimensions 3, 14, 23–25, 28, 30, 31, 34–35, 40, 42–43, 48, 51, 58, 61, 69, 70, 72, 74, 76, 85, 87–88, 90, 95, 118, 126, 135, 142, 148, 151, 161–162, 164–169, 175–176, 194, 219, 229; as a field of knowledge 12, 46, 66, 68, 78, 89, 100, 217; as a function of the nervous system 40, 56, 60, 116, 126–127, 129–130; metapsychology 181; psychologist 67, 253; (psychological) schema 42; (psychological) schools 9; *see also* group psychology *and* trauma
psychopathology: as a field of knowledge 2, 4, 9, 12, 17, 67, 112, 176, 223, 239, 243, 246, 250; as a morbid dimension of psychological processes 7, 15, 97, 127, 238
psychotherapy 7, 10, 45, 58, 67, 98, 102, 119–120, 162–165, 193

railway (or train): accident 5, 13–14, 23, 25–29, 32–39, 41, 77, 80, 161, 164, 174, 228, 238, 243; spine 28–30, 35, 58
reality: in contrast to phantasy 3, 4, 8, 14, 16, 114–117, 142, 144–146, 150–155, 239, 252; in contrast to simultion 27; linked with discourse 147, 149, 233; loss of 182; (reality) testing 248
remember (or remembering): as a psychological function 5, 15–16, 66, 71, 73, 83, 86, 90, 92–96, 98–104, 115, 128, 141, 143, 150, 154, 171, 187, 193, 201, 207, 230–233, 243, 246–247
reparation *see* compensation
repetition: in contrast to remembering 13, 17, 73, 78, 83–84, 86, 93–96, 101, 103–104, 129, 141, 166–167, 172–173, 194, 203, 205–208, 215, 219, 221, 230, 232, 234–235, 239, 242–243, 245–247, 250
representation 17, 23, 55–57, 66, 86, 177, 194, 215, 223, 226, 234, 238, 241, 250–251; *see also* limits of representation *and* web of representation
repression: as a defence mechanism 68–69, 84, *91*, 95, 102, 104, 113, 116, 120, 127–134, 137–138, 140–142, 165, 167, 176–177, 184, 193–194, 201–202, 220, *229*, *231*, 232–234, 242, 244, 247, 250

Salpêtrière 24, 45–46, 48–49, 51, 59, 74–76, 78–79, 84, 105–106, 117, 120–121, 162
Seduction Theory 8, 10, 16, 24, 101, 113–116, 130, 134–135, 142, 153, 164–165; *see also Neurorica*
Shoah 2, 6, 239, 250–251, 253
shock: mechanical (shock) 27, 30, 34–36, 55, 57, 59, 88; nervous (shock) 25, 31, 37–41, 43, 48, 53–54, 66, 162; psychological (or emotional) 24, 35, 37, 51, 60, 88, 162, 171–172, 182, 189–190, 202; sexual 133; shell (or war) 167, 175–177, 193–194
simulation 5, 10, 15, 25, 27, 29, 35, 37, 46, 53, 61, 75, 168–169, 192, 200
splitting (or splitt off) 54, *55*, 57, 72–73, 79, 81, *82*, 83, 86–92, 94, 96, 104, 112, 118–119, 132, 140, 180, 183, 200, 244, 246–247
stigmata 84, 97
subjective (or internal) particularities 4, 13, 16, 36, 41, 44, 61, 136, 165, 173, 185–187, 189, 191, 207, 238, 243–244
suggestion: auto- 57, 60; suggestibility 49; as a synonym for psychic influence or process 8, 45, 49, 79, 82, 84, 86, 93, 95, 115, 143, 149, 151, 176, 186–187; as technique 5, 10, 16, 48, 50, 53–54, 58, 66, 69–70, 73, 77–78, 83, 86, 93–94, 98–99, 103, 117, 161–163, 168, 170, 174, 177, 191–193, 195–197, 246; traumatic 55

Tausk, V. 171, 175, 180–181
temporality of trauma 10, 11, 16, 116–117, 128, 137–138, 141–142, 145, 151, 205, 215, 228, 238, 241, 244; *see also nachträglich*
terror 2, 37, 51, 68, 87, 92, 178, 181
therapy: (therapeutic) approach 2, 8, 10, 16, 53, 56, 58, 68, 76, 82, 162, 166; (therapeutic) effect (or proposal) 33, 74, 92, 150; electrotherapy 166, 191, 197; in the sense of treatment 4, 5, 9, 10, 70, 83–84, 92, 94–97, 103–104, 117, 119, 126, 130, 133, 135, 163, 165, 169–170, 177, 179, 186, 189, 191–197, 199, 239, 243, 246–247; of trauma 5, 14; *see also* psychoterapy
topographical point of view (or conception) 89
traces (of past or traumas) 5, 13, 67, 78–79, 94, 113–114, 127, 138–141, 148, 173, 201, 208, 216, 221, 224–226, 230, *231*, 232–234, 242, 251; *see also* memory
transference 13, 103, 196, 207; (transference) neuroses 179, 183–184, 202, 224
trauma: as agent provocateur 47, 74, 118; anatomical 162, 165, 240; childhood (trauma) 6, 73, 102, 113–116, 128, 130–131, 134–141, 143–149, 152–154, 164, 201, 207, 215, 218, 244; collective (trauma) 2, 4, 12, 14, 17, 117, 215–235, 239, 242, 246, 250–253; as an etiological factor 74–77, 96–97, 146–148, 150–151, 153, 163; as event, experience or situation 4, 6, 43, 58, 61, 68, 73, 82, 84, 87, 90, 95, 99, 103, 113–114, 135–136, 138–142, 164–165, 170–174, 182, 185–190, 194, 200, 204, 206–208, 225, 228, 230–235, 239, 242, 251, 253; mechanical (trauma) 23–25, 47, 54, 58, 60; memorialisation of 58; narratives or testimonies of 4, 16, 17, 99, 114, 129, 135, 144, 146–149, 151–155, 201, 218, 226, 239, 245–246, 251; as nosographic category 25, 52–53, 58–59, 80, 164, 167, 169–170, 173, 175, 183–184, 202–203, 206–207; notion of 1–17, 23–25, 27–29, 31, 34–37, 40–41, 44–48, 50–51, 58, 60–61, 66–70, 80, 88, 104, 117, 128, 134, 137–138, 156, 161–162, 168, 179–181, 191, 197, 199–201, 205, 208, 215, 223, 228–229, 231–232, 238–250; post-traumatic stress disorder (PTSD) 2, 6, 9, 29, 31, 68, 135; psychical or psychological (trauma) 5, 15, 16, 23, 55–57, 60, 78, 81, 83, 88, 195; psychologization of 4, 10, 15, 23–25, 40, 42, 44, 55–58, 61, 142, 165–166; as relantionship 13, 15, 84, 91, 96, 100, 104, 136, 138, 140, 141, 187, 191, 199, 201, 207, 238, 241, 243–245, 247, 249; and sexuality 4, 5, 8, 13, 16, 17, 24, 77, 113, 115–116, 119–121, 128, 130–131, 138, 143–144, 147, 164, 171, 176, 178–184, 188–190, 215–217, 243; slight nature of 47; somatic (trauma) 1, 4, 5, 15, 23–25, 27, 30, 57, 59, 61, 66, 164, 167–170, 174–176, 185–187, 191, 243; transgenerational transmission of 12, 13, 14, 17, 117, 142, 155, 215–216, 218, 221, 223, 225, 228, 229, 231, 233, 239, 242, 243, 251–252; traumatology 1; *see also* economic, memory *and* temporality

unbound drives (or sum of affect) 13, 194, 204, *205*, 207, 241
unconscious: brain or cerebral 42, 70–71, 76, 78; conflict 13, 215; memory 141; process 57, 131, 170, 180, 182–183, 189, 198–199, 201, 217, 233–234; as a system 104, 151–152, 157, 171, 173–176, 243; transmission 142; unconsciousness 38, 70

victim 10–11, 26–29, 31, 36–38, 44–45, 54, 56–58, 95, 138, 141, 185–186, 189–190, 243, 251

war 5, 13, 16, 17, 26, 135, 240, 243; First World War 5, 8–9, 16, 61, 161, 164–208, 216, 223, 241, 245; Second World War 6, 224; Vietnam War 5, 6; *see also* neuroses
web 3, 7; of process 13, 14; of problems 3, 9; of representations 4, 17, 201, 204–205, 207–208, 239, 241–242, 244–245; of theories or practices 3, 13, 14

For Product Safety Concerns and Information please contact our EU
representative GPSR@taylorandfrancis.com
Taylor & Francis Verlag GmbH, Kaufingerstraße 24, 80331 München, Germany

www.ingramcontent.com/pod-product-compliance
Ingram Content Group UK Ltd.
Pitfield, Milton Keynes, MK11 3LW, UK
UKHW020149200926
475702UK00016B/2628
9781032460826